Controversies in the Treatment of Lung Cancer

Frontiers of Radiation Therapy and Oncology

Vol. 42

Series Editors

J.L. Meyer San Francisco, Calif.
W. Hinkelbein Berlin

12th International Symposium on Special Aspects of Radiotherapy
Berlin, October 3–4, 2008

Controversies in the Treatment of Lung Cancer

Volume Editors

J. Heide Berlin
A. Schmittel Berlin
D. Kaiser Berlin
W. Hinkelbein Berlin

34 figures, 4 in color, and 27 tables, 2010

KARGER

Basel · Freiburg · Paris · London · New York · Bangalore · Bangkok · Shanghai · Singapore · Tokyo · Sydney

Frontiers of Radiation Therapy and Oncology

Founded 1968 by J.M. Vaeth, San Francisco, Calif.

Dr. Jürgen Heide
Department of Radiooncology and Radiotherapy
Charité – Campus Benjamin Franklin
Berlin, Germany

Prof. Dr. Dirk Kaiser
Department of Thoracic Surgery
Helios Klinikum Emil von Behring
Chest Hospital Heckeshorn
Berlin, Germany

PD Dr. Alexander Schmittel
Department of Medical Oncology
Charité – Campus Benjamin Franklin
Berlin, Germany

Prof. Dr. Wolfgang Hinkelbein
Department of Radiooncology and Radiotherapy
Charité – Campus Benjamin Franklin
Berlin, Germany

Library of Congress Cataloging-in-Publication Data

International Symposium on Special Aspects of Radiotherapy (12th: 2008: Berlin, Germany)
Controversies in the treatment of lung cancer / 12th International
Symposium on Special Aspects of Radiotherapy, Berlin, October 3–4, 2008;
volume editors, J. Heide ... [et al.].
p. ; cm. – (Frontiers of radiation therapy and oncology, ISSN 0071-9676; v. 42)
Includes bibliographical references and indexes.
ISBN 978-3-8055-9298-7 (hard cover: alk. paper)
1. Lungs – Cancer – Radiotherapy – Congresses. I. Heide, J. (Jürgen) II. Title.
III. Series: Frontiers of radiation therapy and oncology, v. 42. 0071-9676;
[DNLM: 1. Lung Neoplasms – Radiotherapy – Congresses. 2. Lung
Neoplasms – Surgery – Congresses. W3 FR935 v.42 2010 / WF 658 I612c 2010]
RC280.L8I58 2008
616.99'424–dc22 2009038886

Bibliographic Indices. This publication is listed in bibliographic services, including Current Contents® and PubMed/MEDLINE.

www.karger.com
Printed in Switzerland on acid-free and non-aging paper (ISO 9706) by Reinhardt Druck, Basel
ISSN 0071–9676
ISBN 978–3–8055–9298–7
e-ISBN 978–3–8055–9299–4

Contents

Heide J, Schmittel A, Kaiser D, Hinkelbein W (eds): Controversies in the Treatment of Lung Cancer.
Front Radiat Ther Oncol. Basel, Karger, 2010, vol 42, pp 1–14

Prognostic Factors in Histopathology of Lung Cancer

Annette Fisseler-Eckhoff

Institute of Pathology and Cytology, Dr. Horst-Schmidt Clinic, Wiesbaden, Germany

Abstract

Carcinoma of the lung is the most common cause of cancer-related death in men and women. Prognosis correlates strongly with stage of disease at presentation and to some degree with the histological subtype of the tumor. Histological classifications of lung cancer were somewhat arbitrary and a matter of convenience. However, multiple lines of differentiation are often found within a single tumor, if it is sufficiently sampled. The new therapeutic approaches especially of non-small cell lung cancer place high demands on pathologists: a clear histological diagnosis with information on the predominant histological subtype is required, obtained by using additional immunohistochemical methods. Using molecular methods, predictive and prognostic factors for adjuvant and neoadjuvant therapies can be identified in tumor cells of small cell lung cancer and non-small cell lung cancer. Biological and molecular factors known in this regard include the epidermal growth factor family and its receptors, K-RAS mutations, neuroendocrine tumor differentiation, and nucleotide-excision-repair proteins (ERCC1 and RRM1). Thymidilate synthase is an interesting target for anticancer agents such as the antifolate pemetrexed. Given the aspect of individualized lung cancer therapy, the collective term small cell/non-small cell lung cancer introduced by the groups of Chuang in1984 and Thomas in 1993 can be regarded as no longer sufficient.

Carcinoma of the lung is the leading cause of cancer-related death in both men and women. Concerning lung cancer incidence in five continents, it was demonstrated by Parkin et al. [1] that non-small cell lung cancer (NSCLC) accounts for almost 75% of cases, small cell carcinomas (SCC) comprise about 15% and large cell/undifferentiated carcinomas about 9%. Lung cancer is a dynamic and diverse disease associated with numerous somatic mutations, deletions, and amplification events. Patients with the same stage of disease can have markedly different clinical outcomes. Currently, surgery is the major treatment option for patients

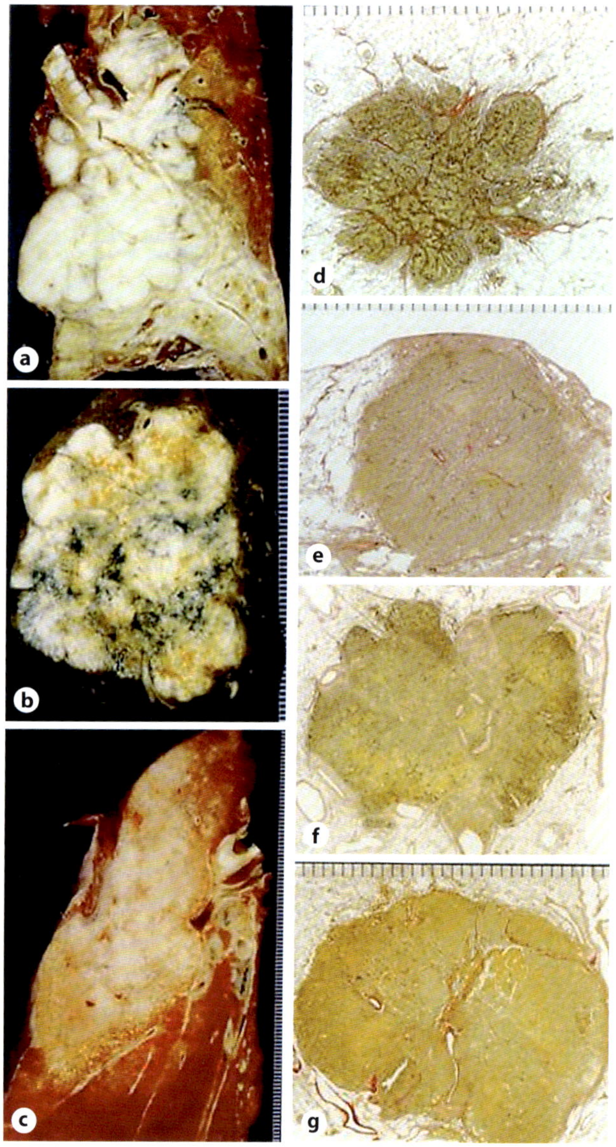

Fig. 1. Macroscopic and microscopic appearance of NSCLC at time of diagnosis. **a** Central localised squamous cell carcinoma with destruction of main bronchus and tumor propagation in adjacent lung parenchyma. **b** Peripheral localized adenocarcinoma. **c** Pneumonic growth pattern of bronchiolo-alveolar cell carcinoma. **d** Cross-section of squamous cell carcinoma in lung periphery. **e** Cross-section of a subpleural localized adenocarcinoma. **f**, **g** Cross-sections of intrapulmonal localized adenocarcinoma consisting of epithelial tumor components and necrosis. Invasion and destruction of pulmonary arteries.

in stage I NSCLC. Even in stage I only 60–65% of NSCLC patients are still alive after 5 years even if the tumor was resected completely. The main reason for this bad prognosis is the fact that the tumor is mainly clinically diagnosed at the time when the tumor is already larger than 2 cm (fig. 1a–g).

Tumor Size: An Essential Prognostic Factor in Lung Cancer

Tumor size matters and is an important prognostic factor for both small cell lung cancer (SCLC) and NSCLC [2]. When using the new TNM classification concerning the pT1 stage lymph node metastases can even be found in tumors with a size up to 1 cm corresponding to pT1a (tumor size up to 2 cm). With increasing tumor size the number of N1 and N2 lymph node metastases increased in number (fig. 2a, b) [unpubl. data]. Primary invasive NSCLC >2 cm is twice more likely to have nodal metastases than carcinomas <2 cm. The new TNM classification 2009 contributes to further subclassification by tumor size within stage I, with tumors <2 cm in size (T1a) and up to 3 cm in size (T1b) contained in a separate substage. Further classification of T2 in T2a (tumor size up to 5 cm) and T2b (tumor size up to 7 cm) may help clarify which patients might benefit from novel adjuvant or neoadjuvant chemotherapy [3].

The prognosis of patients correlates strongly with stage of disease at presentation. In stage I, 5-year survival is about 65% whereas in stage III survival rate is only 13%. However, 35–50% of stage I NSCLC patients will relapse within 5 years indicating that a subgroup of these patients might benefit from adjuvant chemotherapy [4]. On the other hand, patients with clinical stage IB, IIA, IIB or IIIA NSCLC receive adjuvant chemotherapy and some may unnecessarily receive potentially toxic chemotherapeutic treatment.

Small Cell Lung Cancer

SCLC accounts for about 15% of all cases of lung cancer. Of the four major histological types of lung cancer, SCLC has been highly associated with smoking. It is characterized by rapid growth and early extra-thoracic spread and cytotoxic chemotherapy is the cornerstone of any therapeutic strategy. Combined SCC variant refers to the admixture of non-SCC elements including adenocarcinoma, squamous cell or large cell carcinoma and less commonly spindle cell or giant cell carcinoma. For combined small cell and large cell carcinoma there should be at least 10% large cells present. SCLC and pulmonary carcinoids are neuroendocrine (NE) tumors with characteristic features of NE cells. SCLC have high rate of p53 mutations, amplification of MYC, methylation of caspase-8, which is a key

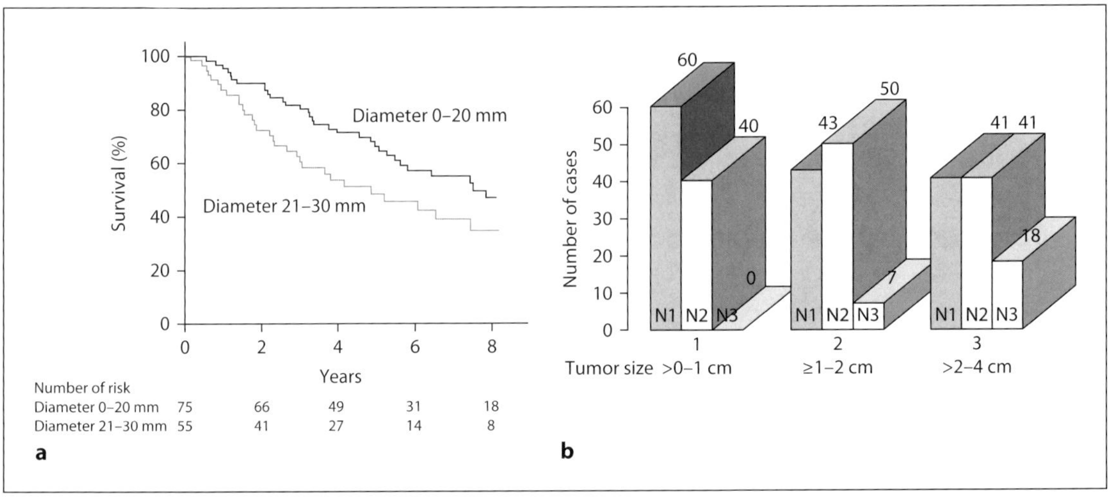

Fig. 2. **a** Tumor size is a determinant of stage distribution in T1 NSCLC [4] and is correlated with clinical outcome. **b** With increasing tumor size in pT1 NSCLC the number of N1 and N2 lymph node metastases increased in number [unpubl. data].

anti-apoptotic gene, inactivation of the retinoblastoma gene and overexpression of E2F1. These are almost universal in SCLC: Multiple other changes occur frequently in SCLC, including upregulation of the proapoptotic molecule Bcl-2, activation of autocrine loops, upregulation of telomerase and expression of vascular growth factors.

Prognosis and Predictive Factors in Small Cell Lung Cancer

A positive history of smoking, socioeconomic status and extensive stage of disease are independent poor prognostic factors in SCLC [5]. Never-smokers had higher median survival (13.6 vs. 9.9 months) and 2-year survival rate (17% versus 7%) than smokers with SCLC. Female gender should be a favorable prognostic factor in extensive disease SCLC, as it has been shown that female SCLC patients survived longer than male and that female patients had higher complete and overall response rates to chemotherapy [6]. ERCC1 and topo IIalpha are candidate markers in predicting clinical outcome and response to treatment in low disease SCLC patients and are worth further investigations in a prospective study. No histological or genetic factors are predictive of prognosis till now [7].

Histological Subtype: A Prognostic Factor in NSCLC

New chemotherapeutic regimens for the treatment of NSCLC have demonstrated that histology is a prognostic and predictive factor for special combined chemotherapy [8].

According to the WHO criteria, stage for stage survival rate is significantly better for squamous cell carcinoma than for adenocarcinoma. Approximately 80% of patients with resected stage I (T1N0M0) squamous cell carcinoma are alive 5 years after diagnosis compared to approximately 70% of similarly staged adenocarcinoma. Stages of disease and performance status at diagnosis remain the most powerful prognostic indicators for survival.

The importance of the histological subtype as a prognostic factor within the groups of NSCLC is documented by the new WHO classification of 1999 and modified in 2004. Further histological subtypes within the single groups of squamous cell carcinomas and adenocarcinomas, which are associated with poor prognosis were ruled out in the new WHO classification [9].

Squamous Cell Carcinoma Histological Subtypes Associated with Poor Prognosis

Papillary variants of squamous cell carcinoma (SCC), which show exophytic and endobronchial growth with or without invasion.

Clear cell variants of SCC, which have to be separated from large cell carcinoma, adenocarcinoma with clear cell changes and metastatic clear cell carcinoma from the kidney.

Small cell variants of SCC, which lack the characteristic nuclear features of SCC having coarse or vesicular chromatin, more prominent nucleoli, more cytoplasm and more distinct cell borders.

Basaloid variants of SCC, which show prominent peripheral palisading of nuclei.

When squamous cell carcinomas are poorly differentiated, the distinction from large cell carcinoma is quite difficult, with poor interobserver and even intraobserver agreement. The smaller the specimen (i.e. bronchial biopsies or cytologic specimens) the greater the difficulty in making such a distinction [10, 11]. If the pathologist can adhere to the WHO criteria for SCC i.e. either keratin pearls, intercellular bridges, or individual cell keratinization are present, then the distinction is seldom a problem. However, these criteria are often absent. As new chemotherapeutic agents like pemetrexed in combination with cisplatin therapy are allowed only in those cases, in which a predominant squamous cell differentiation is ruled out, in doubtful cases, a combination of immunohistochemical stains (TTF 1, CK5/6, p63 and CK7) can assist in making the correct diagnosis.

Adenocarcinoma Histological Subtypes Associated with Poor Prognosis

Adenocarcinoma is the most common subtype of NSCLC. It is mainly diagnosed as a subpleural coin lesion, the central area underlying pleural puckering with a V-shaped area of desmoplastic fibrosis associated with anthracotic pigmentation. Adenocarcinomas demonstrate different growth patterns like central or endobronchial tumor growth or diffuse pneumonia-like lobar consolidation with preservation of underlying architecture, typical of mucinous bronchioloalveolar cell carcinoma (BAC) with disseminated growth along the visceral pleura, resulting in a ring-like thickening mimicking malignant mesothelioma (pseudo-mesotheliomatous carcinoma).

Major histological subtypes of adenocarcinomas are acinar, papillary, bronchioloalveolar and solid adenocarcinoma with mucin production. Further subtypes are fetal adenocarcinoma, mucinous adenocarcinoma, clear-cell adenocarcinoma (fig 3a–e). In 70%, different histological growth patterns can be found within one tumor leading to the classification adenocarcinoma mixed type.

Solid growth pattern with mucin production, *clear cell* and *papillary subtypes* (fig. 3c–e) are correlated with worse prognosis. The papillary growth pattern is characterized by papillae with secondary and tertiary papillary structures. A micropapillary pattern of adenocarcinoma, in which tufts lack a central fibrovascular core, may be prognostically unfavorable [12, 13]. Histological grading has prognostic implications. In general, poorly differentiated adenocarcinomas have more local recurrence and lymph node metastases than patients with well or moderately differentiated tumors. High histological grade, vascular invasion, mitotic activity, lymphangiosis and extensive tumor necrosis are correlated with unfavorable prognosis [14].

Watanabe et al. [15] showed that the ground-glass component in CT correlates with the bronchioloalveolar carcinoma component in the histological specimen.

Tumors having a larger ground-glass component in CT than a solid component have a better prognosis with a long-term survival rate of up to 100%.

Bronchioloalveolar Cell Carcinoma Growth Pattern: A Favorable Prognostic Factor

Bronchioloalveolar cell carcinomas (BAC) (fig. 3f) are morphologically characterized by a lepidic growth pattern of tumor cells along the alveoli. Based on WHO criteria stromal, vascular, lymphatic or pleural invasion must be ruled out. Based on this criterion the diagnosis BAC is no longer possible in bioptically obtained specimens. It is only possible by investigation of surgically obtained tumor [9]. BAC is not an invasive carcinoma but a carcinoma in situ, with better prognosis compared to other histological subtypes. The bronchioloalveolar subtype is of special therapeutic interest concerning targeted therapies.

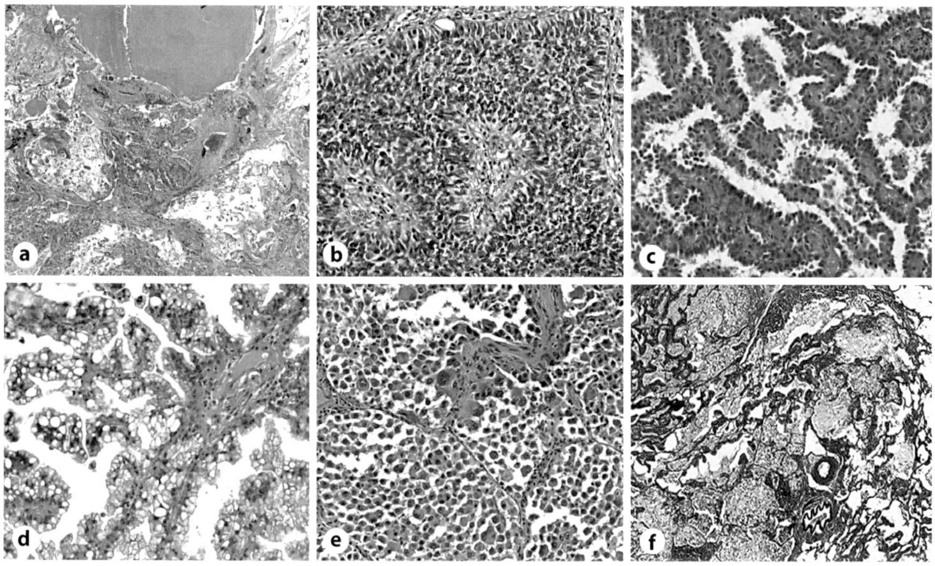

Fig. 3. Histological subtypes of NSCLC associated with prognosis (**a–e**) or favorable prognosis (**f**). ×420. **a**: Squamous cell carcinoma with papillary growth pattern. ×420. **b** Basaloid variant of SCC showing prominent peripheral palisading of nuclei. ×420. **c** Papillary growth pattern of adenocarcinoma with secondary and tertiary papillae. ×420. **d** Clear cell and papillary subtype of adenocarcinoma. ×420. **e** Large cell carcinoma pleomorphic subtype. ×420. **f** Bronchioloalveolar cell carcinoma characterized by a lepidic growth pattern of tumor cells along the alveoli correlated with favorable prognosis. ×420.

Adenocarcinomas with predominant BAC growth pattern and central scarring less than 0.5 cm in tumors of 3 cm or less in diameter (pT1) have a similar, very favorable prognosis. Therefore, pathologists should point out in the morphological diagnosis of adenocarcinomas, whether a bronchioloalveolar growth pattern exists within the tumor or not.

Large Cell Carcinomas

Large cell carcinoma (LCC) is an undifferentiated non-SCC that lacks the cytological and architectural features of SCC and glandular or squamous differentiation. LCC has sometimes been referred to as a 'waste basket' category, and includes several variants like large cell neuroendocrine carcinoma, combined large cell neuroendocrine carcinoma, basaloid carcinoma, lymphoepithelioma-like carcinoma, clear cell carcinoma, and large cell carcinoma with rhabdoid phenotype of clinical importance.

LCC accounts for approximately 9% of all lung cancers in most studies. Large cell neuroendocrine tumors account for 3% of lung cancer. Giant cell carcinoma and pleomorphic carcinomas have a very poor prognosis (fig. 3e). It was shown that this pattern usually occurs in association with adenocarcinoma [11] that can be treated by Pemetrexed, too, but a neuroendocrine feature has to be ruled out by additional immunohistochemical investigations with neuroendocrine markers [15].

Prognostic Implication of Molecular Markers

A wide range of genetic and phenotypic abnormalities have been identified in lung cancer. However, only a few are known to have an impact on patient outcome and thus may influence choice of therapy:

EGFR and K-RAS in Lung Cancer

Mutations of genes in the epidermal growth factor receptor (EGFR) signaling pathway, such as EGFR, K-RAS, HER2 BRAF, and phosphatidyl inositol 3 kinase catalytic alpha (PIK3Ca), are critical to the pathogenesis of a large number of adenocarcinomas and play a prognostic and predictive role concerning therapy. EGFR mutations are more prevalent in females, never-smokers, patients of Asian ethnicity, and those with histology of adenocarcinoma. Tumors with EGFR mutations are highly sensitive to small molecule EGFR-specific tyrosine kinase inhibitors (TKIs), such as Gefitinib or Erlotinib. There is an antagonism between these EGFR TKIs and chemotherapy in tumor cells with wild-type EGFR. Mutations in EGFR occur mainly in exon 18 or exon 21, or deletions occur in exon 19 and exon 21 L858R substitutions. In these adenocarcinomas high EGFR gene copy numbers can be found by FISH analysis and have been associated with response to EGFR-TKI (fig. 4a). These mutations were found in 13% of unselected USA populations, 33% of unselected East Asian populations and overall in 30% of adenocarcinomas [12].

Analyses looking specifically at those subgroups show significantly longer survival times with Gefitinib group than in placebo group for never-smokers (n = 375; median survival time 8.9, vs. 6.1 months) and patients of Asian origin (n = 342, median survival time 9.5 vs. 5.5 months) [16]. In most patients with longer survival times and higher response rates pathological diagnosis revealed mainly adenocarcinoma subtype especially adenocarcinomas with bronchiolo-alveolar growth pattern. In these adenocarcinomas high EGFR gene copy numbers were found.

According to the published data for 1,335 patients, the response rate of NSCLCs with EGFR mutations for EGFR-TKI was about 70%, whereas those without mutations was about 10%. Furthermore, several retrospective studies showed that patients with EGFR mutations have a significantly longer survival than those

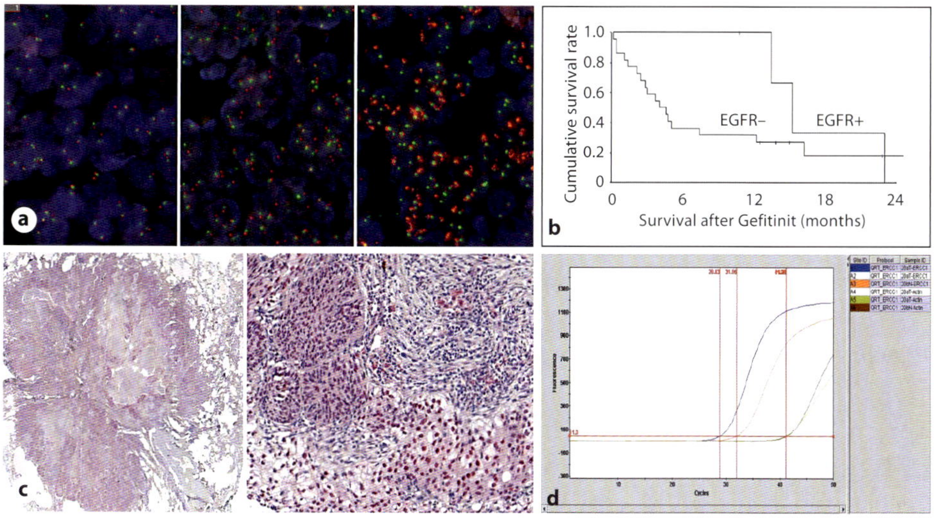

Fig. 4. a EGFR amplification in adenocarcinoma demonstrated by FISH analysis: 2 signals/nucleus, more than 4 signals/nucleus (**b**) and cluster amplification (**c**). ×420. **b** Between 2002 and 2005 68 patients were treated with tyrosine kinase inhibitor therapy in the HSK Clinic Wiesbaden. Patients with EGFR mutations demonstrate a better progression free interval and a better long time survival rate (data unpublished). **c** Immunohistochemical demonstration of ERCC1 expression in adenocarcinoma with heterogeneous staining pattern. Cross-section/detail, ×420. **d** Determination of ERCC1 level in tumor tissue in comparison to normal tissue by real time PCR.

without mutations when treated with EGFR-TKIs. These results indicate that the EGFR mutations are important predictive factors for successful treatment with EGFR-TKIs [17].

Between 2002 and 2005, 68 patients were treated at the HSK Clinic Wiesbaden with tyrosine kinase inhibitor therapy, and the histological subtypes were adenocarcinomas in 55 cases, squamous cell carcinomas in 8 cases, large cell carcinomas in 2 cases, mixed type in 2 cases and undifferentiated type in 1 case. All patients with EGFR mutations demonstrate a better progression-free interval and a better long-term survival rate (fig. 4a, b). EGFR mutations were more prevalent in females, in never smokers or in well-to-moderately differentiated tumors. In those patients in whom tyrosine kinase therapy no longer works, KRAS mutations were found in the tumor cells. Mutations in KRAS are found in approximately 30% of human lung adenocarcinomas [unpubl. data].

However, the prognostic impact of EGFR gene mutations in lung adenocarcinomas remains controversial. Some investigators claim that EGFR mutations are prognostic rather than predictive, because reports showed that patients with NSCLCs harboring EGFR mutations survived for a longer period than those without mutations irrespective of therapy (chemotherapy with EGFR-TKIs or placebo) [18].

Activating mutation of the KRAS gene was one of the earliest discoveries of genetic alteration in lung cancers and about 10% NSCLCs of Japanese patients harbored KRAS mutations. Several meta-analyses revealed that KRAS mutations may be associated with shortened survival in patients with NSCLCs, although sufficient confirmation in well-designed multivariate analysis has not been obtained. KRAS mutations were more prevalent in males or in smokers, which are thought to be predictors of worse survival [18].

Prognostic Implication of Excision Repair Cross-Complementing I

The excision repair cross-complementing 1 (ERCC1) gene is a structure-specific DNA repair endonuclease required to resolve DNA interstrand crosslink-induced double-strand breaks. This enzyme belongs to the nucleotide excision repair (NER) system and has been extensively investigated because of its ability to repair platinum intrastrand DNA adducts. The expression levels of ERCC1 transcripts are associated with survival in cancer patients treated with cisplatin-based chemotherapy. ERCC1 was confirmed to be an independent prognostic factor for survival in low disease SCLC. In NSCLC patients treated with adjuvant cisplatin, ERCC1 protein expression should be a predictive and prognostic factor [19]. Due to the results of different studies on NSCLC, ERCC1-negative patients benefit from cisplatin-based chemotherapy, whereas patients with ERCC1-positive tumors without chemotherapy will have a better overall survival [7, 20]. ERCC1 can be investigated on protein and mRNA level in paraffin-embedded tumor tissue (fig. 4c). Correlations of both methods have not been investigated until now. By real time PCR, it is possible to determine the ERCC1 level in tumor tissue in comparison to normal tissue so that one can get quantitative levels as a basis for the decision for chemotherapy (fig. 4d). In vitro results on human lung cancer cell lines demonstrate significantly higher RRM1 mRNA expression in SCLC compared with NSCLC. However, no correlation between mRNA expression of either the ERCC1, ERCC2 and RRM1 genes, nor chemosensitivity to cisplatin, carboplatin or gemcitabine was found [21]. These in vitro results suggest that further studies are needed to evaluate the expression of the RRM1, ERCC1 and ERCC2 genes as predictive biomarkers for sensitivity to platinum agents and gemcitabine in SCLC as well as in NSCLC.

Prognostic Implication of Ribonucleotide Reductase M1

The ribonucleotide reductase M1 (RRM1) gene codes for an enzyme necessary for DNA synthesis, catalyzing the biosynthesis of deoxyribonucleotides. Different investigators showed that upregulation of RRM1 mRNA levels are generally associated with chemoresistance to gemcitabine-based therapies. A significant correlation between RRM1 and ERCC1 in terms of transcript levels was found in NSCLC patients treated with cisplatin and gemcitabine [22]. With these results, a decision-tree type diagram with the combination of different therapeutic agents was ruled out based on the results of ERCC1 and RRM1 levels.

In first line therapy of NSCLC cisplatin and pemetrexed were not worse than cisplatin and gemcitabine with regard to hazard ratio (HR). Cisplatin and pemetrexed were significantly better in adenocarcinomas and large cell carcinomas concerning survival, whereas cisplatin and gemcitabine were found to be prognostically better in squamous cell carcinomas.

Prognostic Implication of Thymidylate Synthase

The enzyme thymidylate synthase (TS) catalyses the methylation of 2'-deoxyuridine-5-monophosphate-8 (dUMP) to 2'-deoxythymidine-5'-monophosphate (dTMP), an essential precursor during DNA synthesis. TS is usually elevated in tumors and is therefore an interesting target for anticancer agents such as the antifolate pemetrexed (multitargeted antifolate, Alimta), which inhibits activity of TS by competition with the binding site of CH2 – THF of TS. TS mRNA levels were investigated in NSCLC and SCLC by Ceppi et al. [7] 2008. TS levels were increased at mRNA, protein and activity level in squamous cell carcinomas of the lung. Increased TS levels should be responsible for resistance to the TS based antifolate pemetrexed in squamous cell carcinomas, whereas patients with adenocarcinomas and large cell carcinomas should benefit from pemetrexed therapy. The survival rate in patients with NSCLC was better in patients with low TS levels, and these low TS levels were mainly found in adenocarcinomas and large cell carcinomas [20, 23].

Considering the special aspects of individualized chemotherapeutical approaches depending on histological subtypes it is absolutely essential that pathologists give a correct histological diagnosis concerning the subtypes. The primary diagnosis of lung cancer is mainly based on the investigation of a small biopsy.

The new therapeutic agents require a clear differentiation between adenocarcinomas and predominant non-squamous cell carcinoma. The specificity of diagnosis for squamous cell carcinoma in biopsy compared to resection specimens varied between 66 and 95%. As pemetrexed combined with cisplatin therapy and as bevacicumab (Avastin) are allowed only in those cases in which a predominant squamous cell differentiation is ruled out, in doubtful cases, immunohistochemical stains (CK5/6, p63) can assist in making the correct diagnosis. There is a typical immunohistochemical staining pattern for squamous cell carcinomas, as well as one for adenocarcinomas. All undifferentiated G3 carcinomas should be investigated further by immunohistochemistry (fig. 5).

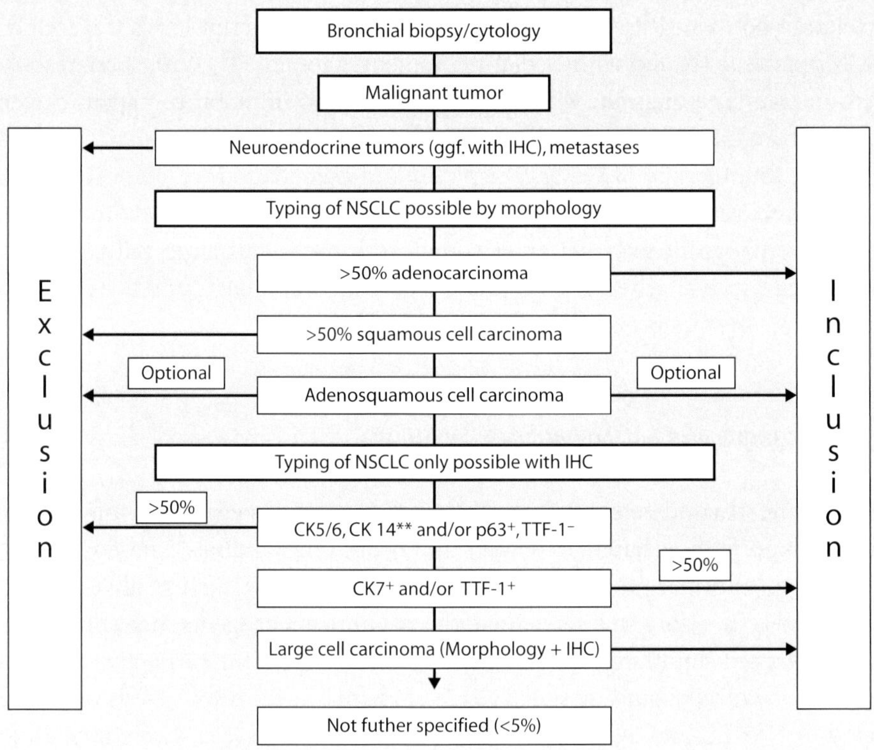

Fig. 5. Algorithm for the diagnosis of NSCLC with exclusion of predominante non-SCC as the basis for individualized chemotherapeutic approaches (pemetrexed, bevacicumab) with the help of immunohistochemistry.

Conclusion

Over the last decades, histological classifications of lung cancer were often somewhat arbitrary and a matter of convenience, although multiple lines of differentiation are often found within a single tumor if it is sufficiently sampled. Historically, histology has not been clearly or consistently described in the literature as a prognostic or predictive factor in advanced NSCLC studies. While some studies suggest a more favorable outcome for adenocarcinomas or nonsquamous histologies, others suggest benefits for patients with squamous cell morphology. Until now, the substantial differences in study design and analyses make such specific conclusions regarding the prognostic and predictive role of histology difficult. The main reasons for these difficulties might be the fact that the morphological diagnosis of the pathologist is mainly concentrated on the differentiation between small cell and non-SCCs. In those cases where adenocarcinomas were diagnosed, further subtyping of growth pattern are often missed, although the new WHO classification pointed out that different histological subtypes within the main tumor entities are correlated with worse prognosis, e.g. papillar, basaloid or sarcomatoid differentiation, whereas, for example, bronchioloalveolar growth pattern are associated with favorable prognosis. Under this aspect within a morphological defined histological subtype such as adenocarcinoma multiple subtypes can exist and these subtypes should be described in the pathological diagnosis. Because each associated subtype might be associated with a different prognosis and/or responsiveness to a particular drug. As BAC and BAC-like growth pattern is associated with better outcome and might response to tyrosine kinase therapy pathologist should give clear information whether bronchioloalveolar growth pattern is present in adenocarcinoma or whether it is absent. This fact might give implication to further molecular pathological investigations. As squamous cell tumors are at risk for hemorrhagic complications when treated with bevacizumab further studies should also include an analysis of the association between histologic subtypes and clinically relevant toxicities. The new therapeutic approaches in the treatment of NSCLC place high demands on pathologists: a clear histological diagnosis with information on the predominant histological subtype is required, if necessary by using additional immunohistochemical methods. Using molecular methods predictive and prognostic factors for adjuvant and neoadjuvant therapies can be identified in tumor cells of NSCLC. To assess treatment-by-histology interactions, large studies are needed to detect an interaction compared with a main treatment effect. For individualized lung cancer therapy, the collective term SCLC/NSCLC [24, 25] can no longer be considered sufficient and should therefore no longer be used. The development of targeted therapies and the refinement of histologic classifications, more studies should include an analysis of histologic subtypes and their association with efficacy outcomes.

References

1 Parkin DM,Whelan SL, Ferlay J, Teppo L, Thomas DB: Cancer Incidence in Five Continents, vol VIII, IARC Scientific Publications No 155. Lyon, IARC Press, 2002.

2 Flieder DB, Port JL, Korst RJ, Christos PJ, Levin MA, Becker DE, Altorki NK: Tumor size is a determinant of stage distribution in t1 non-small cell lung cancer. Chest 2005;128:2304–2308.

3 TNM Staging System of the International Association for the Study of Lung Cancer, 2009;in press.

4 Huber RM: Lungenkarzinom. Internist (Berl) 2006;47:611–620.

5 Wolf M, Holle R, Hans K, Drings P, Havemann K: Analysis of prognostic factors in 766 patients with small cell lung cancer (SCLC): the role of sex as a predictor of survival. Br J Cancer 1991;63:986–992.

6 Ignatius S-H, Ziogas A, Jason A, Zell DO: Prognostic factors for survival in extensive stage small cell lung cancer (ED-SCLC). J Thorac Oncol 2009; 4:1.

7 Ceppi P, Longo M, Volante M, Novello S, Cappia S, Bacillo E, Selvaggi G, Saviozzi S, Calogero R, Papotti M, Scaliotti G: Excision repair cross complementing-1 and topoisomerase iialpha gene expression in small-cell lung cancer patients treated with platinum and etoposide. J Thorac Oncol 2008; 3:583–589.

8 Simon G, Sharma A, Li X, Hazelton T, Walsh F, Williams CH, Chiappori A, Haura E, Tanvetyanon T, Antonia S, Cantor A, Bepler G: Feasibility and efficacy of molecular analysis-directed individualized therapy in advanced non-small-cell lung cancer. J Clin Oncol 2007;25:2741–2746.
9 Travis, WD, Brambilla E, Müller-Hermelink HK, Harris CC: Tumours of the lung, pleura, thymus and heart: World Health Organization Classification of Tumours. Lyon, IARC Press, 2004, pp 9–56.
10 Edwards SL, Roberts C, Mc Kean ME, Cockburn JS, Jeffrey RR, Kerr KM: Preoperative histological classification of primary lung cancer: accuracy of diagnosis and use of the non-small cell category. J Clin Pathol 2000;53:537–540.
11 Roggli VL, Vollmer RT, Greenberg SD, Mc Gavran MH, Spjut HJ, Yesner R: Lung cancer heterogeneity: a blinded and randomized study of 100 consecutive cases. Hum Pathol 1985;16:569–579.
12 Miyoshi T, Satoh Y, Okumura S, Nakagawa K, Shirakusa T, Tsuchiya E, Ishikawa Y: Early-stage lung adenocarcinomas with a micropapillary pattern, a distinct pathologic marker for a significantly poor prognosis. Am J Surg Pathol 2003:27: 101–109
13 Silver SA, Askin FB: True papillary carcinoma of the lung: a distinct clinicopathologic entity. Am J Surg Pathol 1997;21:43–51.
14 Swinson DE, Jones JL, Richardson D, Cox G, Edwards JG, O'Byrne KJ : Tumor necrosis is months)an independent prognostic marker in non-small cell lung cancer: correlation with biological variables. Lung Cancer 2002;37:235–240.
15 Watanabe S, Watanabe T, Arai K, Kasai T, Haratake J, Urayama H: Results of wedge resection for focal bronchioloalveolar carcinoma showing pure ground-glass attenuation on computed tomography. Ann Thorac Surg 2002;73:1071–1075.
16 Silvestri GA, Rivera MP: Target therapy for the treatment of advanced non-small cell lung cancer: a review of the epidermal growth factor receptor antagonists. Chest 2005;128:3975–3984.
17 Kosaka T, Yatabe Y , Onozato R, Kuwano H, Mitsudomi T : Prognostic implication of EGFR, KRAS, and TP53 gene mutations in a large cohort of Japanese patients with surgically treated lung adenocarcinoma. J Thorac Oncol 2009;4:22–29.
18 Massarelli E, Varella-Garcia M, Tang X, Xavier AC, Ozburn NC, Liu DD, Bekele BN, Herbst RS, Wistuba II: KRAS mutation is an important predictor of resistance to therapy with epidermal growth factor receptor tyrosine kinase inhibitors in non-small-cell lung cancer. Clin Cancer Res 2007;13:2890–2896.
19 Olaussen KA, Dunant A, Fouret P, Brambilla E, André F, Haddad V, Taranchon E, Filipits M, Pirker R, Popper HH, Stahel R, Sabatier L, Pignon JP, Tursz T, Le Chevalier T, Soria JC; IALT Bio Investigators: DNA repair by ERCC1 in non-small-cell lung cancer and cisplatin-based adjuvant chemotherapy. N Engl J Med 2006;355: 983–991.
20 Soria J-C: ERCC1 – tailored chemotherapy in lung cancer: the first prospective randomized trial. J Clin Oncol 2007;25:2648–2649.
21 Shimizu J, Horio Y, Osada H, Hida T, Hasegawa Y, Shimokata K, Takahashi T, Sekido Y, Yatabe Y: mRNA expression of RRM1, ERCC1 and ERCC2 is not associated with chemosensitivity to cisplatin, carboplatin and gemcitabine in human cancer cell lines. Respirology 2008;13:510–517.
22 Rosell R, Felip E, Paz-Ares L: How could pharmacogenomics help to improve patient survival? Lung Cancer 2007;57;535–541.
23 Squamous cell carcinoma of the lung compared with other histotypes shows higher messenger RNA and protein levels for thymidilate synthase. Cancer 2006;107:1589–1596.
24 Chuang MT, Marchevsky A, Teirstein AS, Kirschner PA, Kleineman J: Diagnosis of lung cancer by fiberoptic bronchoscopy: problems in the histological classification of non-small cell carcinomas. Thorax 1984;39:175–178.
25 Thomas JS, Lamb D, Ashcroft T, Corrin B, Edwards CW, Gibbs AR, Kenyon WE, Stephens RJ, Whimster WF: How reliable is the diagnosis of lung cancer using small biopsy specimens? Report of a UKCCCR Lung Cancer Working Party. Thorax 1992;48:1135–1139.

Prof. Dr. med. Annette Fisseler-Eckhoff
Institute of Pathology and Cytology, Dr. Horst-Schmidt Clinic (HSK)
Ludwig-Erhard-Strasse 100
DE–65199 Wiesbaden (Germany)
Tel. +49 611 432540, Fax +49 611 433301, E-Mail annette.fisseler-eckhoff@hsk-wiesbaden.de

Heide J, Schmittel A, Kaiser D, Hinkelbein W (eds): Controversies in the Treatment of Lung Cancer.
Front Radiat Ther Oncol. Basel, Karger, 2010, vol 42, pp 15–45

FDG-PET/CT in Lung Cancer: An Update

Richard P. Baum · Cyprian Świętaszczyk · Vikas Prasad

Department of Nuclear Medicine/Center for PET, Zentralklinik Bad Berka, Bad Berka, Germany

Abstract

The prognosis of lung cancer patients mostly depends on the stage at which the disease is diagnosed. Contrast-enhanced CT (ceCT) and MRI play a significant role in initial staging, but often the morphological information is insufficient when compared to the metabolic or molecular information obtained by positron emission tomography (PET). ^{18}F-fluorine deoxyglucose (FDG) is based upon the increased demand of ATP leading to increased consumption of glucose in the tumor tissues. FDG-PET/CT has been proven to be of immense value in the initial diagnosis, evaluation of therapy reponse, detection of recurrent tumor, radiation therapy planning and in the multidisciplinary management of patients with non-small cell lung cancer as well as in patients with small cell lung cancer. The aim of this article is to present a concise summary of the present status of FDG-PET/CT.

Histologically, lung cancer is classified into two main categories: non-small cell lung cancer (NSCLC) and small cell lung cancer (SCLC). NSCLC accounts for roughly 80% of the lung cancer cases, the rest being SCLC. Although there are many histological variants of NSCLC (such as squamous cell carcinoma, adenocarcinoma, large cell carcinoma, adenosquamous carcinoma, etc.), the broader classification SCLC/NSCLC mainly determines clinical management and prognosis.

The average survival time for untreated NSCLC and SCLC is only 6 months and 2 months, respectively. If diagnosed at an early stage, NSCLC can be cured by surgical resection. Locally advanced disease is treated by preoperative chemoradiotherapy followed by surgical resection. In contrast, the primary therapy of SCLC is systemic chemotherapy, since this tumor type is highly sensitive to chemotherapy and is usually metastasized at the time of diagnosis. Because of this difference in the treatment strategies, it is essential to correctly diagnose, stage and restage the patients using various diagnostic modalities [1, 2].

Non-Small Cell Lung Cancer

Imaging Modalities

Various imaging modalities play an important role in the management of lung cancer, depending on the tumor stage and the available therapeutic options. This chapter will outline the role of imaging in relation to patient management focusing on nuclear medicine procedures.

Lung Nodules

By definition, a solitary pulmonary nodule (SPN) is opacity in the lung parenchyma measuring up to 3 cm that is not associated with mediastinal adenopathy or atelectasis. Lesions greater than 3 cm are categorized as masses [3]. Approximately 75% of pulmonary nodules are found incidentally during chest radiographs. Signs and symptoms (coughing, hemoptysis or thoracic pain) suggesting a lung problem are found in only 20–25% of patients with SPN. A German study has shown that there is an average delay of 7 months before a definitive diagnosis is reached [4]. The same study has documented that the younger the patient and the smaller the lesion, the longer is the delay for reaching the final diagnosis.

There are numerous etiologies (approximately 80) for lung nodules ranging from infections to inflammation and malignancies [5]. Approximately 130,000 SPN are diagnosed per year in the USA with an incidence of 52 per 100,000 populations. Invasive techniques like bronchoscopy have a sensitivity of only 65%, whereas transbronchoscopic biopsy reaches a sensitivity of 79% [6]. Although transthoracic fine-needle biopsy (TTFB) has a very high sensitivity (94–98%) and specificity (91–96%), the risk factors associated with its use (mainly pneumothorax) reaches 19–26%, with approximately 10–15% of patients requiring pleural drainage after TTFB resulting in hospital stay and increased expenditure [7].

Conventional imaging (CT scan) and metabolic imaging (PET scan) play a complementary role in the diagnosis of lung cancer and the combination of both modalities (PET/CT) is a very useful diagnostic test.

Morphological Imaging

The evaluation (additional work-up) of a SPN starts (usually after its incidental detection on a chest radiograph) to rule out malignancy. Uniformly dense calcified nodules on chest radiograph are mostly benign in nature. Serial chest radiographs – taken over a longer period of time (2 years or more) showing no signs of change in the appearance – also make the diagnosis of a benign nodule very likely.

Prior to the integration of PET, a radiographically indeterminate SPN was best evaluated using CT [8]. Although CT remains an integral part of the workup of SPN, other options are available. CT is used for the evaluation of shapes, borders, and densities of nodules. With the use of CT densitometry, calcifications can be detected within the nodules. Calcified nodules are mostly benign; however, the list of differential diagnosis includes metastasis from primary tumors (e.g. bone tumor, mucin-producing adenocarcinomas and soft-tissue sarcomas) or internal hemorrhage in metastases (e.g. chorioncarcinoma and melanoma). A nodule is presumably benign only, if the calcification is diffuse, i.e. present in the majority of the region of the nodule. The calcification – measuring more than 300 HU – has to be present in the centre of the nodule to be considered as benign [2, 3]. The pattern of contrast enhancement can also help to differentiate between benign and malignant nodules. Nodules showing less than 15 HU enhancement in the center are more likely to be benign, whereas those showing enhancement greater than 25 HU are more likely to be malignant [9, 10]. A report from the Early Lung Cancer Action Program (ELCAP) study has documented that 20% of pulmonary nodules on baseline screening are ground glass or sub-solid (they are less dense than the solid nodules and the surrounding pulmonary vasculature and thus, do not obscure the lung parenchyma). Ground glass opacities are associated with bronchioloalveolar carcinoma, whereas other adenocarcinomas present more frequently as solid nodules [11].

Apart from the calcification and ground glass appearance, certain morphological characteristics of pulmonary nodules like speculated outer margin, a hazy and indistinct margin, extension to pulmonary veins, focal retraction of adjacent pleura, and endobronchial extension are also suggestive of malignancies. Inhomogeneous internal composition and the evidence of central necrosis point towards malignant nature of the lesion. Some of the malignant lesions sometimes create air bronchograms, commonly associated with pneumonia. Sometimes CT scan features of lymphoma and bronchioalveolar cell carcinoma can be confused with benign lung lesions [2, 3].

In spite of all these morphologic criteria, 25–39% of malignant nodules are inappropriately classified as benign [12]. Although constancy of the nodule in terms of its morphologic characteristic over time is reliable for labeling a nodule benign, the predictive value of stability in size may be only 65%, probably because doubling in volume amounts to only 26% increase in nodular diameter, a change very hard to perceive [13, 14]. Clinical information combined with the radiographic characteristics can be used to calculate the likelihood ratio of malignant disease. This strategy, having its origin in the Bayesian analysis, is also a way to choose the appropriate management protocol. If the probability of cancer is less than 5%, then the patient is monitored over time, if the probability is between 5 and 60% the lesion is biopsied. For a likelihood ratio greater than 60%, resection

Table 1. Evaluation of solitary pulmonary nodules using ^{18}F-FDG-PET

First Author	Year	Cases	Prevalence, %	Sensitivity, %	Specificity, %
Pitman [28]	2002	36	58	90	93
Lowe [26]	1998	89	67	91	89
Gupta [170]	1996	61	73	93	87
Bury [37]	1996	50	66	100	88
Duhaylongsod [40]	1995	47	65	100	81

of the nodule is recommended [15, 16]. However, 50% of the patients undergoing surgical biopsy of an indeterminate SPN have benign disease. Because of the inadequacy of these radiographic characteristics, there was a need to find a better alternative, resulting in the rapid stride of PET in lung cancer diagnosis.

[18]F-Fluorine Deoxyglucose PET

There is a strong relationship between the glucose metabolism – measured as standardized uptake value (SUV) of ^{18}F-fluorine deoxyglucose (FDG) – and the chances of malignancy. Bryant et al. [17] have shown in a large prospective series in 585 patients, that, if the indeterminate pulmonary nodule is less than 2.5 cm, a maximum standardized uptake value (SUV_{max}) between 0 and 2.5 suggested 24% chance of malignancy. If the SUV_{max} is between 2.6 and 4, the chances of the nodule being malignant is 80% which increases to 96% for a SUV_{max} greater than 4.1. However, for solid pulmonary lesions with low FDG uptake (SUV_{max} <2.5), semi-quantitative approaches do not improve the accuracy of ^{18}F-FDG-PET over that obtained with visual analysis. The probability of malignancy is very low if the pulmonary lesion visually has no uptake. On the other hand, the probability of malignancy in any visually evident lesion is about 60% [18].

The results of the PET study should always be analyzed in conjunction with a CT image, because of the poor anatomic localization on PET images alone. The use of PET/CT and the possibility of image fusion has been heralded as a major breakthrough in oncologic PET imaging [19].

For characterization of SPN, ^{18}F-FDG-PET (tables 1, 2) alone better predicts malignancy than a combination of clinical and morphologic criteria. A meta-analysis [20–22] covering the results of numerous studies in approximately 1,400 patients [21, 23–41], proved that ^{18}F-FDG-PET can differentiate between benign and malignant SPN with a sensitivity and specificity of approximately 96.8 and

Table 2. Recommendations related to the FDG-PET in the evaluation of indeterminate lung lesions

Modality	Statement	Level of evidence
Indication for FDG	SPN >8–10 mm in diameter with indeterminate etiology: Patients with low-to-moderate (5–60%) pretest probability of malignancy should undergo FDG-PET/CT	1
No Indication for FDG	SPN <8–10 mm in diameter: patients with high pretest probability of malignancy (>60%)	2
Indication for CT alone	Patients with indeterminate SPN >8–10 mm in diameter, which are potentially curative: serial CT for observing the SPN is an acceptable management strategy if: Very low clinical probability of malignancy (> 5%) Low clinical probability (>30–40%) and the lesion is not hypermetabolic on FDG-PET or does not enhance >15 HU on dynamic ceCT Non-diagnostic needle biopsy and the lesion is not hypermetabolic on FDG-PET A fully informed patient prefers this nonaggressive approach	2
Indication for transthoracic needle biopsy or bronchoscopy	Patients with indeterminate SPN >8–10 mm in diameter which are potentially curative and if the: Clinical pretest probability and findings on imaging tests are discordant Benign diagnosis requiring specific treatment Patients are fully informed and want to prove or disprove the malignancy before surgery, specially when the risk of surgical complications are high	2
Surgical diagnosis	Patients with indeterminate SPN >8–10 mm in diameter which are potentially curative and if the: Clinical pretest probability of malignancy is moderate to high (>60%) SPN is hypermetabolic on FDG-PET A fully informed patient prefers undergoing a definitive diagnostic procedure	1

77.8%, respectively [20]. The counter argument put forward is the relatively high cost of a PET study. A group from Italy compared the traditional SPN work-up using CT, fine-needle aspiration cytology, and thoracoscopic biopsy with a diagnostic work-up including FDG-PET [77]. This study demonstrated a reduction in cost of approximately 50 Euros per patient, if PET was included in the work-up. Lejeune et al. [42] compared the cost-effectiveness ratio of three management strategies for SPN: wait and watch with periodic CT, PET, and a combination of CT plus PET. It was concluded that CT plus PET is the most cost-effective strategy in those patients having a risk of malignancy in the range of 5.7–87%, whereas patients having a risk of 0.3–5% should be followed up under the wait and watch strategy.

In ground glass nodules, preliminary PET studies have found a sensitivity of only 10% and a specificity of only 20% [79]. The ELCAP report has suggested a limited role of FGD-PET in the evaluation of these nodules because of the small size of the nodules and the potential for false negative findings in focal bronchioalveolar cell carcinoma [24]. Chhajed et al. [43] demonstrated the significant role of FDG-PET when combined with bronchoscopy in the diagnosis of noncalcified chest radiologic lesions ≤3 cm in size.

An important issue that determines the diagnostic accuracy of an imaging modality in the evaluation of SPN is the size of the nodule. Pulmonary nodules having a diameter of less than 5 mm on CT scan were found to be nonmalignant in 378 patients monitored with CT in the NY-ELCAP study. Bastarikka et al. [44] found a sensitivity of 69% for the detection of malignancy in nodules measuring 5–10 mm in size and a sensitivity of 95% in nodules greater than 10 mm in size applying ^{18}F-FDG-PET. The authors also observed a reduction in the apparent uptake of FDG in the nodules if the size of the nodule was less than 2 times the system resolution (7–8 mm) underlining the need for generating different criteria for determination of malignancy in patients having SPN smaller than 15 mm. The inability of PET to reliably detect nodules smaller than 7 mm has also been documented in a phantom study by Coleman et al. [45].

A meta-analysis of 5 prospective studies by Hellwig et al. [22], including at least 35 patients per study and fulfilling the quality criteria as specified by the German Consensus Conference, has shown that ^{18}F-FDG-PET has a sensitivity and specificity of 93 and 87%, respectively. The positive and negative predictive values are 94 and 89%, respectively; the probability to miss a malignant nodule is 11%. This risk has to be weighed against possible life threatening complications of surgery.

The method of interpretation of a PET study is also a matter of debate [24]. Hübner et al. [46] have shown that there is an improvement of approximately 10% in specificity of FDG-PET if Patlak analysis is applied for quantitation. Cerfolio et al. [47] – in their retrospective analysis to evaluate the role of maximum SUV in prediction of stage, recurrence, and survival in NSCLC patients – clearly demonstrated that the maximum SUV of a pulmonary nodule on ^{18}F-FDG-PET is an independent predictor of aggressiveness of NSCLC. The maximum SUV predicted more accurately the recurrence rate for stages IB and II NSCLC and the survival for patients with stage IB, II or IIIA than the TNM stage. A recent study by Yi et al. [48] proved that integrated PET/CT is more sensitive and accurate than helical dynamic CT for malignant nodule characterization; therefore, PET/CT should be performed as the first-line evaluation tool for SPN characterization. The authors also concluded that since helical dynamic CT has high specificity and acceptable sensitivity and accuracy, it may be a reasonable alternative for nodule characterization when PET/CT is unavailable.

Fletcher et al. [49] studied 532 subjects with untreated SPNs between 7 and 30 mm in size (average 16 mm) and newly diagnosed on radiography by ^{18}F-FDG-PET and CT. A definitive diagnosis was established for 344 participants. The prevalence of malignancy was 53%. PET inter- and intraobserver reliability was superior to CT. Definitely and probably benign results on PET and CT strongly predict benign SPN. However, such results were 3 times more common with PET. Definitely malignant results on PET were much more predictive of malignancy than were these results on CT. A malignant final diagnosis was approximately 10 times more likely than a benign final diagnosis in participants with PET results rated definitely malignant.

Paul et al. [50] prospectively evaluated 276 patients with newly diagnosed lung lesions whether ^{18}F-FDG-PET/CT is more accurate for determination of malignancy in newly diagnosed pulmonary lesions compared to separate interpretation of CT and FDG-PET. Histopathology was considered the gold standard in all patients; in addition 60 patients with benign lesion were followed-up for a mean duration of 1,040 days. Based upon their observations, the authors concluded that for differentiation of benign from malignant lung lesions, integrated FDG-PET/CT imaging was significantly more accurate than CT, but not ^{18}F-FDG-PET. In summary, the addition of metabolic imaging to morphological imaging leads to an increase in specificity, significantly reduces equivocal findings and is therefore recommended to further specify newly diagnosed lung lesions.

Lymph Node Staging

Prognosis of patients and therapeutic options available in NSCLC heavily depend upon whether mediastinal lymph nodes are involved or not.

A prospective Radiological Diagnostic Oncologic Group Study has shown that CT and MRI have low sensitivity and specificity (approximately 50 and 65%, respectively) in the detection of mediastinal lymph node metastases [77]. 30–40% of enlarged lymph nodes (2–4 cm in diameter) exhibit no tumor cells in histopathology [78]. CT has high false negative (7–39%) and very high false-positive (20–50%) values for the detection of mediastinal lymph nodes [3]. The presence of fat in an enlarged lymph node suggests a benign lesion. The introduction of spiral CT has not significantly improved the accuracy of mediastinal lymph node staging, as shown by a meta-analysis on mediastinal staging using CT and FDG-PET [22].

Table 3. Studies comparing CT and FDG-PET for mediastinal lymph node staging. Cumulative sensitivity and specificity were found to be 87% and 87%, respectively for FDG-PET in 1039 patients and 69 and 65%, respectively for CT in 504 patients

First Author	Year	Number of cases	CT		PET	
			% sensitivity	% specificity	% sensitivity	% specificity
Valk [98]	1995	76	63	54	83	94
Bury [77]	1997	66	79	72	88	87
Vansteenkiste [99]	1998	68	75	63	92	95
Marom [92]	1999	79	64	78	97	87
Liewald [90]	2000	80	n.r.	n.r.	92	76
Pieterman [61]	2000	102	75	66	90	85
Roberts [94]	2000	100	n.r.	n.r.	87	90
Poncelet [59]	2001	61	56	68	66	84
Kernstine [88]	2002	237	n.r.	n.r.	81	81
Vesselle [171]	2002	118	n.r.	n.r.	80	96
von Haag [101]	2002	52	50	65	66	91

Modified from Baum et al. [104].
n.r. = Not reported.

Several studies have investigated the role of FDG-PET and PET/CT in mediastinal lymph node staging [21, 30, 31, 41, 59, 61, 77–101] (table 3). Results of three meta-analyses have proven that FDG-PET is significantly more accurate than CT in the staging of lymph nodes in NSCLC, irrespective of the instrumentation for CT scan [22, 102, 103]. Tables 3 and 4 summarize studies (having more than 35 patients) on mediastinal lymph node staging (N0/1 vs. N2/3) in patients with NSCLC. Pooled data from these 11 studies in 1039 patients demonstrate that FDG-PET has an overall sensitivity of 87% and a specificity of 87% as compared to a sensitivity and specificity of 69 and 65%, for CT scan (7 studies with a total of 505 patients), respectively.

False-negative findings may occur in small-sized lymph nodes (table 5). False-positive findings are also possible (table 6). In order to decrease the impact of false-positive findings on patient management, lymph nodes showing increased FDG uptake on PET (and by that inducing a change in management of the patient, e.g. altering planned surgery) should be verified histologically, e.g. by endobronchial

Table 4. Comparison of different modalities in the mediastinal staging of lymph node metastases

	% sensitivity	% specificity	NPV %	PPV %	Prevalence %
PET	84	89	93	79	32
CT	57	82	83	56	28
Blind TBNA	76	96	71	100	70
EUS-FNA	88	91	77	98	69
Mediastinoscopy	81	100	91	100	37

Data from De Leyn et al. [168].

Table 5. Factors responsible for reduced sensitivity in lymph node assessment by FDG-PET

Low FDG uptake into primary tumor
Hyperglycaemia
Lymph nodes next to the primary tumour especially with central tumours
Short post FDG injection time (less than 60 minutes)
High SUV threshold for the evaluation of mediastinal lymph nodes

ultrasound-guided transbronchial needle aspiration (TBFNA) or mediastinoscopy [104].

The best approach for assessment of patients with stage IIIA-N2 after induction therapy remains a matter of debate specifically when it comes to deciding upon potential surgical treatment [80]. The performance of PET alone has not been as satisfactory in restaging as it was for the baseline lymph node staging. Studies have documented the superiority of PET/CT as compared to PET alone in lymph node staging [105]. PET/CT facilitates the identification of FDG uptake by normal structures such as brown adipose tissue or skeletal muscles. Consequently, the number of false-positive findings is significantly reduced. PET/CT has also been found to be more accurate than visual comparison of PET and CT images or software fusion of independently acquired PET and CT images [106–108]. Some studies [10, 109, 110] have demonstrated the superiority of TBFNA as being superior to CT or PET in mediastinum and hilar lymph node staging. In order to stratify

Table 6. Possible causes of false-positive findings in FDG-PET studies in the chest (modified from Bakheet et al. [169])

Physiologic uptake		
Muscle		Hypermetabolism after activation
Thymus		Normal until puberty
		Hyperplasia after chemotherapy
Bone marrow		Hyperplasia after chemotherapy
Brown fat		Non-shivering thermoregulation
Infection/inflammation		
Lung	Bacterial	Pneumonia, nocardiosis, abscess
	Mycobacterial	Active tuberculosis, atypical mycobacteriosis
	Fungal	Aspergillosis, coccidioides-mycosis, cryptococcosis, blastomycosis
	Granuloma	Granuloma, necrotizing granuloma, Wegner' granulomatosis, sarcoidosis, histoplasma granuloma, rheumatoid arthritis-associated lung disease, plasma cell granuloma
	Interstitial fibrosis	Fibrosing alveolitis, radiation pneumonitis
	Allergic	Airway inflammation with asthma
	Occupational	Inflammatory anthracosilicosis
	Nonspecific	Acute inflammation with bronchiectasis and atelectasis, tumor necrosis, reactive mesothelial cell, histiocytic infiltrate, fibrous histiocytic infiltrate, aspiration pneumonia with barium, aspiration pneumonia with salivary and tracheal secretions, inflammatory pseudotumor, organizing pneumonia
Mediastinum	Esophagus	Esophagitis
	Lymph node	Chronic nonspecific lymphadenitis; cryptococcal; tuberculosis; anthracosilicosis; active granuloma
Pleura		Empyema
		Pleural effusion
Nonmalignant tumors		
Lung		Chondrohamartoma
Pleura		Fibrous mesothelioma
Bone		Enchondroma

Table 6. Continued

Nerve root	Schwannoma
	Aggressive neurofibroma
Iatrogenic	
Trachea	Tracheostomy tube
Skin and soft tissue	Open lung biopsy Irradiation

patients for mediastinoscopy or thoracotomy depending upon the test (PET and CT) results, it is essential to establish the relationship between size and likelihood of malignancy. In a recent meta-analysis, de Langen et al. [111] have evaluated the dependency of FDG-PET on the lymph node size; in patients with a negative FDG-PET result, post-test probability for N2 disease was 5% for lymph nodes measuring 10–15 mm on CT, suggesting that these patients should be planned for thoracotomy as the yield of mediastinoscopy will be extremely low. For patients with lymph nodes measuring ≥16 mm on CT and a negative FDG-PET result, the post-test probability for N2 disease is 21%, indicating that these patients should be planned for mediastinoscopy prior to possible thoracotomy to prevent too many unnecessary thoracotomies in this subset.

Yang et al. [112] compared the diagnostic efficacies of integrated ^{18}F-FDG-PET/CT images and contrast-enhanced helical CT images (ceCT) in locoregional lymph node metastases in 122 potentially operable patients with proven or suspected NSCLC and compared the results of preoperative nodal staging with postoperative histopathological staging. Integrated PET/CT improved sensitivity, specificity, accuracy, positive predictive value, and negative predictive value as compared to ceCT in the assessment of locoregional lymph nodes, and provided more efficient and accurate data of nodal staging with a better effect on diagnosis and therapy in NSCLC.

Staging of Lung Cancer – Distant Metastases

Morphological Imaging

At the time of first presentation, occult metastases are present in approximately 30% of patients with adenocarcinoma or large cell carcinoma as compared to 15% in patients with squamous cell carcinoma [51]. Adrenal glands and liver are the most common sites of extrathoracic occult metastases. Without clinical or laboratory

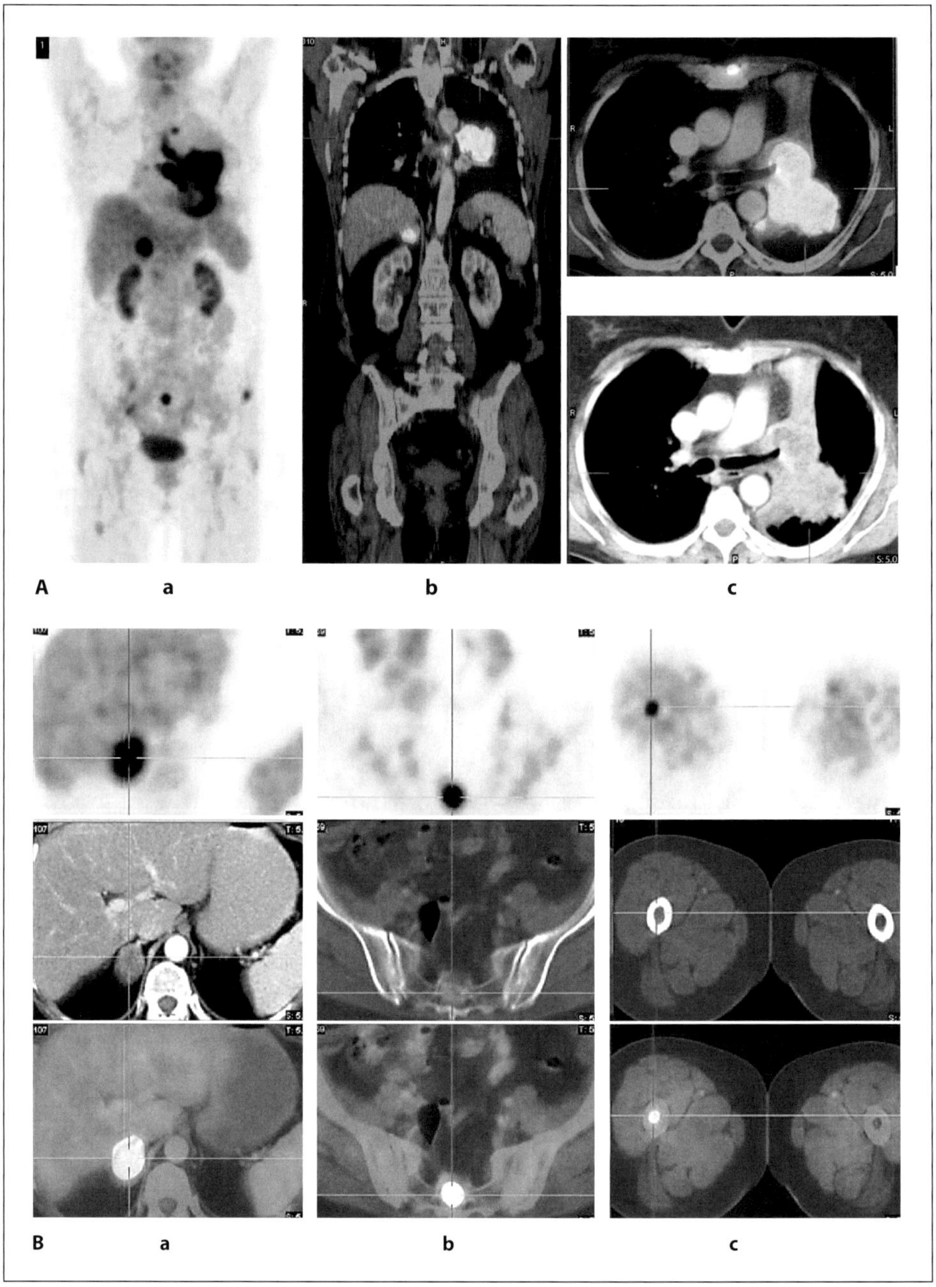

Fig. 1. **A** Whole-body imaging by FDG-PET/CT – a 'one stop shop'. NSCLC (squamous cell carcinoma) of the left lung, centrally located (SUV_{max} 17.9; ϕ 8.8 cm) with right adrenal metastasis (SUV_{max} 12.5, ϕ 3.6 cm), lymph node metastasis and multiple bone lesions which were not appreciable on CT alone. **a** Maximum intensity projection (MIP) image. **b** PET/CT coronal slice. **c** Transversal slice (primary tumor). **B** Accurate localisation of adrenal lesion by fused FDG-PET/CT images (**a**). Often molecular changes precede morphological changes: bone metastasis demonstrated by FDG-PET without appreciable osteoblastic or osteolytic changes on CT (**b, c**).

evidence, routine use of radiology is not advised for the work up of occult metastases. In approximately 10% of patients with lung cancer, an adrenal mass on CT is seen. However, CT alone often fails in differentiating benign adenoma which are present in 3–5% of the overall population from metastases [52, 53]. Non-contrast-enhanced CT followed by MRI has been reported as the most cost-effective morphologic evaluation for assessment of suspected adrenal masses [54]. Adrenal masses less than 10 HU on non-contrast-enhanced CT are generally benign; those adrenal masses which fail to fulfill the CT criteria for a benign lesion are followed up with MRI.

FDG-PET

Li et al. [55] studied 107 newly diagnosed NSCLC patients with clinical T1 stage and definite histologic or cytologic evidence using ^{18}F-FDG-PET/CT and compared the FDG uptake of primary tumors in relation to nodal or distant metastases at presentation. Significant differences were observed in primary tumor SUV_{max} for different stages indicating FDG uptake is a potential indicator of metastases in small primary lesion of NSCLC.

Vessele et al. [56] compared FDG uptake (after correction for partial volume effect) in primary NSCLC to tumor histologic features and Ki-67 proliferation index and found a significant positive correlation between FDG uptake and Ki-67 scores and significant differences in FDG uptake across histologic subtypes and differentiation groups. Bronchioalveolar carcinomas had lower FDG uptake and lower Ki-67 scores than any other histologic subtypes. Non-bronchioalveolar adenocarcinomas had lower FDG uptake and Ki-67 scores than squamous cell carcinomas or large cell undifferentiated carcinomas. Better differentiated NSCLC had lower FDG uptake and Ki-67 scores than more poorly differentiated NSCLC. These differences parallel nearly identical differences in Ki-67 scores, implying that differences in NSCLC tumor cell proliferation may give rise to commensurate differences in tumor glucose metabolism.

Al-Sarraf et al. [57] assessed retrospectively the clinical implication and prognostic significance of the SUV_{max} in 176 consecutive patients with histologically proven primary NSCLC, staged by integrated PET/CT prior to curative intent surgical resection. The SUV_{max} were correlated with tumor characteristics, lymph node involvement, surgical stage, type of surgical resection and survival following resection. Significantly higher SUV_{max} were observed in centrally located tumors, and tumors >4.0 cm in size. It was concluded that SUV_{max} may be a useful preoperative tool, in addition to other known prognostic markers, in allocating patients with potentially poor prognosis preoperatively to neoadjuvant chemotherapy prior to resection to improve their overall survival.

One of the major advantages of PET over other imaging modalities is the feasibility of performing a whole body scan in a single examination thereby

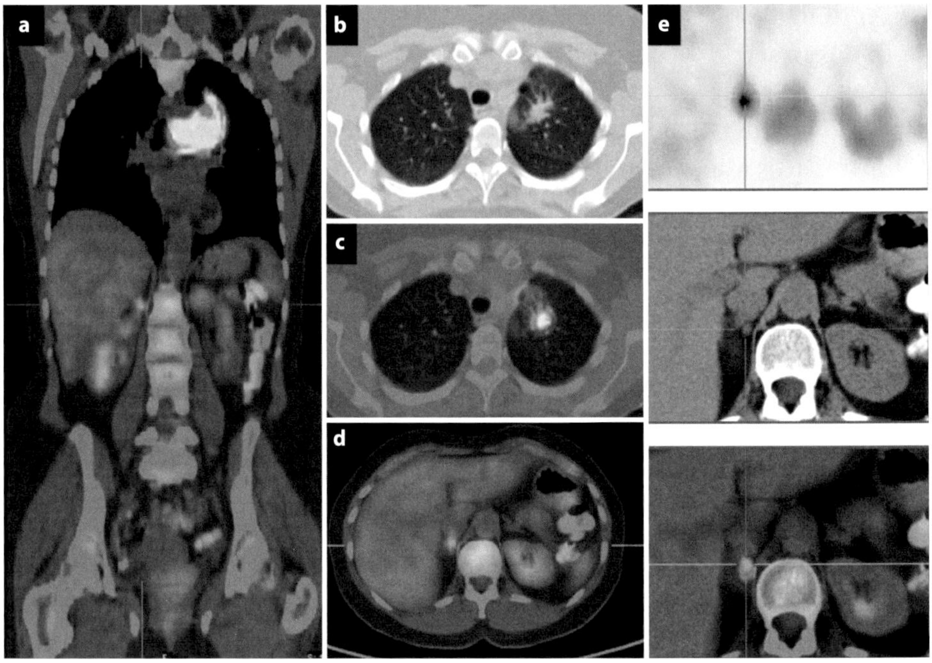

Fig. 2. Small, intense hypermetabolic adrenal metastasis (**a, d**, see also triangulation on image **e**) detected by FDG-PET/CT in a patient with centrally located NSCLC (**a–c**).

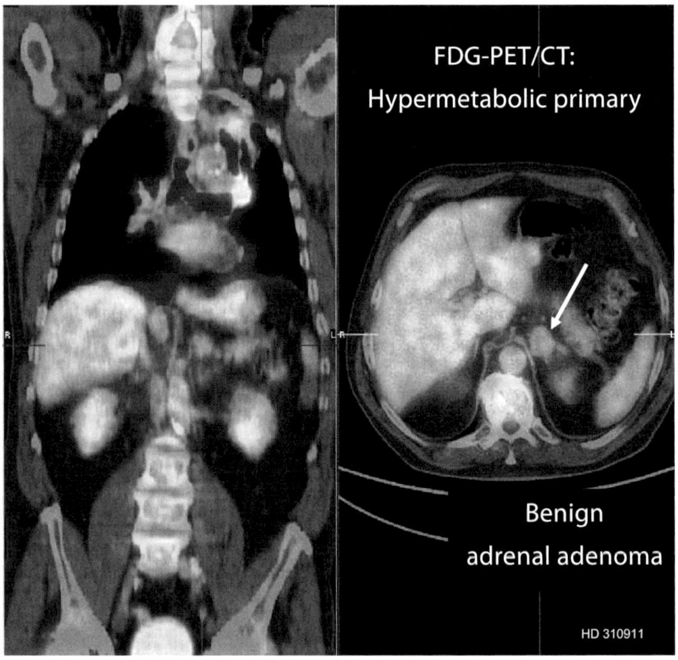

Fig. 3. Enlarged adrenal gland (adenoma) in a patient with lung cancer – a diagnostic challenge for CT. FDG-PET can clearly differentiate between benign changes and metastatic lesions based on the glucose consumption (see also fig. 1B).

allowing detection of distant and lymph node metastases along with the primary tumor (fig. 1). Once distant metastases are diagnosed, palliative treatment is the only available treatment option, except for a single brain metastasis, which, in selected cases can be cured by complete surgical resection followed by stereotactic radiotherapy (e.g. gamma knife) or proton beam radiation. It has been documented in several studies [41, 58–62] that FDG-PET is superior to CT and other conventional imaging techniques in detecting distant metastases in patients with lung cancer. The average frequency of occult extrathoracic metastases in these studies was 13%; FDG-PET resulted in change in treatment management in 18% of all patients studied. A significant correlation was observed between the ISS stage and the frequency of metastases in patients with suspected stage III NSCLC prior to conformational radiotherapy. The frequency of metastases was found to increase with the increase in ISS stage of the disease; 7.5%, 18 and 24% in stage I, stage II and stage III, respectively. Van Tinteren et al. [63] showed that in NSCLC selection of patients for surgical resection can be improved significantly by the addition of FDG-PET. Some studies have shown the superiority of integrated PET/CT over CT or PET alone in staging of lung cancer [64, 65]. In the absence of integrated PET/CT, visually correlated PET and CT is a valuable alternative. Pozo-Rodriquez et al. have found similar performance of FDG-PET and helical CT in the mediastinal staging of NSCLC [66] which contradicts our experience and that of most others.

FDG-PET has been shown to have high sensitivity in detection of adrenal metastases [67] (fig. 2, 3). An enlarged adrenal is present in up to 20% of patients at the time of initial presentation [68]. Pooled data on whole body FDG-PET yielded a sensitivity and specificity of 97 and 98%, respectively [59, 68–70,114–116]. The negative and positive predictive values were 98 and 94%, respectively. These data demonstrate that FDG-PET has a high negative predictive value in the differential diagnosis of small adrenal masses.

In the detection of brain metastases, FDG-PET has no significant role as the positive and negative predictive values are much lower as compared to MRI [22]. For detection of bone metastases, FDG-PET has higher specificity (98% vs. 61%) than skeletal scintigraphy [60, 71].

Kramer et al. [72] have shown that the tumor stage on FDG-PET is the most significant prognostic factor for survival in patients with NSCLC. Nguyen et al. [73] have shown in an important study that FDG tumor uptake is more valuable than Glut-1 or Ki-67 expression in terms of predicting prognosis in patients with resected NSCLC and that SUV_{max} is the only determinant of disease-free survival. Analyzing 498 patients with lung cancer, including surgical and non-surgical cases, Davies et al. [74] concluded that the high tumor uptake of FDG is associated with worse survival. In stage 1 lung adenocarcinoma, FDG uptake was found to be predictive of disease free survival [75].

Yi et al. [76] compared prospectively the diagnostic efficacies of PET/CT and 3.0 T whole-body magnetic resonance imaging (MRI) for determining TNM stages in 165 patients with histologically proven NSCLC and found that both imaging modalities provide acceptable accuracy and comparable efficacy for NSCLC staging, but for M-stage determination, each modality has its own advantages.

Recurrence Detection

Conventional imaging and FDG-PET play a complimentary role in the detection of tumor recurrences. FDG-PET is used to differentiate scar from viable recurrent tumor or residual tissue [113] based upon the increased glucose metabolism in tumor tissue as compared to nonviable fibrotic tissue. FDG-PET detects local recurrences of lung cancer with very high sensitivity (average of 98%) and very good specificity of 87% [68]. False-positive findings may occur especially after external radiation therapy (due to radiation pneumonitis).

Molecular (Metabolic) Radiation Therapy Planning

In patients with lung cancer, radiotherapy is used with curative as well as with palliative intent. For effective radiation therapy, and to increase the therapeutic index, exact staging of disease is essential [114]. The main cause of death after primary radiation therapy of lung cancer is local recurrence, making it necessary to have precise delineation of the extent of tumor and its size. MRI and CT scan often fail to differentiate malignant from normal tissues, particularly when atelectasis, pleural effusion, or normal tissue displacement occurs. During calculation of gross tumor volume (GTV) and ultimately planning target volume this may lead to wide intra-observer variation and radiation exposure to normal and benign tissues [115, 116, 160, 161].

Since in 3D conformational radiation therapy the isodoses can maximally follow the delineated target volume, it is possible to increase the dose without causing damage to normal tissue [79, 117]. The coregistration of planning CT and PET, with the patient in the same treatment position, is an exciting new tool for improving the planning target volume by treating the metabolically active tumor ('biological target volume or BTV) and not – as it is routine today – an anatomical or morphological target volume based only on CT scan [118]. Several studies have shown the importance of incorporating PET (fig. 4) in radiotherapy planning of lung cancer [119–124] and different methods for the delineation of target volume on PET have already been described [125].

In the first prospective study of its kind, describing the use of PET in 3D planning of radiation therapy in 27 patients with NSCLC, Schmücking et al. [114]

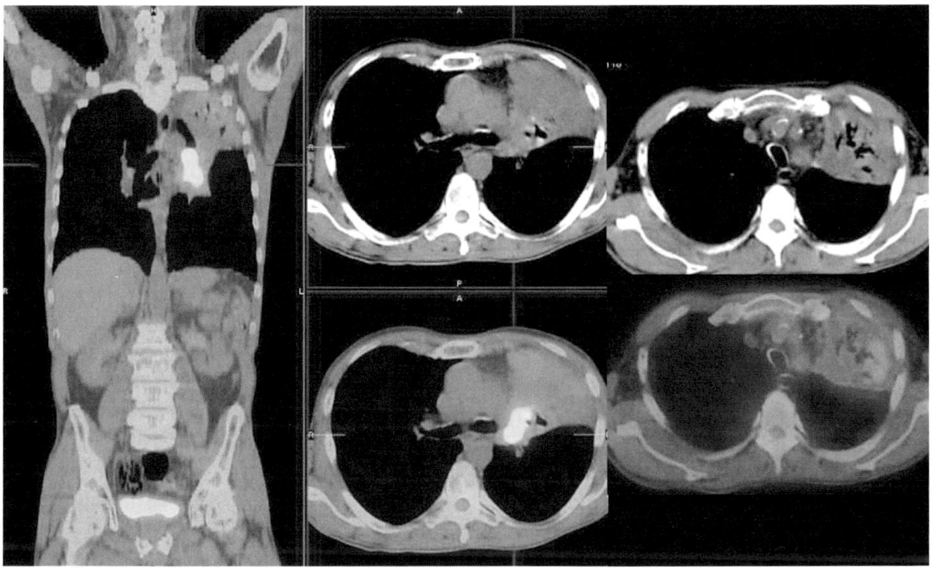

Fig. 4. Differentiating atelectasis (non-FDG-avid) from vital tumor (FDG-avid) and obtructive pneumonitis (non- or only mild FDA-avid) by FDG-PET. This is especially important for patients with functionally inoperable primary tumors before external beam radiation therapy.

concluded that PET is an important complimentary tool to morphological imaging used for exact localization of nodal tumor involvement as well as for determining the extent of the primary tumor; radiation therapy could be delivered with less toxicity in most patients; and better tumor control may be possible by molecular (metabolic) radiation therapy planning.

Recent research has focused on establishing the optimum thresholds for maximum standardized uptake value calculation. The result suggests that 15–20% may be the appropriate threshold value; however, Bihl et al. [126] have shown that there is no single threshold delineating the PET_{GTV} accurate for volume definition when compared with that provided by the CT_{GTV} in the majority of NSCLC patients. In fact, several issues have to be taken into consideration for defining the target volumes [125, 127, 128].

A recent study [129] has shown that glucose metabolic rate derived from dynamic PET/CT were significantly smaller than SUV-based volumes. These findings can be of importance for PET-based radiotherapy planning and therapy response monitoring. The role of PET in radiotherapy is also highlighted in a study by Cherk et al. [127] using ^{18}F-FDG as well as ^{18}F-fluoromisonidazole PET and shows that the hypoxic cell fraction of primary NSCLC is consistently low. Since the response to external beam radiotherapy is highly dependent on the oxygen concentration in the target tissue, this study has far-reaching consequences.

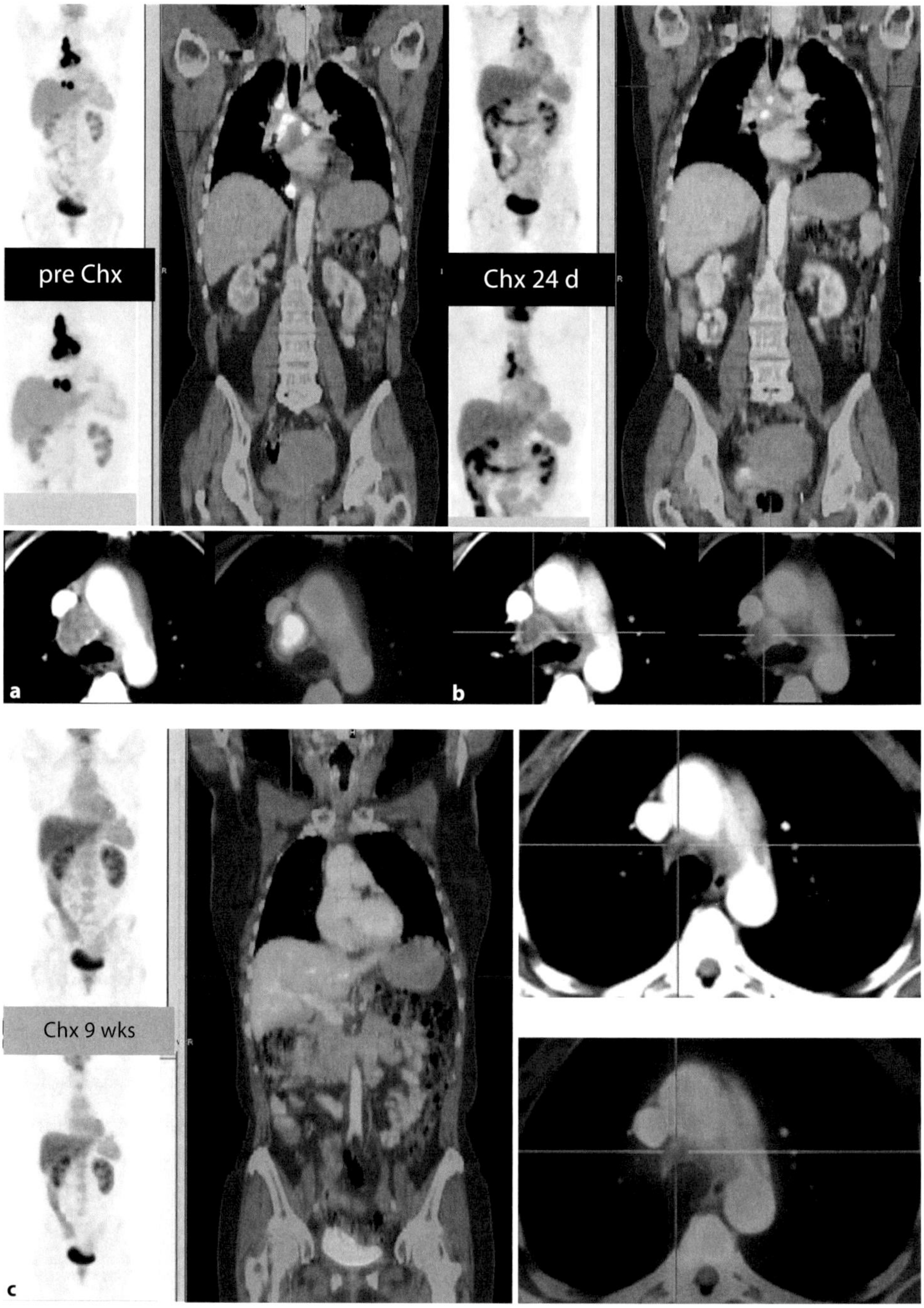

Fig. 5. a–c Response assessment postchemotherapy by FGD-PET/CT: changes in tumor metabolism (PET) precede size changes (CT). Therapy response after one cycle (24 days) chemotherapy demonstrated by FDG-PET (**a**), when CT image still shows enlarged lymph node (**b**), and at 9 weeks (**c**): metabolic complete remission (mCR).

Prediction and Monitoring Response to Therapy

Tumor response is usually assessed according to the WHO or the RECIST criteria. In solid tumors, morphologic changes induced by therapy usually take several weeks to months to occur (fig. 5, 6), thereby subjecting the nonresponding patients to unnecessary side effects of chemotherapy or radiotherapy. Apart from that, the relative inability of morphologic imaging to differentiate scar tissue from viable tumor with high degree of specificity may lead to masking of tumor regression.

In the response assessment of lung cancer patients, PET is used in three main areas: assessment of response to neoadjuvant chemotherapy [130, 131], early assessment of response to therapy and restaging after completion of therapy [6]. The potential of FDG-PET in the evaluation of response to inductive chemotherapy in lung cancer patients has been assessed by Baum et al. [132]. A close correlation between histomorphometric studies and the results of PET imaging was found. In 26 patients treated with neoadjuvant chemotherapy, Ryu et al. [133] found a sensitivity and specificity of FDG-PET of 88 and 67%, respectively, for the diagnosis of tumor viability and of 58 and 97%, respectively, in nodal restaging. Akhurst et al. [134] reported a very high negative predictive value of 98% for the detection of viable residual tumor tissue, but a low diagnostic accuracy (52%) for nodal tumor status. Poettgen et al. [135] concluded that the corrected SUV_{max} from two serial PET/CT scans, before and after three chemotherapy cycles or later, allows prediction of histopathologic response in the primary tumor and mediastinal lymph nodes and have prognostic value.

Su et al. [136] have shown that glucose metabolic activity as measured by FDG-PET reflects the response to gefitnib (endothelial growth factor receptor kinase inhibitor). Weber et al. [137] used FDG-PET for the early assessment of response to chemotherapy in 57 patients with NSCLC 1 and 3 weeks after the first cycle of chemotherapy and found a significant correlation between the metabolic activity and the final outcome after therapy. Whereas the early metabolic response predicted a better survival after the first 3 cycles of chemotherapy, a poor response was associated with disease progression, which opens the possibility of excluding nonresponders from the treatment regime and thereby reducing the morbidity and cost of treatment.

Cerfolio et al. [138] demonstrated that repeat PET/CT is superior to repeat CT for the restaging of patients with stage IIIA NSCLC after neoadjuvant chemoradiotherapy and also concluded that the percent decrease in the SUV_{max} of the primary and of the involved lymph node is predictive of pathology; however, nodal biopsy is required as a persistently high SUV_{max} does not equate to residual cancer.

A high correlation between tumor FDG uptake after chemoradiotherapy and patient outcome was also confirmed by Hellwig et al. [139] in 47 patients after preoperative chemoradiotherapy. Patients were classified as responders, if the SUV

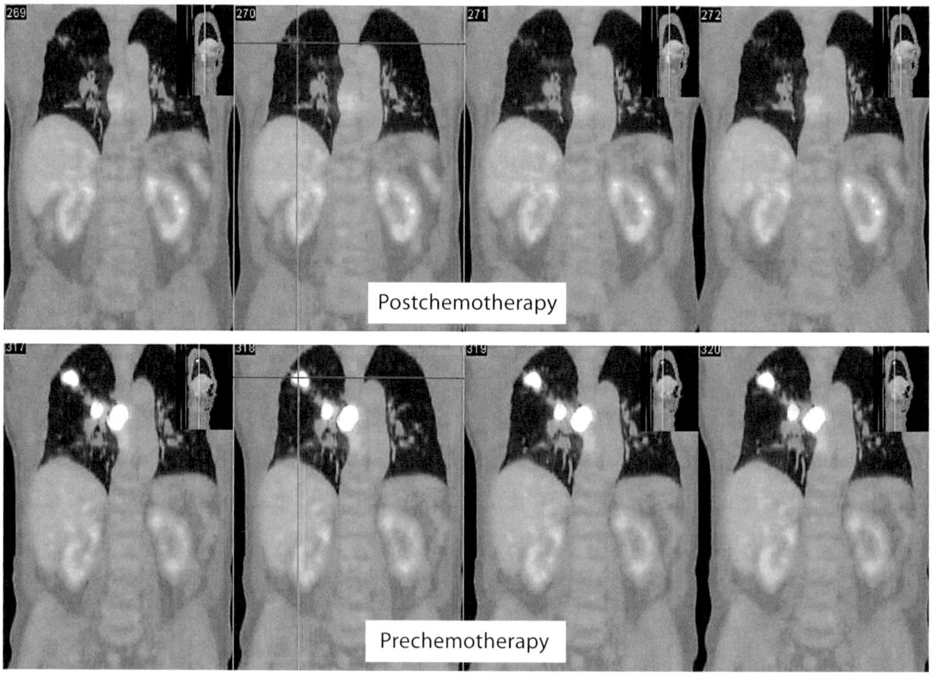

Fig. 6. FDG-PET/CT for evaluation of patients post chemotherapy (3 cycles cisplatinum/paclitaxel): CR (according to PERCIST) on PET whereas CT showed PR. Lobectomy with radical lymphadenectomy was performed and histopathologically revealed complete remission (CR) without evidence of vital tumor tissue confirming the FDG-PET result.

of the primary tumor was <4. Median survival after resection was greater than 56 months for PET responders and 19 months for PET nonresponders ($p < 0.001$). Schmücking et al. [140, 205] have demonstrated a significant correlation between histologic results and the PET findings for tumor regression and survival in locally advanced NSCLC after neoadjuvant treatment.

Nahmias et al. [141] prospectively studied 16 patients with NSCLC weekly for 7 weeks after 2 courses of docetaxel and carboplatin. They observed that the patients with NSCLC, who had a positive outcome, as exhibited by prolonged survival, were those who showed a tumor metabolic response assessed using weekly ^{18}F-FDG-PET studies. ^{18}F-FDG-PET studies performed at 1 and 3 weeks after the initiation of chemotherapy allowed prediction of the response to therapy.

Tanvetyanon et al. [142] reported on a prospective trial that examined the ability of changes in computed tomography (CT) or FDG-PET before and after neoadjuvant chemotherapy for resectable NSCLC to predict survival and to define an appropriate imaging evaluation for these patients so that therapy, and hopefully outcome, could be optimized. CT response, defined by RECIST criteria, seems to predict outcomes only in resectable stage III patients. However, no statistically significant correlation was found between the CT response and survival in resectable stage I and II disease. The investigators also studied whether FDG-PET was a better predictor of survival compared with conventional imaging. Interestingly, the investigators could not find changes in FDG uptake to predicted outcome and serial PET studies did not provide the information needed to guide patient management. This is a different conclusion than reported by other groups. However, one of the limitations of this study was the low number of patients.

Similar caution in evaluating FDG-PET in NSCLC patients after neoadjuvant chemotherapy has been also reported by Poettgen et al. [143]. SUV and residual tumor volumes from FDG-PET/CT were correlated with histopathological parameters of the resection specimens (tumor cell density, necrosis, scar, macrophage infiltration) in patients with locally advanced NSCLC (stage IIIA/IIIB) after neoadjuvant induction chemotherapy (platinum-based doublet) and concurrent chemoradiotherapy (cisplatin/vinorelbine, 45 Gy). Based on their observations in this study, the authors concluded that postinduction FDG uptake should be interpreted with caution in larger residual tumor volumes since high SUV levels may be due to macrophage infiltration and not viable tumor tissue.

Vessele et al. [144] prospectively evaluated the prognostic significance of [18] F-FDG uptake in primary NSCLC in a carefully staged population. In 208 potentially resectable NSCLC patients, the tumor stage was prognostic in NSCLC. However, tumor FDG uptake did not provide additional prognostic information. This prospective study contradicts prior reports.

Pleural Metastases

FDG-PET has also been used for the assessment of pleural mass or pleural effusion for evidence of malignancy [145]. In a study conducted by Erasmus et al. [12, 25] in 25 patients with suspected malignant pleural effusion, the sensitivity, specificity and positive predictive value of FDG-PET were found to be 95, 67 and 95%, respectively, demonstrating that FDG-PET will help in the appropriate staging of NSCLC patients with pleural effusions. Schaffler et al. [146] have compared the utility of FDG-PET with CT in 92 patients for their ability to differentiate benign from malignant pleural effusion. FDG-PET was found to have sensitivity, specificity and positive predictive values of 100, 71 and 63%, respectively. The difference in the positive predictive value from the previous study by Erasmus and coworkers is attributed to the inclusion of a relatively large number of patients with benign pleural disease. This study also demonstrated that CT was indeterminate in 71% of the patients. The pleural dissemination of adenocarcinoma lung is best diagnosed using the CT component of their FDG-PET/CT study, since lesions causing pleural involvement without pleural effusion is beyond the resolution of PET [147]. Research is on-going to find out the role of FDG-PET/CT in pleural mesothelioma and the initial results are very promising [148].

Cost-Effectiveness

One of the major concerns in the routine use of PET in clinical practice are costs associated with FDG-PET studies. However, FDG-PET also has the potential to lead to cost savings by reducing the number of expensive invasive procedures. Several studies have demonstrated the cost-effectiveness of PET in the management of NSCLC patients. Cost of patient care and life expectancy was taken as the criteria for assessment of cost-effectiveness. In spite of differences in medico-economic data due to diversities in the health care structure, various studies from the United States, Europe, Japan and Australia have come to the common conclusion that FDG-PET is cost-effective for the differentiation of lung nodules as well for the pre-operative staging of NSCLC [149–156, 206–216]. A study comparing confirmatory and selective mediastinoscopy in patients with positive FDG-PET has shown approximately double the cost savings per patient (USD 2,267 vs. 1,154) at the cost of missing out 1.7% of patients who might have been cured [152].

Recently, Pompen et al. [157] performed a retrospective medical chart review by collecting data from the time of diagnosis until the time of death or the end of the evaluation period. In addition to the demographic data, they also collected information on the overall management of the patient. Hospital resource utilization data collection included number of outpatient specialist visits, number and length of hospitalizations, type and number of diagnostic and laboratory procedures, type and number of radiotherapy cycles and detailed information on chemotherapy. To evaluate the economic impact of second-line treatment, a distinction was made between patients who received only best supportive care (BSC, group A) and those who received chemotherapy as a second-line treatment in addition to BSC (group B). The study, performed from the hospital perspective and reports on 2005 costs, showed that these patients show high medical resource consumption, with hospitalization being the main cost driver in both groups. As economic arguments are becoming increasingly important in medical decision-making on both national and local levels, this information is relevant for both, policy makers and specialists.

Based upon the multitude of data available on the higher sensitivity and specificity of PET/CT and the ability to predict early response and change management strategies, it can be seen that FDG-PET/CT holds great promise for decreasing the cost burden on the health system.

Small Cell Lung Cancer

SCLC is a tumor of neuroendocrine origin with an aggressive growth pattern, often metastasizing early and proliferating rapidly. The role of FDG-PET in the staging of SCLC is somewhat controversial [158]. According to Detterbeck et al. [159], the clinical presentation and radiographic appearance of the disease are sufficiently characteristic to negate the need for further evaluation. However, the few studies that evaluated the role of FDG-PET as compared to conventional radiographic imaging have demonstrated that PET changed patient management in 8.3–29% of the patients [160, 161]. Patients having extensive disease were treated with chemotherapy whereas those having limited disease received chemoradiotherapy. Kruger et al. [162] have demonstrated low FDG uptake in patients with highly differentiated, low proliferative pulmonary neuroendocrine tumors (so-called typical carcinoids), necessitating biopsy and surgical resection, even if the FDG-PET study does not show any hypermetabolic activity. The recent research in SCLC has shown some promising results on the use of integrated PET/CT in SCLC by simplifying and even improving the accuracy of current staging protocol [163] as well as in response evaluation [164, 165].

A recent study by Kut et al. [166] found that PET is potentially useful for the initial staging and monitoring of patients with SCLC and it may be superior to bone scan in detecting bone metastasis. The cost-effectiveness of PET scan in SCLC remains to be determined.

Niho et al. [167] retrospectively investigated the clinical usefulness of FDG-PET for the evaluation of patients with limited-disease small cell lung cancer (LD-SCLC) diagnosed by conventional staging procedures. They observed that FDG-PET could detect additional lesions in patients diagnosed as having LD-SCLC by conventional staging procedures. The therapeutic strategies were changed in 8% of patients based on the results of FDG-PET. The authors recommended that FDG-PET should be used as the initial staging tool for patients with this disease.

In conclusion, FDG-PET also has a definite role in the initial staging of SCLC patients.

References

1 Spaepen K, Stroobants S, Dupont P, et al: Early restaging positron emission tomography with (18)F-fluorodeoxyglucose predicts outcome in patients with aggressive non-Hodgkin's lymphoma. Ann Oncol 2002;13:1356–1363.

2 Bunyaviroch T, Coleman RE: PET evaluation of lung cancer. J Nucl Med 2006;47:451–469.

3 Lee JKT SS, Stanley RJ, Heiken JP: Computed Body Tomography with MRI Correlation, ed 3. Philadelphia, Lippincott Williams & Wilkins, 1998.

4 Hoffmann H, Dienemann H: Der Pulmonale Rundherd: Prinzipien der Diagnostik. Dt Arzteblatt 2000;97:A1065–A1071.

5 Jeong YJ, Yi CA, Lee KS: Solitary pulmonary nodules: detection, characterization, and guidance for further diagnostic workup and treatment. AJR Am J Roentgenol 2007;188:57–68.
6 Mavi A, Lakhani P, Zhuang H, Gupta NC, Alavi A: Fluorodeoxyglucose-PET in characterizing solitary pulmonary nodules, assessing pleural diseases, and the initial staging, restaging, therapy planning, and monitoring response of lung cancer. Radiol Clin North Am 2005;43:1–21, ix.
7 Gambhir SS, Shepherd JE, Shah BD, et al: Analytical decision model for the cost-effective management of solitary pulmonary nodules. J Clin Oncol 1998;16:2113–2125.
8 Proto AV, Thomas SR: Pulmonary nodules studied by computed tomography. Radiology 1985; 156:149–153.
9 Swensen SJ, Brown LR, Colby TV, Weaver AL, Midthun DE: Lung nodule enhancement at CT: prospective findings. Radiology 1996;201:447–455.
10 Takamochi K, Yoshida J, Murakami K, et al: Pitfalls in lymph node staging with positron emission tomography in non-small cell lung cancer patients. Lung Cancer 2005;47:235–242.
11 Henschke CI, Yankelevitz DF, Mirtcheva R, McGuinness G, McCauley D, Miettinen OS: CT screening for lung cancer: frequency and significance of part-solid and nonsolid nodules. AJR Am J Roentgenol 2002;178:1053–1057.
12 Erasmus JJ, McAdams HP, Rossi SE, Goodman PC, Coleman RE, Patz EF : FDG PET of pleural effusions in patients with non-small cell lung cancer. AJR Am J Roentgenol 2000;175:245–249.
13 Gould MK, Lillington GA: Strategy and cost in investigating solitary pulmonary nodules. Thorax 1998;53(suppl 2):S32–S37.
14 Yankelevitz DF, Henschke CI: Does 2-year stability imply that pulmonary nodules are benign? AJR Am J Roentgenol 1997;168:325–328.
15 Grills IS, Yan D, Black QC, Wong CY, Martinez AA, Kestin LL: Clinical implications of defining the gross tumor volume with combination of CT and (18)FDG-positron emission tomography in non-small-cell lung cancer. Int J Radiat Oncol Biol Phys 2007;67:709–719.
16 Gurney JW: Determining the likelihood of malignancy in solitary pulmonary nodules with Bayesian analysis. I. Theory. Radiology 1993;186: 405–413.
17 Bryant AS, Cerfolio RJ: The maximum standardized uptake values on integrated FDG-PET/CT is useful in differentiating benign from malignant pulmonary nodules. Ann Thorac Surg 2006;82: 1016–1020.
18 Hashimoto Y, Tsujikawa T, Kondo C, et al: Accuracy of PET for diagnosis of solid pulmonary lesions with 18F-FDG uptake below the standardized uptake value of 2.5. J Nucl Med 2006;47:426–431.
19 Slomka PJ, Dey D, Przetak C, Aladl UE, Baum RP: Automated 3-dimensional registration of stand-alone (18)F-FDG whole-body PET with CT. J Nucl Med 2003;44:1156–1167.
20 Gould MK, Maclean CC, Kuschner WG, Rydzak CE, Owens DK: Accuracy of positron emission tomography for diagnosis of pulmonary nodules and mass lesions: a meta-analysis. JAMA 2001; 285:914–924.
21 Albes JM, Lietzenmayer R, Schott U, Schulen E, Wehrmann M, Ziemer G: Improvement of non-small-cell lung cancer staging by means of positron emission tomography. Thorac Cardiovasc Surg 1999;47:42–47.
22 Hellwig D, Ukena D, Paulsen F, Bamberg M, Kirsch CM: Meta-analysis of the efficacy of positron emission tomography with F-18-fluorodeoxyglucose in lung tumors: basis for discussion of the German Consensus Conference on PET in Oncology 2000. Pneumologie 2001;55:367–377.
23 Scott WJ, Schwabe JL, Gupta NC, Dewan NA, Reeb SD, Sugimoto JT: Positron emission tomography of lung tumors and mediastinal lymph nodes using [18F]fluorodeoxyglucose: The Members of the PET-Lung Tumor Study Group. Ann Thorac Surg 1994;58:698–703.
24 Lowe VJ, DeLong DM, Hoffman JM, Coleman RE: Optimum scanning protocol for FDG-PET evaluation of pulmonary malignancy. J Nucl Med 1995;36:883–887.
25 Lowe VJ, Duhaylongsod FG, Patz EF, et al: Pulmonary abnormalities and PET data analysis: a retrospective study. Radiology 1997;202:435–439.
26 Lowe VJ, Fletcher JW, Gobar L, et al: Prospective investigation of positron emission tomography in lung nodules. J Clin Oncol 1998;16:1075–1084.
27 Menda Y, Bushnell DL, Madsen MT, McLaughlin K, Kahn D, Kernstine KH: Evaluation of various corrections to the standardized uptake value for diagnosis of pulmonary malignancy. Nucl Med Commun 2001;22:1077–1081.

28 Pitman AG, Hicks RJ, Binns DS, et al: Performance of sodium iodide based (18)F-fluorodeoxyglucose positron emission tomography in the characterization of indeterminate pulmonary nodules or masses. Br J Radiol 2002;75:114–121.

29 Prauer HW, Weber WA, Romer W, Treumann T, Ziegler SI, Schwaiger M: Controlled prospective study of positron emission tomography using the glucose analogue [18F]fluorodeoxyglucose in the evaluation of pulmonary nodules. Br J Surg 1998; 85:1506–1511.

30 Sazon DA, Santiago SM, Soo Hoo GW, et al: Fluorodeoxyglucose-positron emission tomography in the detection and staging of lung cancer. Am J Respir Crit Care Med 1996;153:417–421.

31 Hagberg RC, Segall GM, Stark P, Burdon TA, Pompili MF: Characterization of pulmonary nodules and mediastinal staging of bronchogenic carcinoma with F-18 fluorodeoxyglucose positron emission tomography. Eur J Cardiothorac Surg 1997;12:92–97.

32 Hain SF, Curran KM, Beggs AD, Fogelman I, O'Doherty MJ, Maisey MN: FDG-PET as a 'metabolic biopsy' tool in thoracic lesions with indeterminate biopsy. Eur J Nucl Med 2001;28: 1336–1340.

33 Halter G, Storck M, Guhlmann A, Frank J, Grosse S, Liewald F: FDG positron emission tomography in the diagnosis of peripheral pulmonary focal lesions. Thorac Cardiovasc Surg 2000;48:97–101.

34 Hung GU, Shiau YC, Tsai SC, Chao TH, Ho YJ, Kao CH: Value of 18F-fluoro-2-deoxyglucose positron emission tomography in the evaluation of recurrent colorectal cancer. Anticancer Res 2001;21:1375–1378.

35 Imdahl A, Reinhardt MJ, Nitzsche EU, et al: Impact of 18F-FDG-positron emission tomography for decision making in colorectal cancer recurrences. Langenbecks Arch Surg 2000;385: 129–134.

36 Knight SB, Delbeke D, Stewart JR, Sandler MP: Evaluation of pulmonary lesions with FDG-PET. Comparison of findings in patients with and without a history of prior malignancy. Chest 1996; 109:982–988.

37 Bury T, Dowlati A, Paulus P, et al: Evaluation of the solitary pulmonary nodule by positron emission tomography imaging. Eur Respir J 1996;9: 410–414.

38 Croft DR, Trapp J, Kernstine K, et al: FDG-PET imaging and the diagnosis of non-small cell lung cancer in a region of high histoplasmosis prevalence. Lung Cancer 2002;36:297–301.

39 Dewan NA, Shehan CJ, Reeb SD, Gobar LS, Scott WJ, Ryschon K: Likelihood of malignancy in a solitary pulmonary nodule: comparison of Bayesian analysis and results of FDG-PET scan. Chest 1997;112:416–422.

40 Duhaylongsod FG, Lowe VJ, Patz EF Jr, Vaughn AL, Coleman RE, Wolfe WG: Detection of primary and recurrent lung cancer by means of F-18 fluorodeoxyglucose positron emission tomography (FDG PET). J Thorac Cardiovasc Surg 1995;110:130–139; discussion 9–40.

41 Gupta NC, Graeber GM, Rogers JS 2nd, Bishop HA. Comparative efficacy of positron emission tomography with FDG and computed tomographic scanning in preoperative staging of non-small cell lung cancer. Ann Surg 1999;229: 286–291.

42 Lejeune C, Al Zahouri K, Woronoff-Lemsi MC, et al: Use of a decision analysis model to assess the medicoeconomic implications of FDG PET imaging in diagnosing a solitary pulmonary nodule. Eur J Health Econ 2005;6:203–214.

43 Chhajed PN, Bernasconi M, Gambazzi F, et al: Combining bronchoscopy and positron emission tomography for the diagnosis of the small pulmonary nodule < or = 3 cm. Chest 2005;128:3558–3564.

44 Bastarrika G, Garcia-Velloso MJ, Lozano MD, et al: Early lung cancer detection using spiral computed tomography and positron emission tomography. Am J Respir Crit Care Med 2005;171: 1378–1383.

45 Coleman RE, Laymon CM, Turkington TG: FDG imaging of lung nodules: a phantom study comparing SPECT, camera-based PET, and dedicated PET. Radiology 1999;210:823–828.

46 Hubner KF, Buonocore E, Gould HR, et al: Differentiating benign from malignant lung lesions using 'quantitative' parameters of FDG PET images. Clin Nucl Med 1996;21:941–949.

47 Cerfolio R, Bryant A, Ohja B: The maximum standardised uptake values on positron emission tomography of non-small cell lung cancer predict stage,recurrence and survival. J Thorac Cardiovasc Surg 2005;130:151–159.

48 Yi CA, Lee KS, Kim BT, et al: Tissue characterization of solitary pulmonary nodule: comparative study between helical dynamic CT and integrated PET/CT. J Nucl Med 2006;47:443–450.

49 Fletcher JW, Kymes SM, Gould M, et al: A comparison of the diagnostic accuracy of 18F-FDG PET and CT in the characterization of solitary pulmonary nodules. J Nucl Med 2008;49:179–185.

50 Pauls S, Buck AK, Halter G, et al: Performance of integrated FDG-PET/CT for differentiating benign and malignant lung lesions: results from a large prospective clinical trial. Mol Imaging Biol 2008;10:121–128.

51 Sider L, Horejs D: Frequency of extrathoracic metastases from bronchogenic carcinoma in patients with normal-sized hilar and mediastinal lymph nodes on CT. AJR Am J Roentgenol 1988; 151:893–895.

52 Oliva JP, Pimentel G, Borron M, et al: Pilot study with the monoclonal antibody IOR-C5 as a potential agent of radioimmunoscintigraphy in colorectal cancer. Rev Esp Med Nucl 2001;20: 282–288.

53 Sandler MA, Pearlberg J, Madrazo B, Gitschlag K, Gross S: Computed tomography evaluation of the adrenal gland in the preoperative assessment of bronchogenic carcinoma. Radiology 1982;145: 733–736.

54 Remer EM, Obuchowski N, Ellis JD, Rice TW, Adelstein DJ, Baker ME: Adrenal mass evaluation in patients with lung carcinoma: a cost-effectiveness analysis. AJR Am J Roentgenol 2000;174: 1033–1039.

55 Li M, Liu N, Hu M, et al: Relationship between primary tumor fluorodeoxyglucose uptake and nodal or distant metastases at presentation in T1 stage non-small cell lung cancer. Lung Cancer 2009;63:383–386.

56 Vesselle H, Salskov A, Turcotte E, et al: Relationship between non-small cell lung cancer FDG uptake at PET, tumor histology, and Ki-67 proliferation index. J Thorac Oncol 2008;3:971–978.

57 Al-Sarraf N, Gately K, Lucey J, et al: Clinical implication and prognostic significance of standardised uptake value of primary non-small cell lung cancer on positron emission tomography: analysis of 176 cases. Eur J Cardiothorac Surg 2008;34:892–897.

58 Vansteenkiste JF: Imaging in lung cancer: positron emission tomography scan. Eur Respir J Suppl 2002;35:49s–60s.

59 Poncelet AJ, Lonneux M, Coche E, Weynand B, Noirhomme P: PET-FDG scan enhances but does not replace preoperative surgical staging in non-small cell lung carcinoma. Eur J Cardiothorac Surg 2001;20:468–474;discussion 74–75.

60 Kao CH, Hsieh JF, Tsai SC, Ho YJ, Yen RF: Comparison and discrepancy of 18F-2-deoxyglucose positron emission tomography and Tc-99m MDP bone scan to detect bone metastases. Anticancer Res 2000;20:2189–2192.

61 Pieterman RM, van Putten JW, Meuzelaar JJ, et al: Preoperative staging of non-small-cell lung cancer with positron-emission tomography. N Engl J Med 2000;343:254–261.

62 Collins BT, Lowe VJ, Dunphy FR: Initial evaluation of pulmonary abnormalities: CT-guided fine-needle aspiration biopsy and fluoride-18 fluorodeoxyglucose positron emission tomography correlation. Diagn Cytopathol 2000;22:92–96.

63 van Tinteren H, Hoekstra OS, Smit EF, et al: Effectiveness of positron emission tomography in the preoperative assessment of patients with suspected non-small-cell lung cancer: the PLUS multicentre randomised trial. Lancet 2002;359: 1388–1393.

64 De Wever W, Ceyssens S, Mortelmans L, et al: Additional value of PET-CT in the staging of lung cancer: comparison with CT alone, PET alone and visual correlation of PET and CT. Eur Radiol 2007;17:23–32.

65 Shim SS, Lee KS, Kim BT, et al: Non-small cell lung cancer: prospective comparison of integrated FDG PET/CT and CT alone for preoperative staging. Radiology 2005;236:1011–1019.

66 Pozo-Rodriguez F, Martin de Nicolas JL, Sanchez-Nistal MA, et al : Accuracy of helical computed tomography and [18F] fluorodeoxyglucose positron emission tomography for identifying lymph node mediastinal metastases in potentially resectable non-small-cell lung cancer. J Clin Oncol 2005;23:8348–8356.

67 Kumar R, Xiu Y, Yu JQ, et al: 18F-FDG PET in evaluation of adrenal lesions in patients with lung cancer. J Nucl Med 2004;45:2058–2062.

68 Nestle U, Hellwig D, Schmidt S, et al: 2-Deoxy-2-[18F]fluoro-D-glucose positron emission tomography in target volume definition for radiotherapy of patients with non-small-cell lung cancer. Mol Imaging Biol 2002;4:257–263.

69 Eschmann SM, Friedel G, Paulsen F, et al: FDG PET for staging of advanced non-small cell lung cancer prior to neoadjuvant radio-chemotherapy. Eur J Nucl Med Mol Imaging 2002;29:804–808.

70 Mac Manus MP, Hicks RJ, Ball DL, et al: F-18 fluorodeoxyglucose positron emission tomography staging in radical radiotherapy candidates with nonsmall cell lung carcinoma: powerful correlation with survival and high impact on treatment. Cancer 2001;92:886–895.

71 Bury T, Barreto A, Daenen F, Barthelemy N, Ghaye B, Rigo P: Fluorine-18 deoxyglucose positron emission tomography for the detection of bone metastases in patients with non-small cell lung cancer. Eur J Nucl Med 1998;25:1244–1247.

72 Kramer H, Post WJ, Pruim J, Groen HJ: The prognostic value of positron emission tomography in non-small cell lung cancer: analysis of 266 cases. Lung Cancer 2006;52:213–217.
73 Nguyen XC, Lee WW, Chung JH, et al: FDG uptake, glucose transporter type 1, and Ki-67 expressions in non-small-cell lung cancer: correlations and prognostic values. Eur J Radiol 2007; 62:214–219.
74 Davies A, Tan C, Paschalides C, et al: FDG-PET maximum standardised uptake value is associated with variation in survival: analysis of 498 lung cancer patients. Lung Cancer 2007;55:75–78.
75 Ohtsuka T, Nomori H, Watanabe K, et al: Prognostic significance of [(18)F]fluorodeoxyglucose uptake on positron emission tomography in patients with pathologic stage I lung adenocarcinoma. Cancer 2006;107:2468–2473.
76 Yi CA, Shin KM, Lee KS, et al: Non-small cell lung cancer staging: efficacy comparison of integrated PET/CT versus 3.0-T whole-body MR imaging. Radiology 2008;248:632–642.
77 Bury T, Dowlati A, Paulus P, et al: Whole-body 18FDG positron emission tomography in the staging of non-small cell lung cancer. Eur Respir J 1997;10:2529–2534.
78 Berlangieri SU, Scott AM, Knight SR, et al: F-18 fluorodeoxyglucose positron emission tomography in the non-invasive staging of non-small cell lung cancer. Eur J Cardiothorac Surg 1999; 16(suppl 1):S25–S30.
79 Vanuytsel LJ, Vansteenkiste JF, Stroobants SG, et al: The impact of (18)F-fluoro-2-deoxy-D-glucose positron emission tomography (FDG-PET) lymph node staging on the radiation treatment volumes in patients with non-small cell lung cancer. Radiother Oncol 2000;55:317–324.
80 Vansteenkiste J, Dooms C: Positron emission tomography in nonsmall cell lung cancer. Curr Opin Oncol 2007;19:78–83.
81 Chin R Jr, Ward R, Keyes JW, et al: Mediastinal staging of non-small-cell lung cancer with positron emission tomography. Am J Respir Crit Care Med 1995;152:2090–2096.
82 Diederich S, Das M: Solitary pulmonary nodule: detection and management. Cancer Imaging 2006;6:S42–S46.
83 Farrell MA, McAdams HP, Herndon JE, Patz EF Jr: Non-small cell lung cancer: FDG PET for nodal staging in patients with stage I disease. Radiology 2000;215:886–890.
84 Guhlmann A, Storck M, Kotzerke J, Moog F, Sunder-Plassmann L, Reske SN: Lymph node staging in non-small cell lung cancer: evaluation by [18F] FDG positron emission tomography (PET). Thorax 1997;52:438–441.
85 Gupta NC, Graeber GM, Bishop HA: Comparative efficacy of positron emission tomography with fluorodeoxyglucose in evaluation of small (<1 cm), intermediate (1 to 3 cm), and large (>3 cm) lymph node lesions. Chest 2000;117:773–778.
86 Gupta NC, Tamim WJ, Graeber GG, Bishop HA, Hobbs GR: Mediastinal lymph node sampling following positron emission tomography with fluorodeoxyglucose imaging in lung cancer staging. Chest 2001;120:521–527.
87 Higashi K, Nishikawa T, Seki H, et al: Comparison of fluorine-18-FDG PET and thallium-201 SPECT in evaluation of lung cancer. J Nucl Med 1998;39:9–15.
88 Kernstine KH, McLaughlin KA, Menda Y, et al: Can FDG-PET reduce the need for mediastinoscopy in potentially resectable nonsmall cell lung cancer? Ann Thorac Surg 2002;73:394–401;discussion 402.
89 Kernstine KH, Stanford W, Mullan BF, et al: PET, CT, and MRI with Combidex for mediastinal staging in non-small cell lung carcinoma. Ann Thorac Surg 1999;68:1022–1028.
90 Liewald F, Grosse S, Storck M, et al: How useful is positron emission tomography for lymphnode staging in non-small-cell lung cancer? Thorac Cardiovasc Surg 2000;48:93–96.
91 Magnani P, Carretta A, Rizzo G, et al: FDG/PET and spiral CT image fusion for medistinal lymph node assessment of non-small cell lung cancer patients. J Cardiovasc Surg (Torino) 1999;40:741–748.
92 Marom EM, McAdams HP, Erasmus JJ, et al: Staging non-small cell lung cancer with whole-body PET. Radiology 1999;212:803–809.
93 Patz EF Jr, Connolly J, Herndon J: Prognostic value of thoracic FDG PET imaging after treatment for non-small cell lung cancer. AJR Am J Roentgenol 2000;174:769–774.
94 Roberts PF, Follette DM, von Haag D, et al: Factors associated with false-positive staging of lung cancer by positron emission tomography. Ann Thorac Surg 2000;70:1154–1159; discussion 9–60.

95 Scott WJ, Gobar LS, Terry JD, Dewan NA, Sunderland JJ: Mediastinal lymph node staging of non-small-cell lung cancer: a prospective comparison of computed tomography and positron emission tomography. J Thorac Cardiovasc Surg 1996;111:642–648.

96 Steinert HC, Hauser M, Allemann F, et al: Non-small cell lung cancer: nodal staging with FDG PET versus CT with correlative lymph node mapping and sampling. Radiology 1997;202:441–446.

97 Tatsumi M, Yutani K, Watanabe Y, et al: Feasibility of fluorodeoxyglucose dual-head gamma camera coincidence imaging in the evaluation of lung cancer: comparison with FDG PET. J Nucl Med 1999;40:566–573.

98 Valk PE, Pounds TR, Hopkins DM, et al: Staging non-small cell lung cancer by whole-body positron emission tomographic imaging. Ann Thorac Surg 1995;60:1573–1581; discussion 81–82.

99 Vansteenkiste JF, Stroobants SG, De Leyn PR, et al: Lymph node staging in non-small-cell lung cancer with FDG-PET scan: a prospective study on 690 lymph node stations from 68 patients. J Clin Oncol 1998;16:2142–2149.

100 Eubank WB, Mankoff DA, Vesselle HJ, et al: Detection of locoregional and distant recurrences in breast cancer patients by using FDG PET. Radiographics 2002;22:5–17.

101 von Haag DW, Follette DM, Roberts PF, Shelton D, Segel LD, Taylor TM: Advantages of positron emission tomography over computed tomography in mediastinal staging of non-small cell lung cancer. J Surg Res 2002;103:160–164.

102 Dwamena BA, Sonnad SS, Angobaldo JO, Wahl RL: Metastases from non-small cell lung cancer: mediastinal staging in the 1990s: meta-analytic comparison of PET and CT. Radiology 1999; 213:530–536.

103 Weber WA, Dietlein M, Hellwig D, Kirsch CM, Schicha H, Schwaiger M: PET with (18)F-fluorodeoxyglucose for staging of non-small cell lung cancer. Nuklearmedizin 2003;42:135–144.

104 Baum RP, Hellwig D, Mezzetti M: Position of nuclear medicine modalities in the diagnostic workup of cancer patients: lung cancer. Q J Nucl Med Mol Imaging 2004;48:119–142.

105 Bruzzi JF, Munden RF: PET/CT imaging of lung cancer. J Thorac Imaging 2006;21:123–136.

106 Halpern BS, Schiepers C, Weber WA, et al: Presurgical staging of non-small cell lung cancer: positron emission tomography, integrated positron emission tomography/CT, and software image fusion. Chest 2005;128:2289–2297.

107 Lardinois D, Weder W, Hany TF, et al: Staging of non-small-cell lung cancer with integrated positron-emission tomography and computed tomography. N Engl J Med 2003;348:2500–2507.

108 Kayani I, Groves AM, Ell PJ, George PJ, Bomanji J: Imaging bronchial carcinoma in situ: possible roles for combined positron emission tomography (PET)-CT. Lancet Oncol 2005;6:190.

109 Eloubeidi MA, Cerfolio RJ, Chen VK, Desmond R, Syed S, Ojha B: Endoscopic ultrasound-guided fine needle aspiration of mediastinal lymph node in patients with suspected lung cancer after positron emission tomography and computed tomography scans. Ann Thorac Surg 2005;79:263–268.

110 Yasufuku K, Nakajima T, Motoori K, et al: Comparison of endobronchial ultrasound, positron emission tomography, and CT for lymph node staging of lung cancer. Chest 2006;130:710–718.

111 de Langen AJ, Raijmakers P, Riphagen I, Paul MA, Hoekstra OS: The size of mediastinal lymph nodes and its relation with metastatic involvement: a meta-analysis. Eur J Cardiothorac Surg 2006;29:26–29.

112 Yang W, Fu Z, Yu J, et al: Value of PET/CT versus enhanced CT for locoregional lymph nodes in non-small cell lung cancer. Lung Cancer 2008;61:35–43.

113 Gilman MD, Aquino SL: State-of-the-Art FDG-PET imaging of lung cancer. Semin Roentgenol 2005;40:143–153.

114 Schmucking M, Baum RP, Griesinger F, et al: Molecular whole-body cancer staging using positron emission tomography: consequences for therapeutic management and metabolic radiation treatment planning. Rec Results Cancer Res 2003;162:195–202.

115 Bosmans G, van Baardwijk A, Dekker A, et al: Intra-patient variability of tumor volume and tumor motion during conventionally fractionated radiotherapy for locally advanced non-small-cell lung cancer: a prospective clinical study. Int J Radiat Oncol Biol Phys 2006;66:748–753.

116 Mah K, Caldwell CB, Ung YC, et al: The impact of (18)FDG-PET on target and critical organs in CT-based treatment planning of patients with poorly defined non-small-cell lung carcinoma: a prospective study. Int J Radiat Oncol Biol Phys 2002;52:339–350.

117 Rosenman J, Chaney EL, Sailer S, et al: Recent advances in radiotherapy treatment planning Cancer Invest 1991;9:465–481.

118 Touboul E, Deniaud-Alexandre E, Moureau-Zabotto L, Lerouge D: The impact of integrating images of positron emission tomography with computed tomography simulation on radiation therapy planning. Cancer Radiother 2004;8(suppl 1):S29–S35.
119 Lavrenkov K, Partridge M, Cook G, Brada M: Positron emission tomography for target volume definition in the treatment of non-small cell lung cancer. Radiother Oncol 2005;77:1–4.
120 Messa C, Ceresoli GL, Rizzo G, et al: Feasibility of [18F]FDG-PET and coregistered CT on clinical target volume definition of advanced non-small cell lung cancer. Q J Nucl Med Mol Imaging 2005;49:259–266.
121 Brianzoni E, Rossi G, Ancidei S, et al: Radiotherapy planning: PET/CT scanner performances in the definition of gross tumour volume and clinical target volume. Eur J Nucl Med Mol Imaging 2005;32:1392–1399.
122 De Ruysscher D, Wanders S, Minken A, et al: Effects of radiotherapy planning with a dedicated combined PET-CT-simulator of patients with non-small cell lung cancer on dose limiting normal tissues and radiation dose-escalation: a planning study. Radiother Oncol 2005;77:5–10.
123 De Ruysscher D, Wanders S, van Haren E, et al: Selective mediastinal node irradiation based on FDG-PET scan data in patients with non-small-cell lung cancer: a prospective clinical study. Int J Radiat Oncol Biol Phys 2005;62:988–994.
124 Senan S, De Ruysscher D: Critical review of PET-CT for radiotherapy planning in lung cancer. Crit Rev Oncol Hematol 2005;56:345–351.
125 Nestle U, Schaefer-Schuler A, Kremp S, et al: Target volume definition for (18)F-FDG PET-positive lymph nodes in radiotherapy of patients with non-small cell lung cancer. Eur J Nucl Med Mol Imaging 2006.
126 Biehl KJ, Kong F-M, Dehdashti F, et al: 18F-FDG PET definition of gross tumor volume for radiotherapy of non-small cell lung cancer: is a single standardized uptake value threshold approach appropriate? J Nucl Med 2006;47:1808–1812.
127 Cherk MH, Foo SS, Poon AM, et al: Lack of correlation of hypoxic cell fraction and angiogenesis with glucose metabolic rate in non-small cell lung cancer assessed by 18F-Fluoromisonidazole and 18F-FDG PET. J Nucl Med 2006;47:1921–1926.
128 Nestle U, Kremp S, Grosu AL: Practical integration of [(18)F]-FDG-PET and PET-CT in the planning of radiotherapy for non-small cell lung cancer (NSCLC): The technical basis, ICRU-target volumes, problems, perspectives. Radiother Oncol 2006;81:209–225.
129 Visser EP, Philippens ME, Kienhorst L, et al: Comparison of tumor volumes derived from glucose metabolic rate maps and SUV maps in dynamic 18F-FDG PET. J Nucl Med 2008;49:892–898.
130 Cerfolio RJ, Bryant AS, Winokur TS, Ohja B, Bartolucci AA: Repeat FDG-PET after neoadjuvant therapy is a predictor of pathologic response in patients with non-small cell lung cancer. Ann Thorac Surg 2004;78:1903–1909;discussion 9.
131 Eschmann SM, Friedel G, Paulsen F, et al: Repeat (18)F-FDG PET for monitoring neoadjuvant chemotherapy in patients with stage III non-small cell lung cancer. Lung Cancer 2007;55:165–171.
132 Baum RP, Griesinger F, Niesen A: Correlation of FDG-PET measurements with morphometric tumor response after induction chemotherapy and adjuvant radiotherapz in stage III non-small cell lung cancer (NSCLC). 25th Int Symp Radioactive Isotopes in Clinical Medicine and Research, Bad Gastein, 2002.
133 Ryu JS, Choi NC, Fischman AJ, Lynch TJ, Mathisen DJ: FDG-PET in staging and restaging non-small cell lung cancer after neoadjuvant chemoradiotherapy: correlation with histopathology. Lung Cancer 2002;35:179–187.
134 Akhurst T, Downey RJ, Ginsberg MS, et al: An initial experience with FDG-PET in the imaging of residual disease after induction therapy for lung cancer. Ann Thorac Surg 2002;73:259–264;discussion 64–66.
135 Pottgen C, Levegrun S, Theegarten D, et al: Value of 18F-fluoro-2-deoxy-D-glucose-positron emission tomography/computed tomography in non-small-cell lung cancer for prediction of pathologic response and times to relapse after neoadjuvant chemoradiotherapy. Clin Cancer Res 2006;12:97–106.
136 Su H, Bodenstein C, Dumont RA, et al: Monitoring tumor glucose utilization by positron emission tomography for the prediction of treatment response to epidermal growth factor receptor kinase inhibitors. Clin Cancer Res 2006;12:5659–5667.

137 Weber WA, Petersen V, Schmidt B, et al: Positron emission tomography in non-small-cell lung cancer: prediction of response to chemotherapy by quantitative assessment of glucose use. J Clin Oncol 2003;21:2651–2657.

138 Cerfolio RJ, Bryant AS, Ojha B: Restaging patients with N2 (stage IIIa) non-small cell lung cancer after neoadjuvant chemoradiotherapy: a prospective study. J Thorac Cardiovasc Surg 2006;131: 1229–1235.

139 Hellwig D, Graeter TP, Ukena D, Georg T, Kirsch CM, Schafers HJ: Value of F-18-fluorodeoxyglucose positron emission tomography after induction therapy of locally advanced bronchogenic carcinoma. J Thorac Cardiovasc Surg 2004;128: 892–899.

140 Schmucking M, Baum RP, Bonnet R, Junker K, Muller KM: Correlation of histologic results with PET findings for tumor regression and survival in locally advanced non-small cell lung cancer after neoadjuvant treatment. Pathologe 2005;26:178–189.

141 Nahmias C, Hanna WT, Wahl LM, Long MJ, Hubner KF, Townsend DW: Time course of early response to chemotherapy in non-small cell lung cancer patients with 18F-FDG PET/CT. J Nucl Med 2007;48:744–751.

142 Tanvetyanon T, Eikman EA, Sommers E, Robinson L, Boulware D, Bepler G: Computed tomography response, but not positron emission tomography scan response, predicts survival after neoadjuvant chemotherapy for resectable non-small-cell lung cancer. J Clin Oncol 2008;26:4610–4616.

143 Poettgen C, Theegarten D, Eberhardt W, et al: Correlation of PET/CT findings and histopathology after neoadjuvant therapy in non-small cell lung cancer. Oncology 2007;73:316–323.

144 Vesselle H, Freeman JD, Wiens L, et al: Fluorodeoxyglucose uptake of primary non-small cell lung cancer at positron emission tomography: new contrary data on prognostic role. Clin Cancer Res 2007;13:3255–3263.

145 Talbot JN, Kerrou K, Grahek D, et al: PET in primary pulmonary or pleural cancer. Presse Med 2006;35:1387–1400.

146 Schaffler GJ, Wolf G, Schoellnast H, et al: Non-small cell lung cancer: evaluation of pleural abnormalities on CT scans with 18F FDG PET. Radiology 2004;231:858–865.

147 Shim SS, Lee KS, Kim BT, et al: Integrated PET/CT and the dry pleural dissemination of peripheral adenocarcinoma of the lung: diagnostic implications. J Comput Assist Tomogr 2006;30: 70–76.

148 Truong MT, Marom EM, Erasmus JJ: Preoperative evaluation of patients with malignant pleural mesothelioma: role of integrated CT-PET imaging. J Thorac Imaging 2006;21:146–153.

149 Alzahouri K, Lejeune C, Woronoff-Lemsi MC, Arveux P, Guillemin F: Cost-effectiveness analysis of strategies introducing FDG-PET into the mediastinal staging of non-small-cell lung cancer from the French healthcare system perspective. Clin Radiol 2005;60:479–492.

150 Dietlein M, Moka D, Weber K, Theissen P, Schicha H: Cost-effectiveness of PET in the management algorithms of lung tumors: comparison of health economic data. Nuklearmedizin 2001;40: 122–128.

151 Dietlein M, Weber K, Gandjour A, et al: Cost-effectiveness of FDG-PET for the management of potentially operable non-small cell lung cancer: priority for a PET-based strategy after nodal-negative CT results. Eur J Nucl Med 2000;27:1598–1609.

152 Gambhir SS, Hoh CK, Phelps ME, Madar I, Maddahi J: Decision tree sensitivity analysis for cost-effectiveness of FDG-PET in the staging and management of non-small-cell lung carcinoma. J Nucl Med 1996;37:1428–1436.

153 Nguyen VH, Peloquin S, Lacasse Y: Cost-effectiveness of positron emission tomography for the management of potentially operable non-small cell lung cancer in Quebec. Can Respir J 2005; 12:19–25.

154 Kosuda S, Ichihara K, Watanabe M, Kobayashi H, Kusano S: Decision-tree sensitivity analysis for cost-effectiveness of chest 2-fluoro-2-D-[(18)F] fluorodeoxyglucose positron emission tomography in patients with pulmonary nodules (non-small cell lung carcinoma) in Japan. Chest 2000; 117:346–353.

155 Kosuda S, Ichihara K, Watanabe M, Kobayashi H, Kusano S: Decision-tree sensitivity analysis for cost-effectiveness of whole-body FDG PET in the management of patients with non-small-cell lung carcinoma in Japan. Ann Nucl Med 2002;16:263–271.

156 Scott WJ, Shepherd J, Gambhir SS: Cost-effectiveness of FDG-PET for staging non-small cell lung cancer: a decision analysis. Ann Thorac Surg 1998;66:1876–1883; discussion 83–85.

157 Pompen M, Gok M, Novak A, et al: Direct costs associated with the disease management of patients with unresectable advanced non-small-cell lung cancer in The Netherlands. Lung Cancer 2009;64:110–116.
158 Abrams J, Doyle LA, Aisner J: Staging, prognostic factors, and special considerations in small cell lung cancer. Semin Oncol 1988;15:261–277.
159 Detterbeck FC, Falen S, Rivera MP, Halle JS, Socinski MA: Seeking a home for a PET, part 2:Defining the appropriate place for positron emission tomography imaging in the staging of patients with suspected lung cancer. Chest 2004; 125:2300–2308.
160 Kamel EM, Zwahlen D, Wyss MT, Stumpe KD, von Schulthess GK, Steinert HC: Whole-body (18)F-FDG PET improves the management of patients with small cell lung cancer. J Nucl Med 2003;44:1911–1917.
161 Bradley JD, Dehdashti F, Mintun MA, Govindan R, Trinkaus K, Siegel BA: Positron emission tomography in limited-stage small-cell lung cancer: a prospective study. J Clin Oncol 2004;22: 3248–3254.
162 Kruger S, Buck AK, Blumstein NM, et al: Use of integrated FDG PET/CT imaging in pulmonary carcinoid tumours. J Intern Med 2006;260:545–550.
163 Fischer BM, Mortensen J, Langer SW, et al: PET/CT imaging in response evaluation of patients with small cell lung cancer. Lung Cancer 2006; 54:41–49.
164 Brink I, Schumacher T, Mix M, et al: Impact of [18F]FDG-PET on the primary staging of small-cell lung cancer. Eur J Nucl Med Mol Imaging 2004;31:1614–1620.
165 Fischer BM, Mortensen J, Langer SW, et al: A prospective study of PET/CT in initial staging of small-cell lung cancer: comparison with CT, bone scintigraphy and bone marrow analysis. Ann Oncol 2007;18:338–345.
166 Kut V, Spies W, Spies S, Gooding W, Argiris A: Staging and monitoring of small cell lung cancer using [18F]fluoro-2-deoxy-D-glucose-positron emission tomography (FDG-PET). Am J Clin Oncol 2007;30:45–50.
167 Niho S, Fujii H, Murakami K, et al: Detection of unsuspected distant metastases and/or regional nodes by FDG-PET [corrected] scan in apparent limited-disease small-cell lung cancer. Lung Cancer 2007;57:328–333.
168 De Leyn P, Lardinois D, Van Schil PE, et al: ESTS guidelines for preoperative lymph node staging for non-small cell lung cancer. Eur J Cardiothorac Surg 2007;32:1–8.
169 Bakheet SM, Saleem M, Powe J, Al-Amro A, Larsson SG, Mahassin Z: F-18 fluorodeoxyglucose chest uptake in lung inflammation and infection. Clin Nucl Med 2000;25:273–278.
170 Gupta NC, Maloof J, Gunel E: Probability of malignancy in solitary pulmonary nodules using fluorine-18-FDG and PET. J Nucl Med 1996;37: 943–948.
171 Vesselle H, Pugsley JM, Vallières E, Wood DE: The impact of fluorodeoxyglucose F 18 positron-emission tomography on the surgical staging of non-small cell lung cancer. J Thorac Cardiovasc Surg 2002;124:511–519.

Prof. Dr. Richard P. Baum
Department of Nuclear Medicine/Center for PET, Zentralklinik Bad Berka
Robert-Koch-Allee 9
DE–99437 Bad Berka (Germany)
Tel. +49 364 585 2200, Fax +49 364 585 3515, E-Mail info@rpbaum.de

Heide J, Schmittel A, Kaiser D, Hinkelbein W (eds): Controversies in the Treatment of Lung Cancer.
Front Radiat Ther Oncol. Basel, Karger, 2010, vol 42, pp 46–54

Whole-Body Magnetic Resonance Imaging for Staging of Lung Cancer

Ralf Puls[a] · Jens-Peter Kühn[a] · Ralf Ewert[b] · Norbert Hosten[a]

Departments of [a]Radiology and [b]Internal Medicine, University Medical Center, Ernst-Moritz-Arndt University Greifswald, Greifswald, Germany

Abstract

Accurate staging of lung cancer is requisite to choose the optimal therapeutic strategy and is very important for prognosis. Multimodality diagnostic imaging is currently used for detection, staging, and follow-up. Whole-body FDG PET/CT provides 'anatometabolic' information and improves diagnostic accuracy especially for M-staging. MRI has unrivalled tissue contrast, provides very exact morphological information, and does not involve ionizing radiation compared to PET/CT. MRI is widely used for diagnosing and characterizing pathologies in all regions of the body. The use of multiple receiver channels and parallel imaging enables examination of the whole body with shorter acquisition time while high image quality is maintained. This article gives an overview of initial clinical results obtained with whole-body MRI in staging lung cancer.

Magnetic resonance imaging (MRI) provides excellent soft tissue contrast and high spatial resolution without using ionizing radiation. A large number of studies have proven MRI to be superior in detecting parenchymal and osseous lesions, especially metastases in the liver bone, and brain [1–3].

A new generation of whole-body MRI scanners with field strengths of 1.5 or 3 Tesla allows the examination of the entire human body in an acceptable scan time and we can now make use of the excellent spatial resolution of this modality for examination of all body regions in the clinical setting.

A reliable imaging modality enabling adequate T-, N- and M-staging is necessary for efficient treatment of lung cancer. FDG PET/CT has become the standard for staging lung cancer and several clinical studies have proven its superior diagnostic accuracy [4–6]. First clinical reports on whole-body MRI show its potential to perform accurate and efficient TNM staging of lung cancer.

Technical Aspects of Whole-Body MRI

A standard MRI scanner does not provide enough surface coils to cover the whole body. Performing whole-body MRI on such a scanner would require patient repositioning for imaging of each body compartment, which is very time consuming and would be unacceptable to patients.

The first development toward whole-body MRI (Angio SURF, Body SURF) was made by the University Hospital in Essen, Germany [7]. They designed a rolling table platform enabling stepwise imaging of the body using the standard spine and one surface coil. With this technique it became possible to image the whole body within an acceptable time range but compromised spatial resolution especially in the head/neck region and extremities.

An important recent addition is the total imaging matrix (TIM) system developed by Siemens Medical Solutions (Erlangen, Germany). Multiple coils with up to 76 elements and up to 32 independent receiver channels allow a more differentiated examination of the body because the individual coils are optimized for different body region (fig. 1). The advent of parallel imaging techniques has decreased scan time without loss of image quality [8–10]. Parallel imaging techniques in conjunction with a moving table and multi-element coil systems are used by other manufactures such as GE Healthcare (Milwaukee, Wisc., USA) and Philips Medical Systems (Best, Netherlands).

Staging of Lung Cancer Using Whole-Body MRI

So far, little literature is available on TNM staging of lung cancer using the recently introduced new generation of whole-body MRI scanners (table 1). With the advent of these scanners, fast imaging of the whole body with high spatial and temporal resolution of each body compartment has become feasible. FDG-PET was developed for better staging of distant metastases to lymph nodes and other organs and structures [6]. Staging efficacy has improved further by combining PET and CT for simultaneously obtaining metabolic and morphological data [4, 5].

The first two studies investigating staging of malignant disease with whole-body MRI still found a superiority of PET/CT for T and N staging but similar or better diagnostic accuracy for detection of metastatic spread [11, 12]. Both studies included patients with lung cancer and other malignancies. Antoch et al. [11] investigated 98 patients with various malignancies (29 patients with lung cancer) using a standard 1.5-Tesla MRI scanner with a newly designed rolling table and standard surface coil. This innovation resulted in faster acquisition but lower spatial and temporal resolution, especially of head, neck and extremities, compared

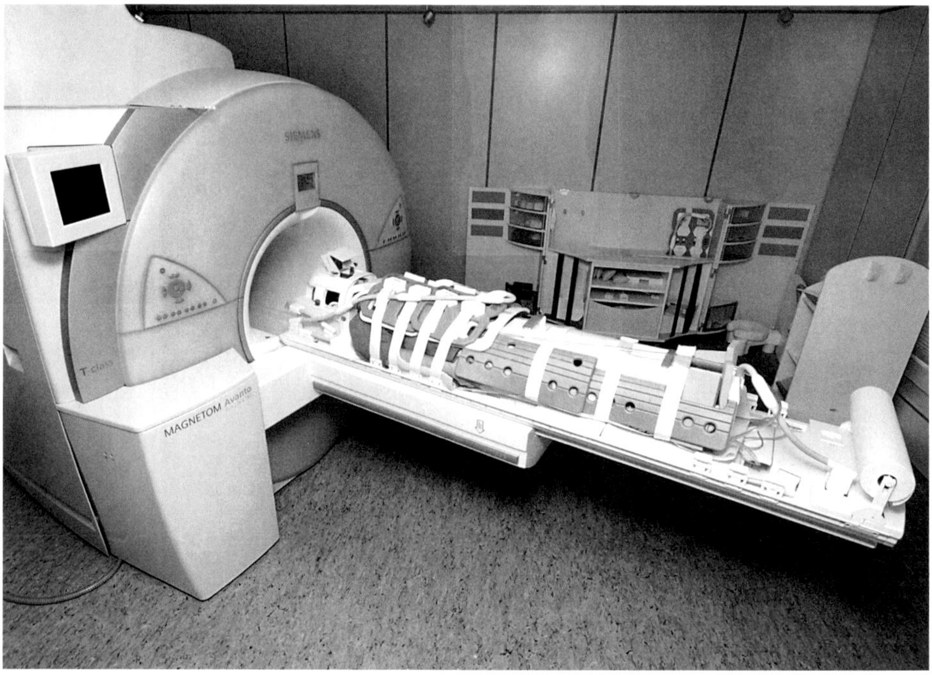

Fig. 1. Multiple coils optimized for each body region and comprising up to 76 elements and up to 32 receiver channels cover the whole human body. With this total imaging matrix (TIM; Siemens, Erlangen, Germany) technology a length of 2.05 m from head to toe can be scanned with sequential or continuous table movement.

with standard examination protocols. The authors performed whole-body MRI using pre- and post-contrast T_1-weighted and T_2-weighted sequences with identical parameters from head to toe and achieved a diagnostic accuracy of 52% for T-staging, 79% for N-staging, and 93% for M-staging compared with 80, 93, and 94% for PET/CT.

Schmidt et al. [10] examined 41 patients with various tumor entities using a new generation of MRI scanner with TIM and parallel imaging. They a found a similar performance of PET/CT and whole-body MRI in T-staging (86% diagnostic accuracy) and a lower accuracy in N-staging (97% PET/CT, 82% WB-MRI). Most notably, WB-MRI missed nearly all lymph nodes smaller than 1 cm.

In contrast, whole-body MRI was found to have superior diagnostic accuracy for M-staging (100%) compared to PET/CT (97%). Bone, liver and brain metastases were better detected with WB-MRI and soft tissue metastases were better seen with PET/CT.

An improved performance in M-staging was also reported by Ohno et al. [13]. They investigated 90 patients with lung cancer and found a diagnostic accuracy

Table 1. Diagnostic accuracies (%) reported for TNM-staging of lung cancer using whole-body MRI in comparison with PET/CT

Study	Year	Scanner type	T	N	M
Antoch et al. [11]	2003	1.5 Tesla, rolling table, body coil	52	79	93
Schmidt et al. [12]	2005	1.5 Tesla, TIM system, parallel imaging	86	82	100
Ohno et al. [13]	2007	1.5 Tesla, rolling table, body coil			80
Yi et al. [14]	2008	3 Tesla, rolling table, multi-elements coils	86	68	86
PET/CT (all studies)			80–86	70–97	73–97

of 80% with whole-body MRI and 73.3% with PET/CT. This investigation used a 1.5-Tesla scanner with moving table and standard body coil and a differentiated sequence protocol comprising pre- and post-contrast T_1-weighted gradient echo (GRE), opposed-phase GRE, and T_2-weighted STIR sequences in coronal and sagittal planes.

A more recent study published by Yi et al. [14] used a 3-Tesla scanner with an advanced coil system. This technique with a higher magnetic field strength promises higher spatial and temporal resolution as a result of improved signal-to-noise ratio. The investigators employed a special cardiac coil with six coil elements for chest scans and a four-element body coil integrated into the bore for whole-body examination. They examined a total of 165 patients with non-small cell lung cancer and found comparable accuracies for PET/CT and whole-body MRI for all T- (86% WB-MRI, 82% PET/CT), N- (68%, 70%) and M-stages (both 86%). Similar to Schmidt et al. [10], they found whole-body MRI to be superior in detecting brain and liver metastases and PT/CT in detecting lymph node and soft tissue metastases. Ohno et al. [15] also investigated the use of diffusion-weighted sequences for whole-body MRI and found a diagnostic accuracy as good as that of integrated PET/CT (87.7% WB-MRI with diffusion-weighted imaging, 88.2 PET/CT).

Based on these insights and our experience with lung cancer imaging, we developed an MRI protocol (table 2) comprising T_2-weighted TIRM sequences for the whole-body scan and optimized sequences for each relevant body region. The TIRM sequence (fig. 2) is used to search for hyperintensities that represent either fluid-containing structures such as the bladder, stomach or spinal fluid or primary and secondary malignancies with an increased cell account. Such tumors are seen as hyperintensities. An example with lesions in the lungs, bones, and liver is shown in figure 2.

Table 2. Sequence protocol for staging lung cancer using whole-body MRI

Body region	Sequence	Plane	TR	TE	Matrix	Time
Whole body	TIRM	coronal	4,891	67	240×320	12:09
Spine	T2-TSE	sagittal	3,760	106	448×448	02:04
Spine	T1-TSE	sagittal	676	12	448×448	02:42
Head	diffusion	axial	8,000	78	154×192	01:36
Head	T1-TSE	axial	500	7.7	192×256	01:40
Head	T2-TSE	axial	5,000	134	230×512	01:27
Thorax	T1–3D GRE	axial	3.08	1.07	208×256	00:21
Thorax	T2-HASTE	axial	550	22	153×256	00:35
Thorax	diffusion	axial	1,700	72	115×192	02:55
Liver	T2-TSE	axial	2,700	116	256×256	01:16
Adrenal gland	T1–3D GRE-DIXON	axial	7.51	2.38	150×320	00:20
Abdomen	T1–2D GRE	axial	251	4.13	129×256	01:17
Pelvis	T1–2D GRE	axial	251	4.13	129×256	00:58
Pelvis	T2-TSE	axial	3,230	34	256×256	02:43
Contrast medium injection (gadobutrol (GADOVIST) at a dose of 0.1 ml/kg/BW)						
Chest	T1–3D GRE	axial	3.08	1.07	208x256	00:21
Abdomen	T1–2D GRE	axial	251	4.13	129x256	01:17
Pelvis	T1–2D GRE	axial	251	4.13	129x256	00:58
Head	T1-TSE	axial	500	7.7	192x256	01:40
Head	T1-TSE	sagittal	580	17	166x256	02:13

Afterwards, each relevant compartment such as the vertebral spine, head, chest, and abdomen will be scanned with an optimized sequence protocol for detection and differentiation of distant metastases (fig. 3). The protocol includes a dual-echo GRE sequence (Dixon), which mainly serves to characterize adrenal masses by estimating fat content and thereby contributing to the differentiation of adenoma from metastasis. Additionally, contrast-enhanced sequences are acquired to detect malignant tumors based on abnormal enhancement. The duration of the examination varies with the patient's condition but the whole procedure will not last longer than 60 min.

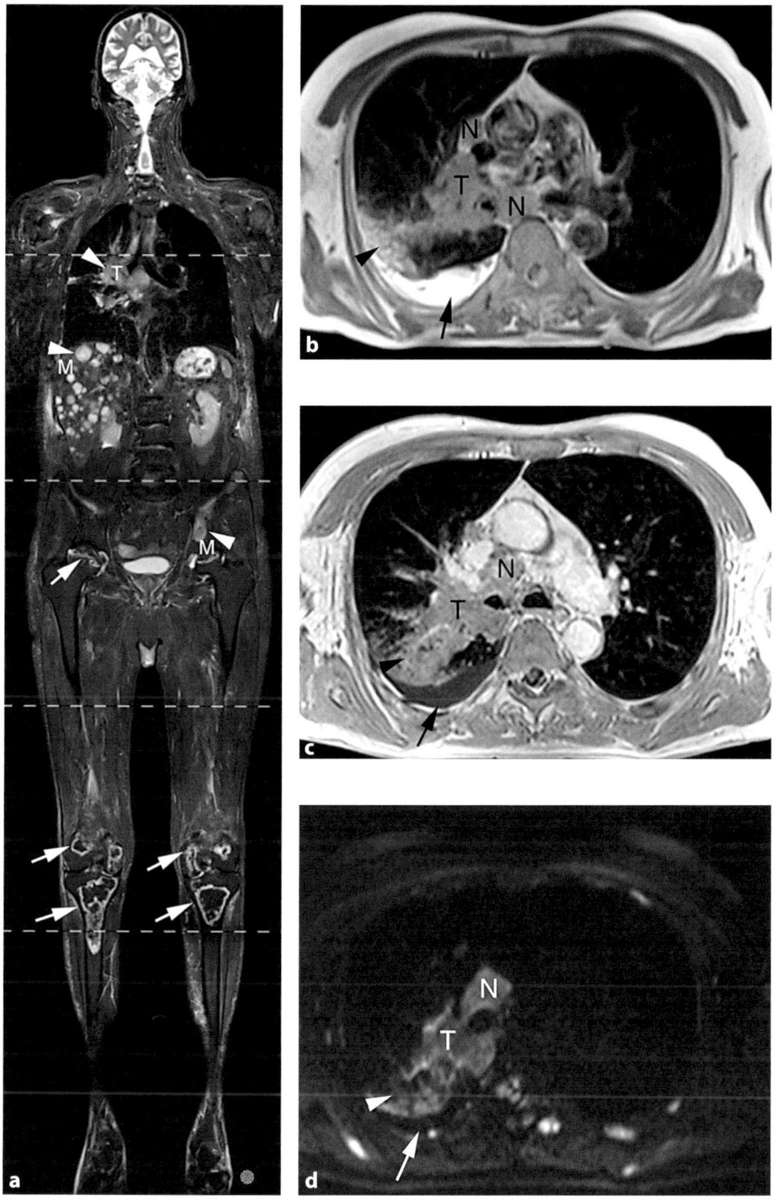

Fig. 2. Whole-body TIRM sequence (**a**) acquired in a 52-year-old man showing right hilar non-small cell lung cancer (T, arrowhead), multiple liver metastases (M, arrowhead), bone metastases (M, arrowhead), and bilateral osteonecrosis of the femur head, distal femur, and proximal tibia (arrows) secondary to chemotherapy. Focused thoracic imaging (T_1-weighted GRE 3D (**b**), T_2-weighted HASTE (**c**), diffusion-weighted (DW) sequence (**d**)) shows the tumor (T3) infiltrating the right hilum with lymph node metastases (N2) in the upper and lower mediastinum. Also detected were poststenotic infiltration (arrowhead) and pleural effusion (arrow).

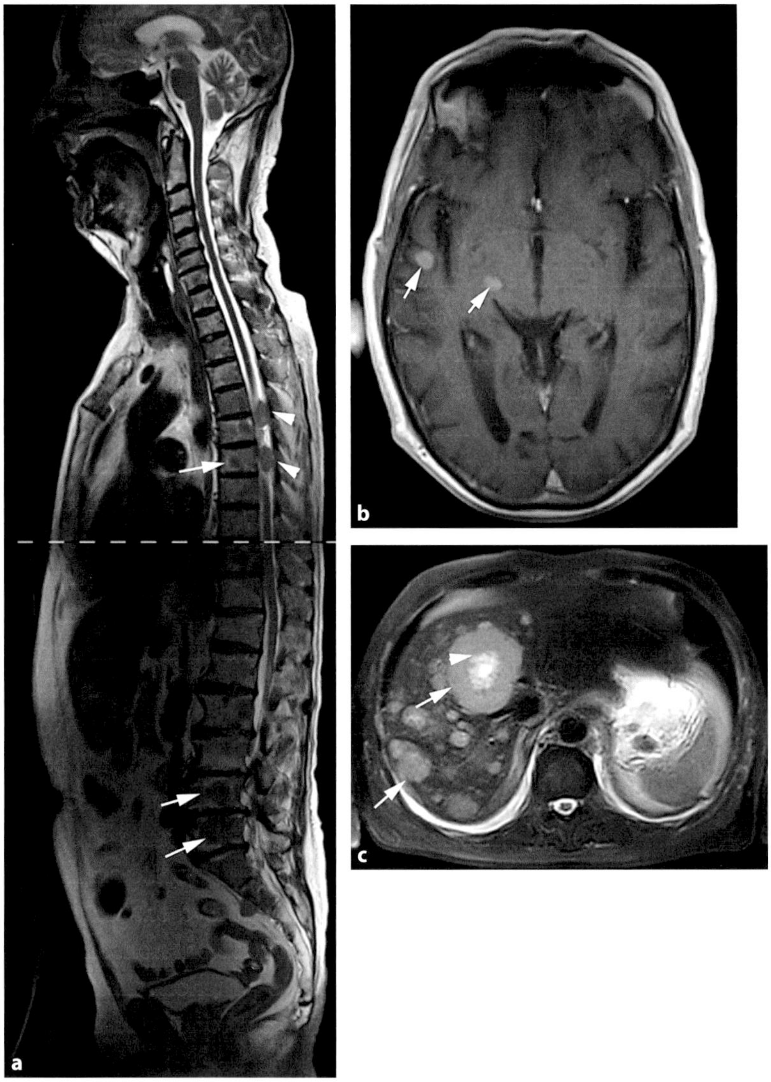

Fig. 3. **a** T_2-weighted TSE sequence of the whole spine demonstrates multiple metastases (arrows) of the vertebral bodies, most of which are located in the lumbar spine, but also intraspinal lesions (arrowhead). **b** Multiple brain metastases (arrows) were seen on post-contrast T_1-weighted TSE images after the intravenous injection of gadolinium-based contrast medium. **c** Abdominal imaging with T_2-weighted TSE sequence demonstrates multiple liver metastases (arrows). The largest metastasis in segment 4b and 8 has a necrotic center (arrowhead).

Conclusions

Initial reports in the literature on TNM staging of lung cancer with whole-body MRI in comparison to PET/CT suggest that both modalities provide sufficient accuracy and efficacy. Whole-body MRI seems to have advantages in detecting brain and liver metastases while PET/CT appears to be superior in detecting lymph node and soft tissue metastases. These results are achieved using new-generation MRI scanners with moving table and multi-elements coil systems. Higher magnetic field strength increases temporal and spatial resolution and may improve detection of small lymph nodes for N-staging. Diffusion-weighted sequences also improve detection and characterization of distant metastases.

Development of an integrated PET/MRI scanner may further increase diagnostic accuracy by combining the advantages of both modalities.

References

1 Takeda T, Takeda A, Nagaoka T, Kunieda E, Takemasa K, Watanabe M, Hatou T, Oguro S, Katayama M: Gadolinium-enhanced three-dimensional magnetization-prepared rapid gradient-echo (3D MP-RAGE) imaging is superior to spin-echo imaging in delineating brain metastases. Acta Radiol 2008;31:1–7.

2 Hamm B, Mahfouz AE, Taupitz M, Mitchell DG, Nelson R, Halpern E, Speidel A, Wolf KJ, Saini S: Liver metastases: improved detection with dynamic gadolinium-enhanced MR imaging? Radiology 1997;202:677–682.

3 Schmidt GP, Schoenberg SO, Schmid R, Stahl R, Tiling R, Becker CR, Reiser MF, Baur-Melnyk A: Screening for bone metastases: whole-body MRI using a 32-channel system versus dual-modality PET-CT. Eur Radiol 2007;17:939–949.

4 Shim SS, Lee KS, Kim BT, Chung MJ, Lee EJ, Han J, Choi JY, Kwon OJ, Shim YM, Kim S: Non-small cell lung cancer: prospective comparison of integrated FDG PET/CT and CT alone for preoperative staging. Radiology 2005;236:1011–1019.

5 Lardinois D, Weder W, Hany TF, Kamel EM, Korom S, Seifert B, von Schulthess GK, Steinert HC: Staging of non-small-cell lung cancer with integrated positron-emission tomography and computed tomography. N Engl J Med 2003;348:2500–2507.

6 Pieterman RM, van Putten JW, Meuzelaar JJ, Mooyaart EL, Vaalburg W, Koëter GH, Fidler V, Pruim J, Groen HJ: Preoperative staging of non-small-cell lung cancer with positron-emission tomography. N Engl J Med. 2000;343:254–261.

7 Lauenstein TC, Freudenberg LS, Goehde SC, Ruehm SG, Goyen M, Bosk S, Debatin JF, Barkhausen J: Whole-body MRI using a rolling table platform for the detection of bone metastases. Eur Radiol 2002;12:2091–2099.

8 Börnert P, Keupp J, Eggers H, Aldefeld B: Whole-body 3D water/fat resolved continuously moving table imaging. J Magn Reson Imaging 2007;25:660–665.

9 Zenge MO, Vogt FM, Brauck K, Jökel M, Barkhausen J, Kannengiesser S, Ladd ME, Quick HH: High-resolution continuously acquired peripheral MR angiography featuring partial parallel imaging GRAPPA. Magn Reson Med 2006;56:859–865.

10 Schmidt GP, Baur-Melnyk A, Tiling R, Hahn K, Reiser MF, Schoenberg SO: Comparison of high resolution whole-body MRI using parallel imaging and PET-CT: first experiences with a 32-channel MRI system. Radiologe 2004;44:889–898.

11 Antoch G, Vogt FM, Freudenberg LS, Nazaradeh F, Goehde SC, Barkhausen J, Dahmen G, Bockisch A, Debatin JF, Ruehm SG: Whole-body dual-modality PET/CT and whole-body MRI for tumor staging in oncology. JAMA 2003;290:3199–3206.

12 Schmidt GP, Baur-Melnyk A, Herzog P, Schmid R, Tiling R, Schmidt M, Reiser MF, Schoenberg SO: High-resolution whole-body magnetic resonance image tumor staging with the use of parallel imaging versus dual-modality positron emission tomography-computed tomography: experience on a 32-channel system. Invest Radiol 2005;40:743–753.

13 Ohno Y, Koyama H, Nogami M, Takenaka D, Yoshikawa T, Yoshimura M, Kotani Y, Nishimura Y, Higashino T, Sugimura K: Whole-body MR imaging vs. FDG-PET: comparison of accuracy of M-stage diagnosis for lung cancer patients. J Magn Reson Imaging. 2007;26:498–509.

14 Yi CA, Shin KM, Lee KS, Kim BT, Kim H, Kwon OJ, Choi JY, Chung MJ: Non-small cell lung cancer staging: efficacy comparison of integrated PET/CT versus 3.0-T whole-body MR imaging. Radiology 2008;248:632–642.

15 Ohno Y, Koyama H, Onishi Y, Takenaka D, Nogami M, Yoshikawa T, Matsumoto S, Kotani Y, Sugimura K: Non-small cell lung cancer: whole-body MR examination for M-stage assessment – utility for whole-body diffusion-weighted imaging compared with integrated FDG PET/CT. Radiology 2008;248:643–654.

PD Dr. med. Ralf Puls
Department of Radiology, University Medical Center, Ernst-Moritz-Arndt University Greifswald
Friedrich-Loeffler-Strasse 23a
DE–17487 Greifswald (Germany)
Tel. +49 3834 866933, Fax +49 3834 866958, E-Mail puls@uni-greifswald.de

Heide J, Schmittel A, Kaiser D, Hinkelbein W (eds): Controversies in the Treatment of Lung Cancer.
Front Radiat Ther Oncol. Basel, Karger, 2010, vol 42, pp 55–62

Bronchoscopy/Endobronchial Ultrasound

Felix J.F. Herth

Pneumologie und Beatmungsmedizin, Thoraxklinik am Universitätsklinikum Heidelberg, Heidelberg, Deutschland

Abstract

Endobronchial ultrasound (EBUS) has emerged as a new diagnostic tool that allows the bronchoscopist to see beyond the airway. The radial probe EBUS was first introduced to evaluate the airway structure, which has been shown to be useful for identifying the extent of tumor invasion in the central airway. The newest development is the convex EBUS-TBNA scope with a curvilinear electronic transducer on the tip of a flexible videoscope. Linear EBUS allows a real-time EBUS-guided TBNA. Although the main indication for EBUS-TBNA is lymph node staging, it can also be used for diagnosis of intrapulmonary tumors, of unknown hilar and/or mediastinal lymphadenopathy, and of mediastinal tumors. To date, there are no reports of complications related to EBUS-guided TBNA. It is a novel approach that has a good diagnostic yield with excellent potential in assisting safe and accurate diagnostic interventional bronchoscopy. The aim of this review is to highlight the current status of the EBUS-TBNA technique and to discuss the future direction of EBUS.

Lung cancer is one of the most common cancers. Despite the advances in surgical treatment and multimodality treatment, lung cancer is still the leading cause of death from malignant disease worldwide [1].

Accurate staging of the disease is important not only to determine the prognosis but also to decide the most suitable treatment plan. During the staging process, mediastinal lymph node staging is one of the most important factors that affect the patient outcome. Mediastinal staging can be divided into noninvasive staging (imaging) and invasive staging (sampling).

Computed tomography (CT), magnetic resonance imaging (MRI), positron emission tomography (PET) and PET-CT are used for noninvasive imaging [2–5].

Other imaging modalities include the use of esophageal ultrasound (EUS) and endobronchial ultrasound (EBUS) using a radial probe for detecting even small mediastinal lymph nodes [6, 7]. Invasive staging provides a definitive tissue diagnosis by surgical biopsy or needle biopsy. Mediastinoscopy is still the gold standard for mediastinal lymph node staging [8, 9].

However, it requires general anesthesia, and complications cannot be ignored. Various needle biopsy techniques exist, including conventional bronchoscopic transbronchial needle aspiration (TBNA), EUS-guided fine-needle aspiration (EUS-FNA), CT fluoroscopy-guided TBNA, and EBUS-guided TBNA using the radial probe [10–14]. Each of these methods has its limitations.

There has been a need for a new modality with a high yield, enabling pulmonologists and thoracic surgeons to assess the mediastinum easily and safely. In 2003, a new endoscope with built-in linear probe ultrasound (US) on the tip enables real-time guidance during TBNA was available.

Compared to the radial probe EBUS, the linear US images are easier to understand. After preliminary studies showing the efficacy of EBUS-TBNA in surgical lung specimens [15], different groups reported the clinical use of EBUS-TBNA for the assessment of mediastinal and/or hilar lymph nodes.

EBUS-TBNA is now being performed in more than 500 centers around the world [16]. Publications concerning the use of EBUS-TBNA in patients with respiratory disease indicate the effectiveness of this new modality. In this article, the role of EBUS-TBNA in the management of lung cancer is reviewed. In particular, its usefulness in the diagnosis and staging of lung cancer is discussed.

EBUS-TBNA: Technique

The EBUS-TBNA scope is a US puncture bronchoscope with a 7.5-MHz convex transducer placed at the tip of a flexible bronchoscope (BF-UC260F-OL8; Olympus, Tokyo, Japan). This EBUS-TBNA is a linear curved array transducer that scans parallel to the insertion direction of the bronchoscope (fig. 1). Images can be obtained by directly contacting the probe to the bronchial wall. The US image is processed in a US scanner and is visualized along with the conventional bronchoscopy image.

The outer diameter of the insertion tube of the EBUS-TBNA is 6.2 mm, and that of the tip is 6.9 mm. The angle of view is 90°, and the direction of view is 35° forward oblique. The inner diameter of the instrument channel is 2.0 mm. A dedicated 22-gauge needle is used to perform EBUS-TBNA. The needle is also equipped with an internal sheath that is withdrawn after passing the bronchial wall, avoiding contamination during TBNA. This internal sheath is also used to clear out the tip of the needle after passing the bronchial wall.

The use of this sheath has significantly increased the yield of EBUS-TBNA. The exit of the needle is at 20° with respect to the outer covering of the insertion

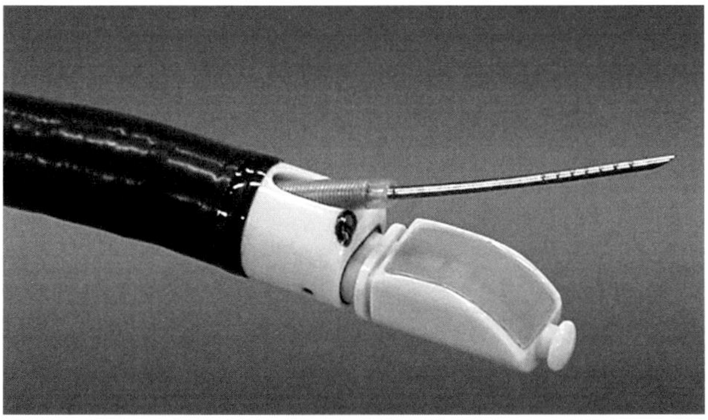

Fig. 1. Tip of the ultrasonic puncture bronchoscope and the 22-gauge transbronchial needle aspiration (TBNA) needle is inserted through the working channel to perform direct real-time endobronchial ultrasound-guided transbronchial needle aspiration (EBUS-TBNA).

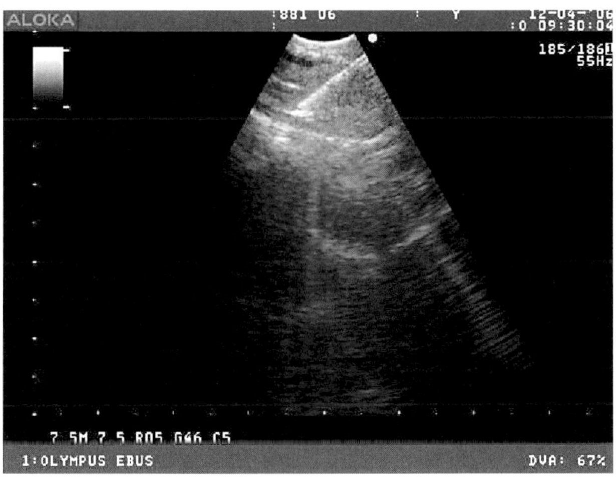

Fig. 2. Representative case of EBUS-TBNA. An EBUS scan demonstrates station 4r lymph node. The 22-gauge needle is seen in the lymph node.

tube. The needle can be visualized through the optics and on the US image (fig. 2) [17].

Because the endobronchial images obtained by the EBUS-TBNA scope is not as clear as the conventional flexible videoscope image, most of the users prefer to examine the tracheobronchial tree using the conventional scopes.

All procedures can be performed under local anesthesia and conscious sedation (midazolam) [18]. Nasal insertion may be difficult owing to the probe on the

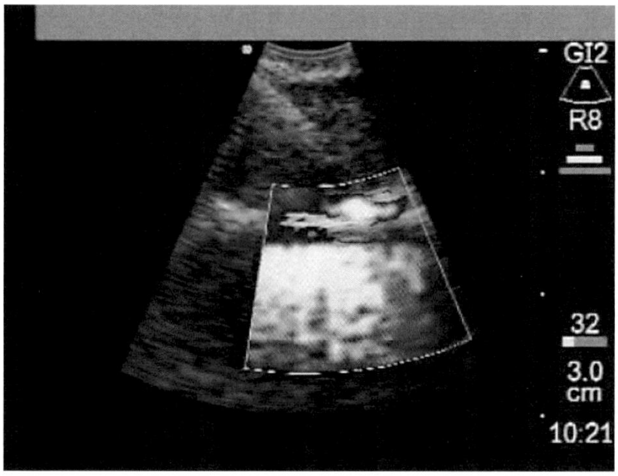

Fig. 3. Puncture of the lymph node in position 10r, the vessel is seen with the help of the Doppler mode.

tip of the scope. After identifying the lesion of interest with EBUS-TBNA, the surrounding structures are visualized with the use of the Doppler mode to confirm blood vessels (fig. 3). The dedicated TBNA needle is inserted through the working channel of the bronchoscope, and the lesion is punctured under direct EBUS guidance (EBUS-TBNA).

Indications for EBUS-TBNA are assessment of mediastinal and hilar lymph nodes, diagnosis of lung tumors, and diagnosis of mediastinal tumors. All of the mediastinal lymph nodes except for the subaortic and paraesophageal lymph nodes (levels 5, 6, 8, and 9) are assessable by EBUS-TBNA. Also the hilar nodes [10–12] are approachable [17].

Clinical Results

To date, several papers have been published on this procedure. Krasnik et al. [15] reported on 11 patients in whom 15 lesions were punctured, without complications. The lesions were located as follows: 4 in region 10L, 4 in region 10R, 1 in region 4L, 3 in region 4R, 1 in region 1, 1 in region 7, and 1 in region 2R. The lesions ranged from 7 to 80 mm. Biopsies obtained through EBUS-FNA showed malignant cells in 13 lesions and benign cells in 2.

Yasufuku et al. [19] published his first experience in a few patients in 2004. In his second trial [20], he examined 70 patients with mediastinal (n = 58) and hilar lymph nodes (n = 12). The sensitivity, specificity, and accuracy of EBUS-TBNA in distinguishing benign from malignant lymph nodes were 95.7, 100, and 97.1%, respectively. There were no complications.

In a European paper by Rintoul et al. [21] EBUS-TBNA was used in 18 patients. Cytology revealed node (N)2/N3 disease in 11 patients and provided a primary diagnosis in 8 patients. Cytology results for EBUS-TBNA samples were negative in 6 patients, and mediastinoscopy or clinical follow-up confirmed this result in 4. Sensitivity, specificity, and accuracy for EBUS-TBNA were 85, 100, and 89%, respectively.

The largest trial reported the results of the method in 502 patients [12]. 572 lymph nodes were punctured, and 535 (94%) resulted in a diagnosis. Biopsies were taken from all reachable lymph node stations (2l, 2r, 3, 4r, 4l, 7, 10r, 10l, 11r and 11l). Mean (SD) diameter of the nodes was 1.6 cm (0.36 cm) and the range was 0.8 to 3.2 cm. Sensitivity was 92%, specificity was 100%, and the positive predictive value was 93%. Like in all other trials no complications occurred.

The Danish-German group [23] examined in addition the accuracy of EBUS-TBNA in sampling nodes less than 1 cm in diameter. Among 100 patients 119 lymph nodes with a size between 4 up to 10 mm were detected and sampled. Malignancy was detected in 19 patients but missed in 2 others; all diagnoses were confirmed by surgical findings. The mean (SD) diameter of the punctured lymph nodes was 8.1 mm. The sensitivity of EBUS-TBNA for detecting malignancy was 92.3%; the specificity was 100%; and the negative predictive value was 96.3%. Again no complications occurred. They summarized, that EBUS-TBNA can sample even small mediastinal nodes, therefore avoiding unnecessary surgical exploration in 1 of 5 patients who have no CT evidence of mediastinal disease. Potentially operable patients with clinically nonmetastatic NSCLC may benefit from presurgical EBUS-TBNA biopsies and staging.

A study comparing EBUS-TBNA, CT, and PET for lymph node staging of lung cancer showed a high yield for EBUS-TBNA [24]. Altogether, 102 potentially operable patients with proven (n = 96) or radiologically suspected (n = 6) lung cancer were included in the study. CT, PET, and EBUS-TBNA were performed prior to surgery for the evaluation of mediastinal and hilar lymph node metastasis. The sensitivities of CT, PET, and EBUS-TBNA for the correct diagnosis of mediastinal and hilar lymph node staging were 76.9, 80.0, and 92.3%, respectively; the specificities were 55.3, 70.1, and 100%, respectively, and the diagnostic accuracies were 60.8, 72.5, and 98.0%, respectively. EBUS-TBNA was proven to have high sensitivity and specificity, compared to CT or PET, for mediastinal staging in patients with potentially resectable lung cancer.

Restaging of the mediastinum is another area of growing interest for the treatment strategy of lung cancer. In cases of advanced lymph node stage lung cancer, induction chemotherapy prior to surgical resection is an option. Mediastinoscopy is considered the gold standard for staging the mediastinum. However, re-mediastinoscopy can be technically difficult and is therefore not commonly performed. The ability to perform multiple, repeat biopsies using EBUS-TBNA allows restaging of the mediastinum after the introduction of chemotherapy.

A group of 124 consecutive patients with tissue-proven IIIA-N2 disease who were treated with induction chemotherapy underwent mediastinal restaging by EBUS-TBNA. The sensitivity, specificity, positive predictive value, negative predictive value, and diagnostic accuracy of EBUS-TBNA for mediastinal restaging following induction chemotherapy were 76, 100, 100, 20, and 77%, respectively. EBUS–TBNA is an accurate, minimally invasive test for mediastinal restaging of patients with NSCLC. However, because of the low negative predictive value, tumor-negative findings should be confirmed by surgical staging [24].

EBUS-TBNA can be also used for the diagnosis of intrapulmonary nodules as well as mediastinal and hilar lymph nodes. The limitation is the reach of EBUS-TBNA, which depends on the size of the bronchus. Usually, the EBUS-TBNA can be inserted as far as the lobar bronchus. Lung tumors located adjacent to the airway within reach of EBUS-TBNA can be diagnosed with EBUS-TBNA. Tornouy et al. [26] have reported their experience is this indication. In 60 patients, who have had a nondiagnostic bronchoscopy before, they were able to establish the definitive diagnosis in 77% without any complication.

Complications

Complications related to the procedure are similar to those of conventional TBNA including bleeding from major vessels, pneumomediastinum, mediastinitis, pneumothorax, bronchospam and laryngospasm. All authors have not encountered complications related to EBUS-TBNA and to date there are no major complications reported in the literature. Although EBUS has enabled the bronchoscopist to see beyond the airway, one must be aware of the possible complications related to the procedure [27, 28].

Conclusion

EBUS-TBNA has emerged as a new instrument that enables real-time TBNA of the mediastinum, hilum, and intrapulmonary nodules. It is a minimally invasive, safe procedure that is useful and effective for the diagnosis and staging of NSCLC. More prospective data describing the diagnostic yield of EBUS-TBNA compared to conventional tools are needed to support the value of this new modality. However, based on the current experience, EBUS-TBNA can be used as the first test for patients with undiagnosed mediastinal lymphadenopathy either with or without a lung mass. It is an attractive procedure that allows simultaneous lymph node staging as well as diagnosis.

References

1 Ferlay J, Bray F, Pisani P, et al: GLOBOCAN 2002: Cancer Incidence, Mortality and Prevalence Worldwide. IARC Cancer Base No. 5 version 2.0. Lyon, IARC Press, 2004.

2 Kramer H, Groen HJM: Current concepts in the mediastinal lymph node staging of non-small cell lung cancer. Ann Surg 2003;238:180–188.

3 De Leyn P, Lardinois D, Van Schil PE, Rami-Porta R, Passlick B, Zielinski M, Waller DA, Lerut T, Weder W: ESTS guidelines for preoperative lymph node staging for non-small cell lung cancer. Eur J Cardiothorac Surg 2007;32:1–8.

4 Silvestri GA, Gould MK, Margolis ML, Tanoue LT, McCrory D, Toloza E, Detterbeck F, American College of Chest Physicians: Noninvasive Staging of Non-Small Cell Lung Cancer: ACCP Evidenced-Based Clinical Practice Guidelines, ed 2. Chest 2007;132:178S–201S.

5 Detterbeck FC, Jantz MA, Wallace M, Vansteenkiste J, Silvestri GA, American College of Chest Physicians: Invasive Mediastinal Staging of Lung Cancer: ACCP Evidence-Based Clinical Practice Guidelines, ed 2. Chest 2007;132:202S–220S.

6 Herth FJ, Eberhardt R, Ernst A: The future of bronchoscopy in diagnosing, staging and treatment of lung cancer. Respiration 2006;73:399–409.

7 Eloubeidi MA: Endoscopic ultrasound-guided fine-needle aspiration in the staging and diagnosis of patients with lung cancer. Semin Thorac Cardiovasc Surg 2007;19:206–211.

8 Hoffmann H: Invasive staging of lung cancer by mediastinoscopy and video-assisted thoracoscopy. Lung Cancer 2001;34(suppl 3):3–5.

9 Yasufuku K, Fujisawa T: Staging and diagnosis of non-small lung cancer: invasive modalities. Respirology 2007;12:173–183.

10 Fritscher-Ravens A, Davidson BL, Hauber HP, et al: Endoscopic ultrasound, positron emission tomography, and computerized tomography for lung cancer. Am J Respir Crit Care Med 2003;168: 1293–1297.

11 Fritscher-Ravens A: Endoscopic ultrasound evaluation in the diagnosis and staging of lung cancer. Lung Cancer 2003;41:259–267.

12 Garpestad E, Goldberg S, Herth F, et al: CT fluoroscopy guidance for transbronchial needle aspiration: an experience in 35 patients. Chest 2001;119:329–332.

13 Herth F, Becker HD, Ernst A: Conventional vs. endobronchial ultrasound-guided transbronchial needle aspiration: a randomized trial. Chest 2004; 125:322–325.

14 Harrow EM, Abi-Saleh W, Blum J, et al: The utility of transbronchial needle aspiration in the staging of bronchogenic carcinoma. Am J Respir Crit Care Med 2000;161:601–607.

15 Krasnik M, Vilman P, Larsen SS, Jacobsen GK: Preliminary experience with a new method of endoscopic transbronchial real time ultrasound guided biopsy for diagnosis of mediastinal and hilar lesions. Thorax 2003;58:1083–1086.

16 Yasufuku K, Nakajima T, Fujiwara T, Chiyo M, Iyoda A, Yoshida S, Suzuki M, Sekine Y, Shibuya K, Yoshino I: Role of endobronchial ultrasound-guided transbronchial needle aspiration in the management of lung cancer. Gen Thorac Cardiovasc Surg 2008;56:268–276.

17 Herth FJF, Krasnik M, Yasufuku K, Rintoul R, Ernst A: Endobronchial ultrasound-guided transbronchial needle aspiration – how I do it. J Bronchol 2006;13:84–91.

18 Sarkiss M, Kennedy M, Riedel B, Norman P, Morice R, Jimenez C, Eapen G: Anesthesia technique for endobronchial ultrasound-guided fine needle aspiration of mediastinal lymph nodes. J Cardiothorac Vasc Anesth 2007;21:892–896.

19 Yasufuku K, Chhajed PN, Sekine Y, Nakajima T, Chiyo M, Iyoda A, Yoshida S, Otsuji M, Shibuya K, Iizasa T, Saitoh Y, Fujisawa T: Endobronchial ultrasound using a new convex probe: a preliminary study on surgically resected specimens. Oncol Rep 2004;11:293–296.

20 Yasufuku K, Chiyo M, Sekine Y, Chhajed PN, Shibuya K, Iizasa T, Fujisawa T: Real-time endobronchial ultrasound guided transbronchial needle aspiration of mediastinal and hilar lymph nodes. Chest 2004;126:122–128.

21 Rintoul RC, Skwarski KM, Murchison JT, Wallace WA, Walker WS, Penman ID: Endobronchial and endoscopic ultrasound-guided real-time fine-needle aspiration for mediastinal staging. Eur Respir J 2005;25:416–421.
22 Herth FJ, Eberhardt R, Vilmann P, Krasnik M, Ernst A: Real-time endobronchial ultrasound guided transbronchial needle aspiration for sampling mediastinal lymph nodes. Thorax 2006;61: 795–798.
23 Herth FJ, Ernst A, Eberhardt R, Vilmann P, Dienemann H, Krasnik M: Endobronchial ultrasound-guided transbronchial needle aspiration of lymph nodes in the radiologically normal mediastinum. Eur Respir J 2006;28:910–914.
24 Yasufuku K, Nakajima T, Motoori K, Sekine Y, Shibuya K, Hiroshima K, Fujisawa T: Comparison of endobronchial ultrasound, positron emission tomography, and computed tomography for lymph node staging of lung cancer. Chest 2006; 130:710–718.
25 Herth FJ, Annema JT, Eberhardt R, Yasufuku K, Ernst A, Krasnik M, Rintoul RC: Endobronchial ultrasound with transbronchial needle aspiration for restaging the mediastinum in lung cancer. J Clin Oncol 2008;26:3346–3350.
26 Tournoy KG, Rintoul RC, van Meerbeeck JP, Carroll NR, Praet M, Buttery RC, van Kralingen KW, Rabe KF, Annema JT: EBUS-TBNA for the diagnosis of central parenchymal lung lesions not visible at routine bronchoscopy. Lung Cancer 2008;Epub ahead of print.
27 Herth FJ, Rabe KF, Gasparini S, Annema JT: Transbronchial and transoesophageal (ultrasound-guided) needle aspirations for the analysis of mediastinal lesions. Eur Respir J 2006;28:1264–1275.
28 Herth FJ, Eberhardt R: Actual role of endobronchial ultrasound (EBUS). Eur Radiol 2007;17: 1806–1812.

Prof. Felix J.F. Herth, MD, FCCP
Pneumologie und Beatmungsmedizin, Thoraxklinik am Universitätsklinikum Heidelberg
Amalienstrasse 5
DE–69126 Heidelberg (Germany)
Tel. +49 6221 396 1200, Fax +49 6221 396 1202, E-Mail Felix.Herth@thoraxklinik-heidelberg.de

Heide J, Schmittel A, Kaiser D, Hinkelbein W (eds): Controversies in the Treatment of Lung Cancer.
Front Radiat Ther Oncol. Basel, Karger, 2010, vol 42, pp 63–70

New Developments in Videomediastinoscopy: Video-Assisted Mediastinoscopic Lymphadenectomy and Mediastinoscopic Ultrasound

Biruta Witte

Sektion Thoraxchirurgie, Lungenzentrum Koblenz, Katholisches Klinikum Koblenz, Koblenz, Germany

Abstract

Background: Mediastinal lymphadenectomy is usually performed at thoracotomy together with lung resection. It is a prerequisite for accurate nodal staging and has an impact on survival. **Methods:** VAMLA (video-assisted mediastinoscopic lymphadenectomy) dissection is guided by anatomical landmarks. It includes en bloc resection of the right and central compartments, and dissection and lymphadenectomy of the left-sided compartment. **Results:** VAMLA harvested significantly more mediastinal lymph nodes than open lymphadenectomy ($p < 0.001$). Mean duration was 54 min, the complication rate 4.6%, sensitivity 93.8%, specificity 100%, and the false-negative rate 0.9%. 16 of 24 cT4 tumors were correctly predicted to be resectable by MUS (mediastinoscopic ultrasound). For minimally invasive oncological lung resections, combined VATS + VAMLA harvested significantly more lymph nodes than VATS alone without impact on operation time and complication rate ($p < 0.05$). **Conclusion:** VAMLA is a well-tolerated minimally invasive method for accurate mediastinal staging and radical mediastinal dissection. VAMLA can be carried out independently from tumor resection. We suggest its application together with neoadjuvant strategies, trials, VATS lobectomy, and radiation therapy for curatively intended involved field radiation. Additional MUS is helpful to detect resectable cT4 cases, and offer them curative treatment.

Evolving technologies of imaging, ultrasound-guided fine-needle aspiration, proteomic and genomic research are incorporated more or less frequently into diagnostic work-up and treatment decisions of lung cancer patients. On the other hand, mediastinoscopy is still considered to be the gold standard for mediastinal staging [1], and complete mediastinal dissection is considered to be an independent prognostic factor [2]. Since its introduction by Carlens [3], mediastinoscopy has developed from a method for inspection and biopsies into a tool for complete mediastinal dissection (video-assisted mediastinoscopic lymphadenectomy; VAMLA) [4–9]. For the first time ever, VAMLA facilitates complete mediastinal dissection independent from major surgery. In the same procedure, radiological T overstaging and consecutive undertreatment of central tumors is addressed by intraoperative ultrasound imaging (mediastinoscopic ultrasound; MUS) [10, 11].

Methods

Prerequisites for VAMLA and MUS are a two-bladed spreadable videomediastinoscope [4], a sterile finger-tip ultrasound probe [10] (fig. 1), and a dedicated thoracic surgeon familiar with conventional mediastinoscopy and minimally invasive surgery. Incision and access are similar to conventional mediastinoscopy [12], whereas the features of mediastinal dissection are similar to open surgery [13]. Dissection (fig. 2) is guided by anatomical landmarks and performed mainly as a compartmental en bloc resection of mediastinal adipose tissue containing the lymph nodes [4, 6, 8]. For routine VAMLA, we adhered to the Naruke map [14] to define a subcarinal compartment (7, upper 8), a central compartment (3, 4R), and a left compartment (4L). The latter is not resected en bloc with regard to the left recurrent nerve. If appropriate, VAMLA can be extended to the 2R+L stations cranial of the annominate artery, to station 10 at the upper hilum and the intermediate bronchus, and via extended mediastinolscopy [15] to the para- and subaortic nodes of station 5 and 6. Alternatively, the latter can be reached by EUS-FNA [16], as well as the lower station 8 (paraesophageal) and 9 (ligamentum pulmonale).

Results

The first description by Huertgen et al. [4] in 2002 defined the principles and standard procedure of videomediastinoscopic lymphadenectomy. It demonstrated that VAMLA harvested significantly more mediastinal adipose tissue containing significantly more mediastinal lymph nodes (20.7 (5–60) vs. 14.3 (2–26) nodes, $p < 0.0001$), comparing 40 VAMLA specimens to 80 open surgery lymphadenectomy specimens from the same institution. Another pilot study of 20 patients from the working party of Linder published in 2003 [5] described the dissection rates of different mediastinal nodal stations (2R: 96%, 4R: 92%, 7:100%, 4L: 100%, 2L: 28%). On its way into clinical routine, VAMLA was evaluated by a prospective feasibility study published in 2006 [6], including 144 patients fit for lung resection with resectable tumors and normal mediastinal findings on CT scan. Under routine clinical conditions, VAMLA had a mean duration of 54.1 min (40–175), a mortality of 0%, a conversion rate of 0%, and a complication rate of 4.6% dropping from 5.3 to 2.6% with growing experience of the three surgeons involved. The complication most frequently observed was temporary left-sided recurrent nerve paralysis. Pleural effusion, chylothorax, mediastinitis

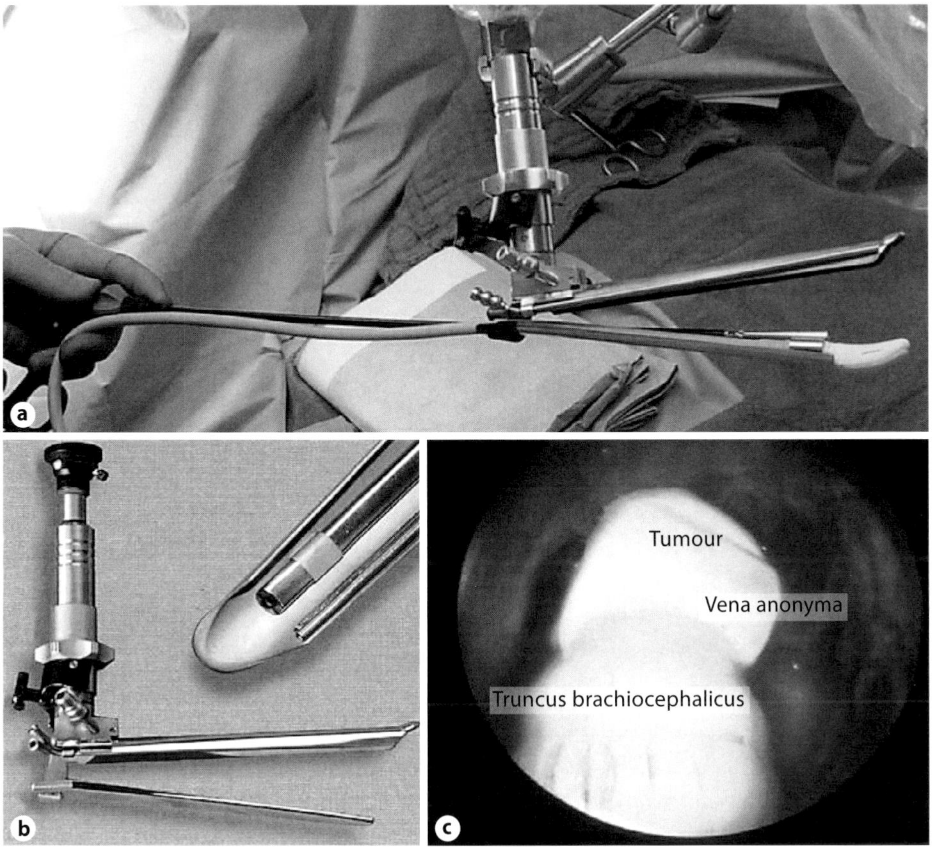

Fig. 1. Unlike other unvariable tubular (video)mediastinoscopes, the Linder-Dahan scope (**a**, **b**) is equipped with a spreadable shaft, providing a wide operation field, being the prerequisite of bimanual dissection and development of videomediastinoscopic surgery (VAMS). Besides VAMLA, the Linder-Dahan scope facilitated techniques like mediastinoscopic ultrasound (MUS, **b, c**), mediastinoscopic excision of mediastinal cysts, and secondary main bronchus stump closure.

and major bleeding were rare complications. Accuracy data derived from 130 patients reexplored at open lung resection being sensitivity, specificity and false-negative rate were 93.8, 100, and 0.9%. In a subset of 24 patients with centrally located cT4 tumors, a sterile fingertip ultrasound probe was introduced intraoperatively into the mediastinum in order to predict technical resectability by the means of MUS. Of 24 cT4 patients investigated by MUS, 8 were not operated on for oncological or functional reasons. The others underwent R0 resection as predicted [10, 11]. The next step was the assessment of other mediastinal staging tools by VAMLA, as we did for 120 patients with negative EUS-FNA findings [16]. EUS-FNA sensitivity was 43.8, 78.1 and 91.7% for normal nodes, enlarged

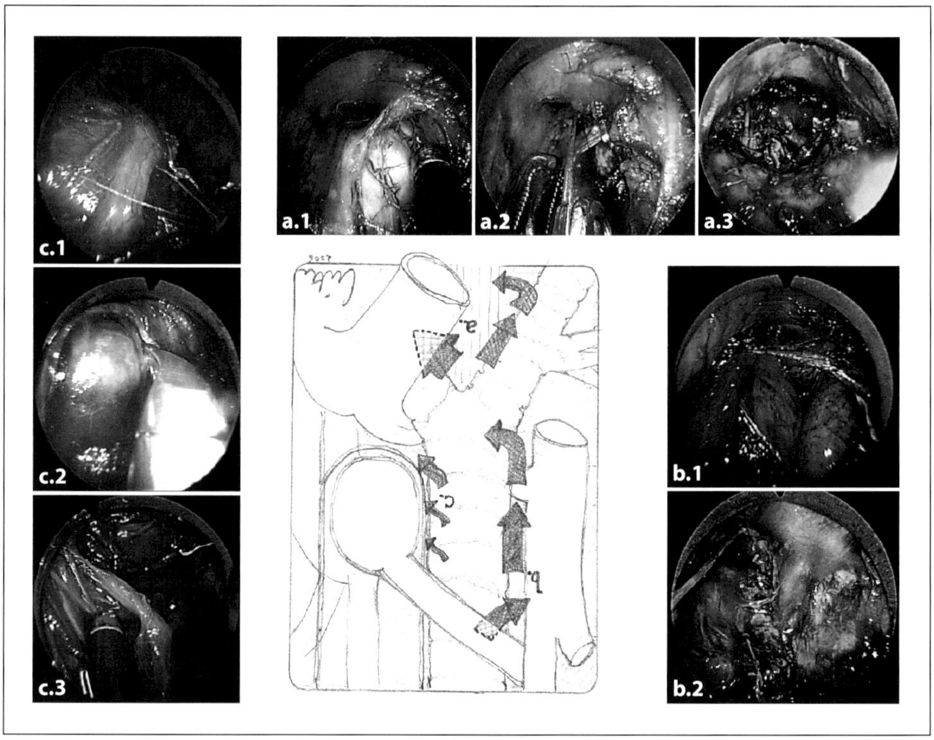

Fig. 2. VAMLA map and screen shots as seen by the surgeon. In the subcarinal compartment (**a**), the pulmonary artery and main carina is defined (**a.1**), the bronchial artery clipped and divided (**a.2**), and the subcarinal nodes excised en bloc (**a.3**). The right compartment (**b**) is removed following the parietal pleura (**b.1**), vena cava and azygos (**b.2**). The left compartment (**c**) is opened between the left tracheobronchial angle and recurrent nerve (**c.1**), carefully dissected, and lymph nodes removed (**c.2**, **3**).

nodes and bulky disease on CT scan, respectively. EUS-FNA sensitivity also was stratified for different mediastinal nodal stations (4R: 23.8%, 7: 80.6%, 4L: 25%, 5 and 6: 78.9%). At present, the role of VAMLA as a fully fledged tool for mediastinal dissection and its free combination with other modalities in different clinical settings is under investigation. A prospective study of a VATS-VAMLA combination for minimally invasive management of early stage lung carcinoma describes 32 stage I lung cancer patients who underwent thoracoscopic resection, either by a combined VATS + VAMLA approach, or by VATS only [17]. The groups were balanced for most epidemiologic and oncologic features. In the combined VATS+VAMLA group, the number of dissected mediastinal stations (6.4 (5–9) vs. 3.6 (2–6), $p < 0.005$) as well as the weight of the mediastinal specimen (10.7 (2.7–1.4) vs. 5.6 (0.6–15), $p < 0.005$) were significantly higher than in the VATS only group. For none of the feasibility parameters, i.e. conversion rate, blood loss, operation time, complications and drainage time, was a significant difference detected. Comprehensive VAMLA long-term survival data for lung cancer patients are not available at the moment. However, looking into our institutional data, we identified 41 stage III patients followed up for more than 4 years, 26 of them stage IIIA, and 36 of them resected. Median overall survival has not yet been reached, and median recurrence-free survival was 2 years. Two thirds of the recurrences have been distant metastases.

Comments

The development of the two-bladed spreadable videomediastinosscope by Linder and Dahan in 1992 allowed increased exposure and bimanual dissection of mediastinal structures. Concurrent with technical progress in mediastinoscopy, neoadjuvant treatment of stage III lung cancer and minimally invasive anatomical resections of stage I lung carcinoma were introduced. In this setting, development of a videomediastinoscopic technique for complete mediastinal lymphadenectomy (VAMLA) was the obvious thing to do [18]. Preliminary studies published in 2002 and 2003 already made clear that the VAMLA technique, being at least as radical as open surgery, has propelled mediastinoscopy from a method of biopsy and staging to a surgical dissection tool [4, 5]. Nevertheless, VAMLA found its first routine clinical application and field of prospective investigation in analogy to conventional mediastinoscopy, replacing it as a staging tool with extraordinary accuracy becoming even more sophisticated with additional extended mediastinoscopy for left-sided and additional MUS for central tumors. This was accomplished without any conversions or morbidity, and, compared to open lymphadenectomy, with a favorable complication profile [6]. The next step was to exploit VAMLA's extraordinary accuracy for assessment of other new staging methods, e.g. EUS FNA [16], and to exploit its minimally invasive radicality for combination with other oncologic modalities regardless of timing and resectability. With regard to fine-needle aspiration techniques, the results [16] suggest approaching the radiologically normal mediastinum by VAMLA and all other cases by EUS-FNA first. The free combination of VAMLA is a comparatively new field of clinical investigation. Preliminary data of a VATS-VAMLA combination for complete minimally invasive resection of early stage lung carcinoma [17], and VAMLA stage III long-term survival showed promising results. To come to a first conclusion, development and implementation of VAMLA as an extremely accurate mediastinal staging tool as well as a minimally invasive method of radical mediastinal dissection has taken place during the last decade, and has been well documented (table 1).

It is probably easier to state who should not be considered to implement VAMLA. From the technical point of view, thoracic surgeons inexperienced with

Table 1. VAMLA: survey on published evidence

Working party	Design	Objective	Results
Huertgen et al. [4], 2001	pilot case-control study, n = 40	VAMLA technique radicality vs. open LA	VAMLA more radical ($p<0.0001$) as open lymphadenectomy
Leschber and Linder [5], 2003	prospective pilot study, n = 20	VAMLA technique radicality vs. open LA	VAMLA dissection rates up to 100%
Witte and Huertgen [6], 2006	prospective study, n = 144	feasibility accuracy	duration 54 min, conversions 0%, mortality 0%, morbidity 4.6%, sensitivity %, specificity 100%, false-negative rate 0.9%
Witte, Neumeister and Huertgen [16], 2007	prospective study, n = 120	EUS-FNA vs. VAMLA	EUS-FNA accuracy dependent on size and location of mediastinal nodes
Witte, Neumeister and Huertgen [17], 2008	pilot prospective study, n = 32	VATS + VAMLA vs. VATS only for stage I lung carcinoma	VATS + VAMLA combination significantly improves mediastinal dissection without impact on feasibility ($p<0,005$)

mediastinoscopy and minimally invasive surgery should certainly not, given this kind of surgeon really does exist. Further, they should ignore that left-sided open procedures preclude a complete bilateral mediastinal dissection for anatomical reasons [13], as well as the fact that VATS mediastinal lymphadenectomy is often cumbersome and incomplete [18]. From the oncological point of view, lung cancer groups feeling comfortable with adjuvant treatment of mediastinal disease, exclusion of mediastinal disease from involved field radiation, and exclusion of resectable cT4 pT2 tumors from surgery and thus curative treatment should certainly not. Working parties considering their rates of false-negative fine-needle aspiration findings and false-positive PET findings to be without impact on treatment decisions and survival should not, and neither should those in doubt whether mediastinal dissection is an independent prognostic factor [2] or whether pretherapy N staging requires a tissue diagnosis. However, these pragmatic approaches have several disadvantages: (1) Mediastinal staging should not only address the N denominator, but describe the real extent of mediastinal disease, especially in studies and trials, as reflected by the forthcoming seventh edition of the lung carcinoma TNM classification [19, 20]. (2) The range of any lymphadenectomy performed together with a lung resection is limited, especially for left-sided tumors and VATS lobectomy. Therefore, there is an inherent

Table 2. VAMLA, suggested indications

Context	Entity	Objective
Research	evaluation of new prognostic factors evaluation of new therapies	VAMLA provides accurate mediastinal staging, being prerequisite for comparability of results and an 'old' prognostic factor
Surgery	left-sided tumors VATS lobectomy	complete mediastinal dissection
Oncology	minor N2/3: mediastinal staging/clearance prior to multimodality treatment apparent FNA-proved N2 /3: mediastinal restaging after neoadjuvant therapy	more neoadjuvant treatment, no re-mediastinoscopies
Radiation oncology	identification of false-negative/positive scans, e.g. PET-CT	involved field radiation; combined limited resection and limited radiation

risk of mediastinal understaging. (3) There is no evidence that adjuvant chemotherapy for stage III disease is superior or even equal to neoadjuvant treatment. (4) Adjuvant treatment is more often administered incompletely than neoadjuvant treatment. The individual patient suitable for VAMLA should be fit for lung resection, have a technically resectable tumor, and normal lymph node size on CT scan. Contraindications against multimodality treatment should be observed. VAMLA is also suitable for nonresectable patients to define the smallest appropriate radiation field, or new combinations of limited minimally invasive surgery and hypofractionated radiation.

Implications for Clinical Practice and Further Research

To conclude, VAMLA is an extremely accurate staging tool as well as definitive mediastinal surgery. However, VAMLA is minimally invasive and therefore independent of surgical resection. Therefore, VAMLA is indicated if neoadjuvant treatment is considered for any even minor mediastinal involvement, to avoid remediastinoscopies after induction therapy, to define the exact involved radiation field in functionally unresectable patients, for highly accurate pretherapy staging in trials, and to improve mediastinal dissection with VATS lobectomy and left-sided tumors (table 2).

References

1 De Leyn P, Lardinois D, Van Schil PE, Rami-Porta R, Passlick B, Zielinski M, Waller DA, Lerut T, Weder W: ESTS guidelines for preoperative lymph node staging for non-small cell lung cancer. Eur J Cardiothorac Surg 2007;32:1–8.
2 Wright G, Manser RL, Byrnes G, Hart D, Campbell DA: Surgery for non-small cell lung cancer: systematic review and meta-analysis of randomised controlled trials. Thorax 2006;61:597–603.
3 Carlens E: Mediastinoscopy: a method for inspection and tissue biopsy in the superior mediastinum. Chest 1959;36:343–352.
4 Huertgen M, Friedel G, Toomes H, Fritz P: Radical video-assisted mediastinoscopic lymphadenectomy (VAMLA) – technique and first results. Eur J Cardiothorac Surg 2002;21:348 – 351.
5 Leschber G, Holinka G, Linder A: Video-assisted mediastinoscopic lymphadenectomy (VAMLA): a method for systematic mediastinal lymph node dissection. Eur J Cardiothorac Surg 2003;24:192–195.
6 Witte B, Wolf M, Huertgen M, Toomes H: Video-assisted mediastinoscopic surgery: clinical feasibility and accuracy of mediastinal lymph node staging. Ann Thorac Surg 2006;82:1821–1827.
7 Huertgen M, Friedel G, Witte B, Toomes H, Fritz P: Systematic video-assisted mediastinoscopic lymphadenectomy (VAMLA). GMS Thoracic Surg Sci 2005;2:DOC02/20051109.
8 Witte B, Huertgen M: Systematic video-assisted mediastinoscopic lymphadenectomy (VAMLA). Multimedia Man Cardiothorac Surg doi:10.1510/mmcts.2006.002576.
9 Witte B, Huertgen M: Video-assisted mediastinoscopic lymphadenectomy (VAMLA). J Thorac Oncol 2007;2:367–369.
10 Huertgen M, Metzler B, Friedel G, Toomes H: Mediastinoscopic ultrasonography (MUS). Eur J Cardiothorac Surg 2004;26:842–844.
11 Huertgen M, Wolf M, Witte B: Mediastinoscopic ultrasonography. J Thorac Oncol 2007;2:362–364.
12 De Leyn P, Lerut T: Videomediastinoscopy. Multimedia Man Cardiothorac Surg doi:10.1510/MMCTS.2004.000166.
13 Lardinois D, De Leyn P, Van Schil P, Rami Porta R, Waller D, Passlick B, Zielinski M, Junker K, Rendina EA, Ris HB, Hasse J, Detterbeck F, Lerut T, Weder W: ESTS guidelines for intraoperative lymph node staging in non-small cell lung cancer. Eur J Cardiothorac Surg 2006;30:787–792.
14 Naruke T, Goya T, Tsuchiya R, Suemasu K: Prognosis and survival in resected lung carcinoma based on the new international staging system. J Thorac Cardiovasc Surg1988;96:440–447.
15 Ginsberg RJ, Rice TW, Goldberg M, Waters PF, Schmocker BJ: Extended cervical mediastinoscopy: a single staging procedure for bronchogenic carcinoma of the left upper lobe. J Thorac Cardiovasc Surg 1987;94:673–678.
16 Witte B, Neumeister W, Huertgen M. Does endoesophageal ultrasound-guided fine-needle aspiration (EUS-FNA) replace mediastinoscopy in mediastinal staging of thoracic malignancies? Eur J Cardiothorac Surg 2008;33:1124–1128.
17 Witte B, Messerschmidt A, Hillebrand H, Groß S, Wolf M, Kriegel E, Neumeister W, Hürtgen M: Combined videothoracoscopic and videomediastinoscopic approach improves radicality of minimally invasive mediastinal lymphadenectomy for early stage lung carcinoma. Eur J Cardiothorac Surg 2009;35:343–347.
18 Witte B, Huertgen M: Videoassistierte mediastinoskopische Chirurgie. Chirurg 2008;79:45–49.
19 Goldstraw P, Crowley J, Chansky K, Giroux DJ, Groome PA, Rami-Porta R, Postmus P, Rusch V, Sobin L: The IASLC Lung Cancer Staging Project: proposals for the revision of the TNM stage groupings in the forthcoming (seventh) edition of the TNM classification of malignant tumors. J Thorac Oncol 2007;2:706–714.
20 Rusch V, Crowley J, Giroux DJ, Goldstraw P, Im JG, Tsuboi M, Tsuchiya R, Vansteenkiste J: The IASLC Lung Cancer Staging Project: proposals for the revision of the N descriptors in the forthcoming seventh edition of the TNM classification for lung cancer. J Thorac Oncol 2007;2:603–612.

Dr. med. Biruta Witte
Sektion Thoraxchirurgie, Lungenzentrum Koblenz, Katholisches Klinikum Koblenz
Rudolf-Virchow-Strasse 7
DE–56073 Koblenz (Germany)
Tel. +49 261 496 4581, Fax +49 261 496 3599, E-Mail b.witte@kk-koblenz.de

Heide J, Schmittel A, Kaiser D, Hinkelbein W (eds): Controversies in the Treatment of Lung Cancer.
Front Radiat Ther Oncol. Basel, Karger, 2010, vol 42, pp 71–77

Resection in Stage I/II Non-Small Cell Lung Cancer

F.M. Smolle-Juettner · A. Maier · J. Lindenmann · V. Matzi · N. Neuböck

Division of Thoracic and Hyperbaric Surgery, Department of Surgery, Medical University of Graz, Graz, Austria

Abstract

In spite of the developments in chemo- and radiotherapy, surgery remains the mainstay of curative treatment of early stage non-small cell lung cancer (NSCLC). In stage Ia/Ib (T1, T2, N0), NSCLC lobectomy offers the best chance for cure, yielding survival rates of between 58 and 76%. Since the extent of mediastinal lymph node dissection does not seem to play a major prognostic role in stage Ia, video-thoracoscopic lobectomy yields equally good results as the open approach. Due to the necessity for a small thoracotomy when harvesting the specimen and the time-consuming lymph-node dissection minimally invasive lobar resections have failed to become routinely used. Minor resections, though sometimes necessary from the functional point of view, have a lower curative potential. They yield the best results if applied in tumors measuring less than 2 cm. Stage II, characterized by involvement of the N1-position and/or a more central tumor growth, has a 5-year survival of 45–52% and requires treatment by lobectomy or pneumonectomy. Sleeve resection may obviate the need for pneumonectomy in central upper-lobe tumors. In interlobar N1, however, pneumonectomy is indicated from the oncological point of view, since even meticulous lymph-node dissection is unable to achieve tumor control in this situation.

With the introduction of the TNM staging, Williams et al. [1] in 1981 reported an 80% 5-year survival rate in T1N0 (stage Ia) after resection. In spite of a variety of efforts concerning staging procedures, selective surgical approaches and attempts of adjuvant treatment the survival rate of stage Ia has remained more or less unchanged with recently published rates ranging between 58 and 76% [2, 3]. In T2N0 (stage Ib) survival reaches 60% at 5 years.

Once the intrapulmonary lymph nodes are affected by the tumor (stage II), there is a drop in prognosis with recently published 5-year survival rates of about 52% [2]. There has been a continuous increase of the survival rates in stage II non-small cell lung cancer (NSCLC) during the last 25 years: In 1983, Carr [4] reported 35% 5-year survival and in 1992 Martini et al. [5] found 39%. Considering the fact that the surgical procedures had remained more or less the same during the period, the better results are most likely due to 'stage migration': high-resolution imaging, PET and more widely used invasive preoperative staging of the mediastinum enabled the identification of advanced stages, formerly misdiagnosed as stage II [6, 7].

On the other hand, pathological investigations at the molecular level are beginning to demonstrate substantial, prognostically relevant differences between morphologically similar lesions. Together with refinements in the staging system these findings may lead to selective surgical and nonsurgical treatment of NSCLC.

Patients with lung cancer often suffer from cardiorespiratory co-morbidity. If the functional possibility for 'standard' lobar resection is not given in the very stages I and II in which the chance for cure is comparatively high, alternatives have to be sought [8]. Their functional benefits, however, have to be weighed against possible oncological disadvantages.

When assessing the definitive therapeutic outcome, long-term follow-up is required: Sorensen [9], in 1982, carried out a well-researched survey evaluating 265 patients of various stages resected between 1942 and 1955: By means of age-adjusting of healthy controls he found that actuarial cure time, i.e. when the age-adjusted survival percentage is constant, is not reached until after 14 years. There are hardly any studies, however, referring to observation times longer than 10 years.

Surgery in Stages I and II

Lobectomy

Lobectomy, the anatomical resection of one or two lobes (so-called bi-lobectomy), is the gold standard for resection in early stage lung cancer [3, 8, 10].

The procedure is not time-consuming and, given a correct preoperative functional assessment, it carries a low rate of morbidity and mortality [10].

The question whether complete mediastinal lymph node dissection should be included in the therapeutic regimen in these stages is still a matter of discussion. Whereas on the one hand actual N0 obviously does not require surgical removal, it is still impossible to define the nodal status in a clear-cut way without systematic lymph node dissection. Further refinement of imaging techniques may allow a preoperative determination of N0, N1 or N2 stages, but for the time being accurate staging relies on histology [6, 11, 12]. There is evidence, however, that in elderly patients aged between 75 and 89 years systematic lymph node dissection might prolong the postoperative in-hospital course and may be omitted without having a negative impact on prognosis [13, 14].

The outcome of lobectomy in early stages depends on more factors than simple stage Ia/Ib or stage II allocation: recent investigations have shown that there is a clear correlation between tumor size and prognosis – patients with tumors of a maximum diameter of 2 cm or less fare significantly better than those with larger ones [2]. This fact, however, seems to be related specifically to adenocarcinomas: in tumors sized 2 cm or less, survival of squamous cell carcinomas and adenocarcinomas was found to be equal, whereas in tumors sized 3 cm and more, adenocarcinomas did significantly worse than squamous cell cancer [3]. Moreover, women had a better outcome than men, and age above 65 years had a positive impact on prognosis [2, 3].

Video-thoracoscopic (VATS) lobectomy has repeatedly been advocated as a method equaling the open technique [15], especially in stages I and II. Throughout more than a decade, however, it has failed to become widely accepted as a routine procedure. There are various reasons for this: due to the necessity for a small thoracotomy when harvesting the specimen, most surgeons prefer resections by 'mini-thoracotomy' to 'truly' minimally invasive lobar resections. Moreover, an exact lymph node dissection via VATS is time-consuming. The possibility of a two-stage approach with initial video-mediastinoscopic complete lymph node dissection followed by VATS lobectomy is theoretically possible, but requires two not too short interventions instead of one. It has not become generally accepted up to this time.

In the presence of interlobar lymph node involvement, lobectomy can no longer be considered curative, even if a meticulous lymph node dissection is performed. In these cases pneumonectomy is indicated even in the presence of a small primary tumor.

Sleeve Resection

If an upper lobe tumor reaches the level of the main bronchus or if it is invading the intermediate section of the pulmonary artery, a classical lobectomy is no longer feasible. Though, for anatomical reasons, pneumonectomy would be the logical consequence, the method is fraught with a high rate of perioperative complications. Though locoregional recurrence is rare in pneumonectomy, long-term survival is reduced due to non-tumor-related cardiorespiratory impairment [16].

Sleeve lobectomy implicates a lobar resection en bloc with a circumferential segment of the intermediate bronchus at the origin of the lobar bronchus. Alternatively, a segment of the pulmonary artery may have to be resected. In some cases both a bronchial and a vascular 'sleeve' have to be removed in order to achieve a complete resection. The method has been used for more than 40 years and has occupied a well-defined place in the array of surgical techniques [17]. The question whether it is equivalent to pneumonectomy from the oncological point of view has not yet been definitely answered, because it is all but impossible to really match identical tumor stages treated by sleeve resection or pneumonectomy, respectively. From the functional point of view, sleeve resection is superior to pneumonectomy, with the re-implanted lobe contributing essentially to function. In stages I/II, however, survival following sleeve resection is not better than after pneumonectomy [16, 18, 19]. As with any procedure, the nodal status determines prognosis and no compromise must be made in achieving tumor-free resection margins [20–22].

Limited Resection

In contrast to lobectomy or sleeve lobectomy, limited resection is not a well-defined type of resection. Two different procedures, i.e. segmental resection and extra-anatomical wedge resection, are applied.

Segmental resection means dissection along the planes of the anatomical lung segments. It requires technical skill and anatomical knowledge. In order to be carried out correctly, it will usually require at least a small thoracotomy, because the resection plane is difficult to discern during VATS.

In contrast, extra-anatomical wedge resection describes the removal of a 'wedge' of – in this case – tumor-bearing lung by means of a stapling device that allows simultaneous suturing of the resection margin and cutting along the stapled suture line. This method is very simple, requires only basic anatomical knowledge and can be easily carried out using video-assisted techniques.

For the last 25 years studies have been fperformed elucidating the question whether limited resection is equal to lobectomy in terms of long-term tumor control. Ginsberg and Rubinstein [10] documented a clear prognostic disadvantage with 75% increase of locoregional recurrence and 30% reduction in survival following limited resection. Other authors did not find significant differences between lobectomy and minor resections [23, 24]. A meta-analysis did not procure further information, because of too much interstudy inhomogeneity [24]. More recent studies corroborated the concept that lobectomy is connected with a better prognosis than limited approaches: Chang et al. [2] performed a retrospective study in more than 10,000 stage Ia lung cancer patients in the US national cancer registry. Whereas survival of was 44% in sublobar resections, lobectomies yielded a 61% survival rate.

Anatomical segmental resections may be regarded as a somewhat different option: due to the resection plane along the anatomical segments there is probably less risk of leaving behind residual microscopic tumor debris in lymph vessels draining from the primary lesion. Sienel et al. [25] were able to prove that segmental resections provided better tumor control than extra-anatomical wedge resections, yet the results were still inferior to lobectomy. Massard [26] stated that anatomic segmentectomy may be an alternative to lobectomy in patients with peripheral tumors measuring less than 2 cm in diameter.

Considering all these aspects, limited resections should be reserved to patients with functional impairment and thus unfit for lobectomy.

Resection of Stage I and II NSCLC in Aged Patients

With increasing life expectancy, more patients are reaching old age in a good general condition. The question is whether lung resection would be advisable in patients aged 75 years and above. In a series of 39 octogenarians and 1 patient aged 90 years, Mizuguchi et al. [14] found a 5-year survival rate of 40%, Mun et al. [27] reported 66% 5-year survival in a group of 55 patients aged 80 years and over. The fact is whether lymph node dissection was performed or not did not affect survival, but lymph node dissection was connected with a higher rate of perioperative complications. Obviously, the rate of minimal resections in aged patients was higher than in younger ones [27], but a considerable number of patients aged over 75 will functionally tolerate lobar resections [13, 27].

Conclusion

There is no actual breakthrough in the treatment of non-small cell lung cancer from the surgical point of view. Prolonged survival rates in stage II are mainly due to improvements in the preoperative staging. On the other hand, video-assisted less-invasive techniques enable minimal resections in well-selected subgroups of functionally impaired or very old patients. Further subclassifications of stage and histopathological properties will enable us to define a better estimation of prognosis and a 'tailored' individual treatment.

References

1 Williams DE, Pairolero PC, Davis CS, Bernatz PE, Payne WS, Taylor WF, Uhlenhopp MA, Fontana RS: Survival of patients surgically treated for stage I lung cancer. J Thorac Cardiovasc Surg 1981;82:70–76.

2 Chang MY, Mentzer SJ, Colson YL, Linden PA, Jaklitsch MT, Lipsitz SR, Sugarbaker DJ: Factors predicting poor survival after resection of stage IA non-small cell lung cancer. J Thorac Cardiovasc Surg 2007;134:850–856.

3 Ost D, Goldberg J, Rolnitzky L, Rom WN: Survival after surgery in stage IA and IB non-small cell lung cancer. Am J Resp Critical Care Med 2008;177:516–523.

4 Carr DT: Is staging of cancer of value? Cancer 1983;51(suppl 12):2503–2505.

5 Martini N, Burt ME, Bains MS, McCormack PM, Rusch VW, Ginsberg RJ: Survival after resection of stage II non-small cell lung cancer. Ann Thorac Surg 1992;54:460–465; discussion 466.

6 Lardinois D, Suter H, Hakki H, Rousson V, Betticher D, Ris HB: Morbidity, survival, and site of recurrence after mediastinal lymph-node dissection versus systematic sampling after complete resection for non-small cell lung cancer. Ann Thorac Surg 2005;80:268–274; discussion 274–275.

7 Kimura H, Yasufuku K, Ando S, Yoshida S, Ishikawa A, Wada Y, Fujisawa T: Indications for mediastinoscopy and comparison of lymph node dissections in candidates for lung cancer surgery. Lung Cancer 2007;56:349–355.

8 Pennathur A, Abbas G, Christie N, Landreneau R, Luketich JD: Video assisted thoracoscopic surgery and lobectomy, sublobar resection, radiofrequency ablation, and stereotactic radiosurgery: advances and controversies in the management of early stage non-small cell lung cancer. Curr Opinion Pulm Med 2007;13:267–270.

9 Sorensen HR: Long-term survival and cure in lung cancer surgery. Thorac Cardiovasc Surg 1982;30: 292–293.

10 Ginsberg RJ, Rubinstein LV: Randomized trial of lobectomy versus limited resection for T1 N0 non-small cell lung cancer. Lung Cancer Study Group. Ann Thorac Surg 1995;60:615–622; discussion 622–623.

11 Whitson BA, Groth SS, Maddaus MA: Surgical assessment and intraoperative management of mediastinal lymph nodes in non-small cell lung cancer. Ann Thorac Surg 2007;84:1059–1065.

12 Doddoli C, Aragon A, Barlesi F, Chetaille B, Robitail S, Giudicelli R, Fuentes P, Thomas P: Does the extent of lymph node dissection influence outcome in patients with stage I non-small-cell lung cancer? Eur J Cardio-Thorac Surg 2005;27:680–685.

13 Iwasaki A, Hamatake D, Hamanaka W, Hamada T, Shirakusa T, Yamamoto S, Shiraishi T: Is systemic node dissection for accuracy staging in clinical stage I non-small cell lung cancer worthwhile in the elderly? Thorac Cardiovasc Surg 2008;56:37–41.

14 Mizuguchi S, Inoue K, Iwata T, Izumi N, Tsukioka T, Morita R, Nishida T, Nishiyama N, Shuto T, Suehiro S: Impact of mediastinal lymph node dissection on octogenarians with non-small cell lung cancer. Jpn J Thorac Cardiovasc Surg 2006;54:103–108.

15 McKenna RJ Jr: Lobectomy by video-assisted thoracic surgery with mediastinal node sampling for lung cancer. J Thorac Cardiovasc Surg 1994;107: 879–881; discussion 881–882.

16 Takeda S, Maeda H, Koma M, Matsubara Y, Sawabata N, Inoue M, Tokunaga T, Ohta M: Comparison of surgical results after pneumonectomy and sleeve lobectomy for non-small cell lung cancer: trends over time and 20-year institutional experience. Eur J Cardio-Thorac Surg 29:276–280.

17 Naruke T, Suemasu K: Bronchoplastic surgery for lung cancer and the results. Jpn J Surg 1983;13: 165–172.

18 Deslauriers J, Gregoire J, Jacques LF, Piraux M, Guojin L, Lacasse Y: Sleeve lobectomy versus pneumonectomy for lung cancer: a comparative analysis of survival and sites or recurrences. Ann Thorac Surg 2004;77:1152–1156; discussion 1156.

19 Balduyck B, Hendriks J, Lauwers P, Van Schil P: Quality of life after lung cancer surgery: a prospective pilot study comparing bronchial sleeve lobectomy with pneumonectomy. J Thorac Oncol 2008;3:604–608.

20 Mehran RJ, Deslauriers J, Piraux M, Beaulieu M, Guimont C, Brisson J: Survival related to nodal status after sleeve resection for lung cancer. J Thorac Cardiovasc Surg 1994;107:576–582; discussion 582–583.

21 Bennett WF, Smith RA: A twenty-year analysis of the results of sleeve resection for primary bronchogenic carcinoma. J Thorac Cardiovasc Surg 1978;76:840–845.

22 Cerfolio RJ, Bryant AS: Surgical techniques and results for partial or circumferential sleeve resection of the pulmonary artery for patients with non-small cell lung cancer. Ann Thorac Surg 2007;83:1971–1976; discussion 1976–1977.

23 Keenan RJ, Landreneau RJ, Maley RH Jr, Singh D, Macherey R, Bartley S, Santucci T: Segmental resection spares pulmonary function in patients with stage I lung cancer. Ann Thorac Surg 2004; 78:228–233.

24 Nakamura H, Kawasaki N, Taguchi M, Kabasawa K: Survival following lobectomy vs limited resection for stage I lung cancer: a meta-analysis. Br J Cancer 2005;92:1033–1037.

25 Sienel W, Dango S, Kirschbaum A, Cucuruz B, Horth W, Stremmel C, Passlick B: Sublobar resections in stage IA non-small cell lung cancer: segmentectomies result in significantly better cancer-related survival than wedge resections. Eur J Cardio-Thorac Surg 2008;33:728–734.
26 Massard G: Criteres de qualite de la chirurgie d'exerese des cancers bronchiques non microcellulaires. Rev Maladies Resp 2007;24:640–649.
27 Mun M, Kohno T: Video-assisted thoracic surgery for clinical stage I lung cancer in octogenarians. Ann Thor Surg 2008;85:406–411.

F.M. Smolle-Juettner, MD
Division of Thoracic and Hyperbaric Surgery, Department of Surgery, Medical University of Graz
Auenbruggerplatz 29
AT–8036 Graz (Austria)
Tel. +43 316 385 3302, Fax +43 316 385 4679, E-Mail freyja.smolle@meduni-graz.at

Heide J, Schmittel A, Kaiser D, Hinkelbein W (eds): Controversies in the Treatment of Lung Cancer.
Front Radiat Ther Oncol. Basel, Karger, 2010, vol 42, pp 78–86

Role of Mediastinal Lymph Node Dissection in Non-Small Cell Lung Cancer

Servet Bölükbas[a] · Michael H. Eberlein[b] · Joachim Schirren[a]

[a]Department of Thoracic Surgery, Dr. Horst-Schmidt Clinic, Wiesbaden, Germany; [b]Division of Pulmonary and Critical Care Medicine, Johns Hopkins University School of Medicine, Baltimore, Md., USA

Abstract

The role of systematic mediastinal lymph node dissection in the staging and treatment of non-small cell lung cancer (NSCLC) is the subject of ongoing debate. Surgical practice varies from simple visual inspection of the unopened mediastinum to radical, systematic lymphadenectomy of all accessible lymph node levels. As the evaluation of mediastinal lymph nodes is a precondition for accurate intraoperative staging of NSCLC we advocate for complete interlobar, hilar and mediastinal lymphadenectomy as compartment dissections in patients with NSCLC. The therapeutic effect of extensive mediastinal lymphadenectomy, however, remains controversial. In this review we discuss the role of mediastinal lymph node dissection in the management of NSCLC.

The lymphatic system of the lungs has a high anatomical variability. The intrapulmonary system consists of lymph vessels and lymphatic tissue. The lymphatic tissue is organized in the form of lymph follicles or in regional lymph nodes. The intrapulmonary lymph vessels include superficial, reticular, subpleural and peribronchial, as well as perivascular lymph vessels. These run to vein branches and unify at the hilus of the lung [1]. The extrapulmonary lymphatic system of the lung consists of mediastinal lymph vessels and lymph nodes (fig. 1) [2]. Segmental and subpleural lymphatics may drain directly to paratracheal or supraclavicular stations which is a possible explanation for skip metastases to these lymph node stations without involvement of intrapulmonary or hilar nodes [3]. This manifestation of lymphatic spread depends on anatomical characteristics, the special abilities of the tumor cells and earlier inflammatory diseases of the lung. Pneumoconiosis, anthrasilicoses, and hyaline changes are also considered as possible causes of this phenomenon. Metastatic spread may not affect all topographical lymph node positions. The cortex and medullary cords usually occupy 70–80%

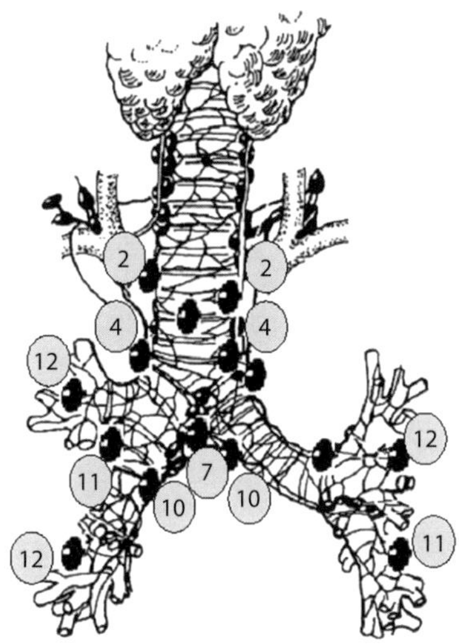

Upper mediastinum:
Level 1: highest mediastinal
Level 2: upper paratracheal
Level 3: pre-vascular and retro-tracheal
Level 4: lower paratracheal
Level 5: subaortic
Level 6: para-aortic

Lower mediastinum:
Level 7: subcarinal
Level 8: paraesophageal
Level 9: pulmonary ligament

N1-Lymph nodes
Level 10: hilar
Level 11: interlobar
Level 12: lobar
Level 13: segmental
Level 14: subsegmental

Fig. 1. Anatomical variability of the lymphatic system and the lymph node levels.

of the node [4]. The pulmonary, hilar and intrapulmonary nodes have a small cortex (almost 30%), whereas cervical, axillary, and upper mediastinal nodes extend to have a large cortex. Variations between individuals are evident. Cortices of the cervical nodes are significantly larger in specimens from elderly white Americans than elderly Japanese. The maximum and average number of lymph nodes in every lymph node station can vary (table 1) [5]. Mediastinal skip metastases can be found in 25% of the cases [6]. Moreover, the incidence of contralateral mediastinal lymph node involvement is high. Therefore, the use of a sentinel lymph node cannot provide reliable and predictable information [7].

Surgical Technique of Systematic Lymph Node Dissection

There is a significant variability in the surgical practice of dissecting all mediastinal N2 lymph nodes and this technique is not well established among all thoracic surgeons [8]. Removal of at least six lymph nodes (UICC) from hilar and mediastinal stations is recommended to define nodal staging accurately and to determine pN0 status [9]. The European Society of Thoracic Surgeons proposes the removal of, at least, three hilar and interlobar nodes and three mediastinal nodes from three stations. The subcarinal lymph node should always be included [10]. In contrast to these recommendations we advocate for complete interlobar,

Table 1. Average number and maximum number of nodes in the lymph node groups of the lung [5]

Lymph node level	% with nodes present	Number of nodes		Short transverse diameter, mm
		maximum	mean	
2R	80	11	2.5	7.8
2L	68	7	2.1	5.8
4R	98	11	4.8	9.2
4L	98	16	4.5	9.2
5	58	6	1.1	8.5
6	85	15	4.7	7.2
7	100	6	2.9	12.3
8R	58	6	1.2	8.2
8L	50	5	1.1	6.1
9R	10	2	0.1	3.9
9L	35	3	0.5	6.5
10R	95	10	3.5	10.8
10L	90	7	2.4	6.8

hilar and mediastinal lymphadenectomy as compartment dissections in patients with non-small cell lung cancer (NSCLC). The compartment of the upper mediastinum consists of the lymph levels 2, 4, 5 and 6, whereas the lower mediastinum is composed of the levels 7, 8, 9 and 10 (fig. 1). Right-sided thoracotomies should include the lymph node stations 2R, 2L, 4R, 4L, 7, 8, 9, 10R, 10L, 11, 12, and left-sided thoracotomies the stations 2L, 4L, 5, 6, 7, 8, 9, 10R, 10L, 11, 12, respectively (R and L define right and left). We published on the principles of systematic lymph node dissection in surgically treated bronchial carcinoma and highlighted the importance of the preparation of the posterior part of the bifurcation which allows best for exposure and dissection of the lymph node stations 10R, 7, and 10L [2]. Furthermore, in left-sided thoracotomies the ligamentum botalli must be cut through and the aorta has to be mobilized to dissect the lymph node station 4L. This technique allows also dissecting the contralateral lymph nodes. This surgical strategy leads to a high number of dissected lymph nodes which facilitates a correct postoperative staging, detects possible micrometastases and ensures a 'real' complete resection (R0).

Role of Nodal Involvement on Survival

In patients with NSCLC treated with standardized lymph node dissection strategies the impact of nodal involvement on survival still remains controversial Fadel et al. [11] noted a 5-year survival rate of 0% in the event of N2 involvement. In contrast, Cerfolio et al. [12] demonstrated a 5-year survival of up to 53% in selected subgroups of N2 disease. The situation of N1 disease also remains controversial. Van Schil et al. [13] noted significant differences between patients with N0 and N1 or N2 disease, but not between N1 and N2 involvement. In the recent published series by Schirren et al. [14] of patients with NSCLC, long-term survival differed between N0 and N1 status ($p = 0.027$) and N0 and N2 status ($p = 0.029$), but not between N1 and N2 status ($p = 0.754$). Furthermore Bölükbas et al. [15] showed that long-term survival was also not affected by nodal status ($p = 0.383$) in 157 elderly patients with NSCLC who underwent complete pulmonary resection. Survival of patients with single-level N2 metastases was not significantly different from that of patients with N1 disease provided that the primary tumors were located in the upper lobes [16]. Isolated N2 metastases without concomitant N1 disease (skip metastases) were associated with significantly better survival than that patients who had both N1 and N2 metastases ($p = 0.001$). At this point, the role of nodal involvement on survival of multimodality treated and completely resected patients with NSCLC remains unclear and continues to be controversial.

Impact of Mediastinal Lymph Node Dissection on Operative Morbidity, Mortality and Quality of Life

Systematic lymph node sampling (SS) and complete mediastinal lymph node dissection (MLND) may be associated with potential complications related to the interruption of the blood supply to the bronchial stump, injury to the recurrent laryngeal nerve, and removal of a large portion of the intrathoracic lymphatics. However Izbicki et al. [17] demonstrated in a randomized controlled clinical trial comparing MLND to conventional node dissection in 182 patients with non-small cell lung cancer that radical MLND was not associated with higher morbidity compared to lymph node sampling. The operative mortality after pulmonary resection varies between 0 and 7% [18, 19]. Even extended MLND in elderly patients is not associated with a higher risk of mortality (3.8%) [15]. Thus, MLND does not increase morbidity and mortality. In general, patients undergoing thoracotomy for a diagnosis of lung cancer experience decreased short-term quality of life (QoL), which returns to baseline 6 months after surgery [20, 21]. There is no evidence that MLND has additional impact on QoL of patients undergoing surgical resection for NSCLC. An argument against an aggressive surgical approach is that, resection is associated with loss of pulmonary function. On the other hand, most of the patients undergoing surgical resection for lung cancer were found to have good long-term pulmonary function, even patients with impaired preoperative pulmonary function [22, 23]. Furthermore, MLND itself is not associated with decrements in pulmonary function. In summary, MLND has no impact on operative morbidity, mortality and QoL after surgical resection and thus should not influence the decision whether to proceed to surgery or not.

Diagnostic Role of Mediastinal Lymph Node Dissection

The assessment of mediastinal lymph nodes is precondition for an exact NSCLC staging. The sensitivity and specificity of computed tomography (CT) of the chest and positron emission tomography (PET) in the staging of mediastinal lymph nodes are 57–82% (CT) and 84–89% (PET [24]. Mediastinoscopy as the most invasive approach has a higher sensitivity (81%) and specificity (100%) [25]. But this diagnostic procedure causes iatrogenic tumor seeding in the mediastinum. The sensitivities and accuracies of endobronchial ultrasound-guided transbronchial needle aspiration (EUS-FNA) in patients without enlarged nodes vary between 35–61% and 76–89%, respectively. The sensitivity (range 72–100%) and specificity (range 88–100%) are higher only in patients with enlarged or PET positive nodes [26]. However, minimal invasive EBUS and EUS should be preferred to avoid tumor seeding in the mediastinum. In this staging evaluation of patients with NSCLC there is the high risk of false pre- and postoperative staging, with the subsequent danger of inappropriate therapeutic approaches. Cerfolio et al. [27] conducted a prospective study with preoperative staging of all patients using 64-slice helical computed tomographic scan and integrated 2-deoxy-2–18-fluoro-d-glucose positron emission tomography computed tomography. All patients with clinically stage I underwent open thoracotomy with palpation of the rest of the lung and mediastinal lymph node dissection. Nonimaged malignant pulmonary nodules could be detected in different lobes in 8–9%. These patients were classified stage IIIB or IV. Twelve of 166 patients (7.2%) had unsuspected N2 disease. Clinically, stage Ia tumors are often understaged. Veeramachaneni et al. [28] reported that 15% of patients staged Ia had occult nodal metastasis. The risk of occult nodal disease increases with tumor size. There was a threefold increase in the risk of having pathologic stage II or stage III disease with every 1.0 cm increase in tumor size. There is the hypothesis of higher tumor cell aggressiveness in case of micrometastases [29]. Micrometastases were associated with poorer survival which was also supported by more cancer-related deaths and the responsiveness to adjuvant treatment observed in that group. These are arguments for MLND of all assessable N2 stations at the time of surgery. The detection of pathologic N1,

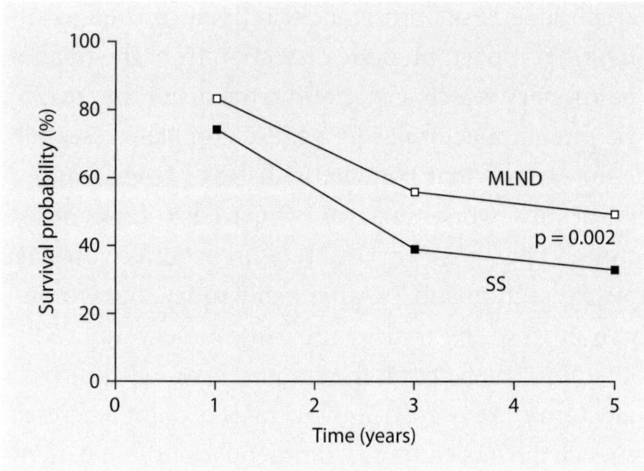

Fig. 2. Patients who underwent complete MLND survived significantly longer than those patients who underwent SS. From Schirren [2], with permission.

N2 or M1 disease after resection can change the postoperative therapeutic concept. Therefore, appropriate intraoperative staging is mandatory. The removal of only suspected or known malignant pulmonary nodules alone is insufficient. Stage migration can be avoided and advanced pathologic tumor stages can be translated over to the appropriate adjuvant therapy regimes.

Therapeutic Role of Mediastinal Lymph Node Dissection

The strongest determinants of survival in oncological surgery for lung cancer are nodal status and complete resection. Lymph node sampling was as efficacious as complete MLND in staging of 373 patients with resected NSCLC [30]. But complete MLND identified significantly more levels of N2 disease. Furthermore, MLND was associated with improved survival (66.4 vs. 24.5 months, $p < 0.001$) in comparison to lymph node sampling in patients with stages II and IIIa. Ma et al. [31] demonstrated for patients with clinical stage IA NSCLC with lesions between 2 and 3 cm that the 5-year overall survival (81.6 vs. 55.8%, $p = 0.041$) and disease-free survival (77.9 vs. 52.5%, $p = 0.038$) were significantly higher in the MLND group compared to the SS group. Also, Lardinois et al. [32] reported a longer disease-free survival after MLND than after SS (60.2 vs. 44.8 months, $p = 0.03$) in patients with stage I disease. Moreover, SS was associated with higher incidence of local recurrence (45 vs. 12.5%, $p = 0.02$) in patients with stage I tumor. In 307 operated patients with stage II NSCLC, MLND was associated with better survival in compared to SS (fig. 2) [2]. Surgical resection after neoadjuvant treatment is technically demanding, especially after chemoradiation or previous mediastinoscopy. A variable degree of fibrosis and scar tissue can be encountered during surgery which can hinder the lymph node dissection from the trachea, bronchi or the branches of the pulmonary vessels, especially in the major fissure [33]. Inevitable consequences may be pneumonectomies to achieve complete resection. However, Simon et al. [34] demonstrated that patients with NSCLC who underwent pneumonectomy had significantly worse survival compared to lesser resections like lobectomy or bilobectomy. The 2-year survival rates in patients with stage III are about 14% after incomplete resection and 7% after exploratory thoracotomy [35]. These assumptions apply to most of the trials comparing surgery and radiotherapy after induction chemotherapy. The fact that the surgical arms of these trials had both high rates of pneumonectomies (44–49%) and low rates of complete resections (47–50%) had as a consequence the misleading recommendations that patients with IIIA-N2 NSCLC should be considered for radiotherapy instead of surgery after induction chemotherapy [36–38]. Albain et al. [39] presented a survival benefit in patients with lobectomy (median survival: 34 months) compared to pneumonectomy (median survival: 22 months) in multimodality treated NSCLC in stage III-N2. Downstaging and complete resections are the prognostic factors for prolonged survival [37]. Downstaging depends on tumor biology but complete resections and the avoidance of pneumonectomy can be strongly influenced by the surgeon. These results point out that better survival following MLND is not only a 'Will Roger phenomenon' which is only an effect of stage migration without influence on survival [40]. MLND has a therapeutic effect in terms of exact staging and 'real' locoregional complete resection which can be strongly influenced by the surgeon [41].

Conclusion

MLND leads to a high number of dissected lymph nodes which facilitates accurate postoperative staging, detects possible micrometastases and ensures complete resection. Complete MLND is associated with improved survival. Therefore, complete resection of the tumor in anatomic units combined with MLND should be aspired in all resectable stages, even after neoadjuvant therapy in the situation of advanced stages of NSCLC.

References

1 Naruke T, Suemasu K, Ishikawa S: Lymph node mapping and curability at various levels of metastases in resected lung cancer. J Thorac Cardiovasc Surg 1978;76:832–839.

2 Schirren J: Die systematische mediastinale Lymphknotendissektion beim Bronchialkarzinom. Indikation, Technik, Ergebnisse; Habsschr medizinische Gesamtfakultät der Ruprecht-Karls-Universität zu Heidelberg, 1995.

3 Riquet M, Hidden G, Debesse B: Direct lymphatic drainage of lung segments to the mediastinal nodes: an anatomic study on 260 adults. J Thorac Cardiovasc Surg 989; 97:623—632.

4 Murakami G, Taniguchi I: Histological heterogeneity and intra nodal shunt flow in lymph nodes from elderly subjects: a cadaveric study. Ann Surg Oncol 2004;11:279–284.

5 Kiyono K, Sone S, Sakai F, Imai Y, Watanabe T, Izuno I, Oguchi M, Kawai T, Shigematsu H, Watanabe M: The number and size of normal mediastinal lymph nodes: a postmortem study. Am J Roentgenol 1988;150:771–776.

6 Hata E, Hayakawa K, Miyamoto H, Hayashida R: Rationale for extended lymphadenectomy for lung cancer. Theor Surg 1990;5:19—25.

7 Schirren J, Bergmann T, Beqiri S, Bölükbas S, Fisseler-Eckhoff A, Vogt-Moykopf I. Lymphatic spread in resectable lung cancer: can we trust a sentinel lymph node? Thorac Cardiov Surg 2006; 54:372–380.

8 Little AG, Rusch VW, Bonner JA, Gaspar LE, Green MR, Webb WR, Stewart AK. Patterns of surgical care of lung cancer patients. Ann Thorac Surg 2005;80:2051–2056.

9 Goldstraw P: Report on the International Workshop on Intrathoracic Staging, London, October 1996. Lung Cancer 1997;18:107—111.

10 Lardinois D, De Leyn P, Van Schil P, Rami Porta R, Waller D, Passlick B, Zielinski M, Junker K, Rendina EA, Ris HB, Hasse J, Detterbeck F, Lerut T, Weder W: ESTS guidelines for intraoperative lymph node staging in non-small cell lung cancer. Eur J Cardiothorac Surg 2006;30:787–792.

11 Fadel E, Yildizeli B, Chapelier AR, Dicenta I, Mussot S, Dartevelle PG: Sleeve lobectomy for bronchogenic cancers: factors affecting survival. Ann Thorac Surg 2002;74:851–858; discussion 858–599.

12 Cerfolio RJ, Maniscalco L, Bryant AS: The treatment of patients with stage IIIA non-small cell lung cancer from N2 disease: who returns to the surgical arena and who survives. Ann Thorac Surg 2008;86:912 – 920.

13 Van Schil PE, Brutel de la Riviere A, Knaepen PJ, van Swieten HA, Reher SW, Goosens DJ, Vanderschueren RG, van den Bosch JM: Long-term survival after bronchial sleeve resection: univariate and multivariate analyses. Ann Thorac Surg 1996; 61:1087—1091.

14 Schirren J, Bölükbas S, Bergmann T, Fisseler-Eckhoff A, Trainer S, Beqiri S: Prospective study on perioperative risks and functional results in bronchial and bronchovascular sleeve resections. Thorac Cardiovasc Surg, Feb 2009;57:35–41.

15 Bölükbas S, Beqiri S, Bergmann T, Trainer S, Fisseler-Eckhoff A, Schirren J: Pulmonary resection of non-small cell lung cancer: is survival in the elderly not affected by tumor stage after complete resection? Thorac Cardiovasc Surg 2008;56:476–481.

16 Keller SM, Vangel MG, Wagner H, Schiller JH, Herskovic A, Komaki R, Marks RS, Perry MC, Livingston RB, Johnson DH: Prolonged survival in patients with resected non–small cell lung cancer and single-level N2 disease. J Thorac Cardiovasc Surg 2004;128:130–137.

17 Izbicki JR, Thetter O, Habekost M, Karg O, Passlick B, Kubuschok B, Busch C, Haeussinger K, Knoefel WT, Pantel K, Schweiberer L: Radical systematic lymphadenectomy in non–small cell lung cancer. Br J Surg 1994;81:229–235.

18 Watanabe S, Asamura H, Suzuki K, Tsuchiya R: Recent results of postoperative mortality for surgical resections in lung cancer. Ann Thorac Surg 2004;78:999–1002.

19 Deneffe G, Lacquet LM, Verbeken E, Vermaut G: Surgical treatment of bronchogenic carcinoma: a retrospective study of 720 thoracotomies. Ann Thorac Surg 1988;45:380–383.

20 Dales RE, Belanger R, Shamji FM, Leech J, Crepeau A, Sachs HJ: Quality-of-life following thoracotomy for lung cancer. J Clin Epidemiol 1994; 47:1443–1449.

21 Nou E, Aberg T: Quality of survival in patients with surgically treated bronchial carcinoma. Thorax 1980;35:255–263.

22 Myrdal G, Valtysdottir S, Lambe M, Ståhle E: Quality of life following lung cancer surgery. Thorax 2003;58:194 –197.

23 Handy JR Jr, Asaph JW, Skokan L, Reed CE, Koh S, Brooks G, Douville EC, Tsen AC, Ott GY, Silvestri GA: What happens to patients undergoing lung cancer surgery? Outcomes and quality of life before and after surgery. Chest 2002;122:21–30.

24 Toloza EM, Harpole L, McCrory DC: Noninvasive staging of non-small cell lung cancer: a review of the current evidence. Chest 2003; 123(suppl 1):137S–146S.

25 Toloza EM, Harpole L, Detterbeck F, McCrory DC: Invasive staging of non-small cell lung cancer: a review of the current evidence. Chest 2003; 123(suppl 1):157S–166S.

26 Herth FJF, Rabe F, Gasparini S, Annema JT: Transbronchial and transoesophageal (ultrasound-guided) needle aspirations for the analysis of mediastinal lesions. Eur Respir J 2006;28:1264–1275.

27 Cerfolio RJ, Bryant AS: Is palpation of the nonresected pulmonary lobe(s) required for patients with non-small cell lung cancer? A prospective study. J Thorac Cardiovasc Surg 2008;135:261–268.

28 Veeramachaneni NK, Battafarano RJ, Meyers BF, Zoole JB, Patterson GA: Risk factors for occult nodal metastasis in clinical T1N0 lung cancer: a negative impact on survival. Eur J Cardiothorac Surg 2008;33:466–469.

29 Riquet M, Bagan P, Barthes FLP, Banu E, Scotte F, Foucault C, Dujon A, Danel C: Completely resected non-small cell lung cancer: reconsidering prognostic value and significance of N2 metastases. Ann Thorac Surg 2007;84:1818–1824.

30 Keller SM, Adak S, Wagner H, Johnson DH: Mediastinal lymph node dissection improves survival in patients with stages II and IIIa non-small cell lung cancer. Ann Thorac Surg 2000;70:358–365.

31 Ma K, Chang D, He B, Gong M, Tian F, Hu X, Ji Z, Wang T: Radical systematic mediastinal lymphadenectomy versus mediastinal lymph node sampling in patients with clinical stage IA and pathological stage T1 non-small cell lung cancer. J Cancer Res Clin Oncol 2008;134:1289–1295.

32 Lardinois D, Suter H, Hakki H, Rousson V, Betticher D, Ris HB: Morbidity, survival, and site of recurrence after mediastinal lymph-node dissection versus systematic sampling after complete resection for non-small cell lung cancer. Ann Thorac Surg 2005;80:268–275.

33 Liptay MJ, Fry WA: Complications from induction regimens for thoracic malignancies: perioperative considerations. Chest Surg Clin North Am 1999;9:79–95.

34 Simón C, Moreno N, Peñalver R, González G, Alvarez-Fernández E, González F-Aragoneses Bronchogenic Carcinoma Cooperative Group of the Spanish Society of Pneumology and Thoracic Surgery: The side of pneumonectomy influences long-term survival in stage I and II non-small cell lung cancer. Ann Thorac Surg 2007;84:952–958.

35 Ratto GB, Fabiano F, Rovida S, Baracco F, De Palma M: Survival after incomplete resection or exploratory thoracotomy in patients with advanced non small cell lung cancer. Ital J Surg Sci 1988;18: 377–383.

36 Van Meerbeeck JP, Kramer GWPM, Van Schil PEY, Legrand C, Smit EF, Schramel F, Tjan-Heijnen VC, Biesma B, Debruyne C, van Zandwijk N, Splinter TAW, Giaccone G: Randomized controlled trial of resection versus radiotherapy after induction chemotherapy in stage IIIA-N2 non–small-cell lung cancer. J Natl Cancer Inst 2007; 99:442–450.

37 Betticher DC, Schmitz SH, Tötsch M, Hansen E, Joss C, von Briel C, Schmid RA, Pless M, Habicht J, Roth AD, Spiliopoulos A, Stahel R, Weder W, Stupp R, Egli F, Furrer M, Honegger H, Wernli M, Cerny T, Ris HB: Mediastinal lymph node clearance after docetaxel-cisplatin neoadjuvant chemotherapy is prognostic of survival in patients with stage IIIA pN2 non–small-cell lung cancer: a multicenter phase II trial. J Clin Oncol 2003;21: 1752–1759.

38 Lorent N, De Leyn P, Lievens Y, Verbeken E, Nackaerts K, Dooms C, Van Raemdonck D, Anrys B, Vansteenkiste J, The Leuven Lung Cancer Group: Long-term survival of surgically staged IIIA-N2 non-small-cell lung cancer treated with surgical combined modality approach: analysis of a 7-year prospective experience. Ann Oncol 2004;15:1645–1653.

39 Albain KS, Swann RS, Rusch VW, Turrisi AT, Shepherd FA, Smith CJ, Gandara DR, Johnson DH, Green MR, Miller RC, North American Lung Cancer Intergroup: Phase III study of concurrent chemotherapy and radiotherapy (CT/RT) vs. CT/RT followed by surgical resection for stage IIIA(pN2) non-small cell lung cancer (NSCLC): outcomes update of North American Intergroup 0139 (RTOG 9309). ASCO Meet Abstr 2005;23: 7014.

40 Feinstein AR, Sosin DM, Wells CK: The Will Rogers phenomenon: stage migration and new diagnostic techniques as a source of misleading statistics for survival in cancer. N Engl J Med 1985;312:1604–1608.

41 Schirren J, Schneider P, Richter W, Trainer C, Muley T, Bulzebruck H, Vogt-Moykopf I: Radical surgery and lymph node dissection in bronchial carcinoma. Langenbecks Arch Chir Suppl Kongressbd 1996;113:790–797.

Dr. Joachim Schirren
Department of Thoracic Surgery, Dr. Horst-Schmidt Clinik (HSK)
Ludwig-Erhard-Strasse 100
DE–65199 Wiesbaden (Germany)
Tel. +49 611 433132, Fax +49 611 433135, E-Mail Joachim.Schirren@hsk-wiesbaden.de

Heide J, Schmittel A, Kaiser D, Hinkelbein W (eds): Controversies in the Treatment of Lung Cancer.
Front Radiat Ther Oncol. Basel, Karger, 2010, vol 42, pp 87–93

Radiation Therapy for Early Stage (I/II) Non-Small Cell Lung Cancer

Branislav Jeremic[a] · Francesc Casas[b] · Luhua Wang[c] · Branislav Perin[d]

[a]Division of Human Health (NAHU), Applied Radiobiology and Radiotherapy (ARBR) Section, International Atomic Energy Agency (IAEA), Vienna, Austria; [b]Department of Radiation Oncology, University Clinic, Barcelona, Spain; [c]Chinese Medical Academy of Sciences, Beijing, China; [d]Institute of Lung Disease, Sremska Kamenica, Serbia

Abstract

For patients with early (stage I/II) non-small cell lung cancer (NSCLC) surgery is considered as the standard treatment of choice, although recent data on additional chemotherapy (CHT) showed that it may be beneficial in this setting. There is, however, a subset of patients that never undergo surgery. These patients are considered technically operable, but medically inoperable, due to existing comorbidities. In addition, frequently elderly patients with early NSCLC are denied surgery due to expected peri- and/or postoperative complications. Finally, in recent years there has been an increase in the incidence of patients refusing surgery. For all these patients, radiation therapy (RT) was traditionally considered as the standard treatment option. Data accumulated over the last 5 decades showed that RT alone can produce median survival times of up to >30 months and 5-year survival of up to 30%. When cancer-unrelated deaths were taken into account, cause-specific survival rates were usually higher for some 10–15%. Accumulated experience seems to suggest that doses of at least 65 Gy with standard fractionation or its equivalent when altered fractionation is used are necessary for control of the disease. Smaller tumors seem to have favorable prognosis, while the issue of elective nodal RT continues to be controversial. Patterns of failure have clearly identified local failure as the predominant one. Although a number of potential pretreatment patient- and tumor-related prognostic factors have been examined, none has been shown to clearly influenced survival. Toxicity was usually low.

For patients with early (stage I/II) non-small cell lung cancer (NSCLC) surgery is considered as the standard treatment of choice. Recent data, however, showed that additional chemotherapy (CHT) may be beneficial in this setting. There is, however, a subset of patients that never undergo surgery. These patients are considered technically operable, but medically inoperable, due to existing comorbidities. In addition, frequently elderly patients with early NSCLC are denied surgery due to expected peri- and/or post-operative complications. Finally, in recent years there has been an increase in the incidence of patients refusing surgery. For all these patients, radiation therapy (RT) was traditionally considered as the standard treatment option.

Patients undergoing RT alone for early stage NSCLC mostly constitute negative selection, not just due to their poor general health characteristics and clinical staging, but insufficient staging as well. Results of RT in this population cannot, therefore, be meaningfully compared to those of surgery, even when clinical staging is used in the latter. Other reasons for the observed bias in reporting RT versus surgical series include institutional/investigator bias as well as differences in the process of decision making (patients versus physicians), the latter one materialized in great variance across the studies with the respect to the proportion of patients refusing surgery.

Radiation Therapy alone in Early Non-Small Cell Lung Cancer

Details of studies that unequivocally document the outcome of patients with operable, mostly those of early (I/II) stage NSCLC; characteristics of patients enrolled into these studies, and their outcome are presented in an earlier comprehensive review [1]. With all caveats of focusing on prolonged periods of time (more than 4 decades) that was used to search the literature, nevertheless, the data showed that RT alone was capable of producing a median survival time (MST) of up to >30 months (>40 months in T1N0) since the mid-1980s, with 5-year survival rates of up to 30% in stage I NSCLC (40% in T1N0) and up to 25% in stage II NSCLC.

These results were achieved in a cohort of substantially differing patient populations. The reason for not undergoing surgery was considerably different across the studies, particularly considering patient refusal. While in the majority of studies it was around 10%, in several studies it was >20% [2–5]. Interestingly, the highest MST (up to 33 months) was observed in the latter studies, and it was coupled with the highest 5-year survival rates (up to 32%). These patients represent the population which seems to resemble surgical candidates at most. They should, therefore, be the ones most likely to give true insight in the effectiveness of RT in this disease, because in this patient population, using overall survival (OS) as an endpoint is more meaningful, due to less cancer-unrelated events. In other patient populations, the use of cancer-specific survival (CSS) or disease-specific survivals (DSS) must be mandatory to correct for events other than cancer-related. Indeed, when 5-year CSS/DSS rates were reported [6–11], they were usually twice as high as those of OS in the same studies, the difference being approximately 10–20%. Importantly, patients' refusal inversely correlates with the incidence of intercurrent deaths (6–16%) [2, 4, 5, 7], which, on the other side, directly correlated with increasing age and pre-existing comorbidity (21–43%) [3, 8, 10, 12, 13].

Of various pretreatment and treatment aspects considered in early NSCLC, age and gender [1] seems no to play an important aspects of RT. Only occasionally Karnofsky performance status (KPS) score and/or weight loss were shown to influence survival in RT series [1]. Tumor stage/size was frequently investigated. Although analyses from the accumulated data sometimes favored even lower doses of RT, it would still be preferable to recommend/use the doses traditionally considered as 'curative', being in the order of >65–70 Gy with standard fractionation or its equivalent when altered fractionation is used. Although it is reasonable to expect impact of tumor stage/size on the outcome, it should first exert its influence at local/regional level. By primarily influencing these endpoints, it may eventually influence OS, which was shown to heavily depend on local/regional tumor control in this disease. One of the obstacles of defining the role of tumor stage/size is staging systems widely used in the last 15 years [14, 15]. These surgical systems did not relate only to a tumor size, but also to a particular tumor location It is expected that recent revision of current international staging system should make both T and N staging more specific/detailed and, therefore, easier to interpret/compare in future RT series in early NSCLC. Regarding histology, only Sibley et al. [10] found an improvement in CSS for squamous histology, while Gauden et al. [16] observed so for the mixed (adenocarcinoma/squamous cell carcinoma) histology using both OS and RFS as endpoints, majority of studies, however, observing no such effect [4, 7, 13, 17–20]. Finally, only Hayakawa et al. [18] observed influence of tumor location (better for tumors located in the upper lobes or the superior segment of the lower lobes) on outcome of these patients, all other studies excluding its possible effect when comparing central versus peripheral locations [4, 6, 11, 13, 21].

Besides a recommended dose of an equivalent to 65 Gy with standard fractionation [1], optimal treatment fields are frequently discussed. Owing to somewhat conflicting results, no reliable recommendations can be made concerning elective nodal RT, as recent editorials [22, 23] and comprehensive review [24] recently summarized. There seems to be a subgroup of patients with increased risk of developing nodal metastasis, identification of which must be one of the priorities of research in this field. Contrary to that, it is reasonable to assume that small peripheral, low-grade tumors would be the best candidates for limited RT (omitting elective RT), due to lowest incidence of occult nodal metastasis. However, more information regarding biology of these tumors is needed because identification of potential factors contributing to higher incidence of subclinical regional lymph node metastasis would help optimize RT fields and enable successful dose escalation at the primary tumor level.

An important and unique observation about proliferative potential of early NSCLC was recently brought up by Jeremic at al. [25] who investigated the impact of treatment delays due to high-grade toxicity on the outcome of patients with early stage NSCLC treated with hyperfractionated RT. While patients who refused surgery did not experience high-grade toxicity, 11 of 72 patients with medical inoperability and comorbidity requested treatment interruptions due to high-grade toxicity. Ten of 11 patients had an interruption of ≥14 days. As a result, patients without treatment interruptions had significantly better outcome than those with interruption. Treatment interruption was shown to be an independent prognostic factor of overall survival, local recurrence free survival and cause-specific survivals.

Results achieved with RT alone must be placed into a context of observed toxicity. In majority of studies, it was judged to be rather low, even in studies including elderly patients and incidence of both acute and late high-grade (3 and 4) toxicity was similar among all age groups [16, 26]. When RT-related deaths occurred [27], again there was no difference between elderly (5%) treated with highest dose levels (80 Gy) and their nonelderly counterparts (4%) treated the same way. A substantial problem with all these reports is a great variety of both pretreatment and RT-related factors, such as the total dose, fractionation or treatment fields, inter- and intra-institutionally. While it is a well-established premise for many years that higher total dose, higher dose per fraction and larger volume of the lung irradiated should lead to more toxicity [28–32], both acute and late, it is unknown to what extent other, RT-unrelated factors such as pre-existing comorbidity, infections, or simply natural processes such as sclerosis present in elderly, may add to the occurrence of toxicity [30, 33–35]. Some, however, have observed that concomitant chronic obstructive pulmonary disease did not increase the risk of radiation pneumonitis [35]. Acute high-grade toxicity may also be interesting from the standpoint of treatment interruptions which may adversely influence treatment outcome [36, 37]. Late high-grade toxicity also becomes interesting from the standpoint of prolonged survival of these patients.

Reporting of toxicity poses an additional problem. Only rarely have scoring systems been used and it was almost always done on an actual (crude) basis, and not on the actuarial one. While the former method may be acceptable, although not preferable, for acute toxicity, it should be strongly discouraged as totally inappropriate for late toxicity. It is, therefore, mandatory to have prolonged follow-up in long-term survivors, as we may become able to observe more of these toxicities. In addition, during prolonged follow-up of long-term survivors of early NSCLC treated with RT alone, Jeremic et al. [38] were the first to observe that there is a chance of developing a second cancer. A total of 26 of 194 patients developed second cancers. The cumulative incidence of second cancer was 21.8% (SE 4.7%) at 5 years and 34.8% (SE 6.7%) at 10 years. For second lung cancers, it was 6.0% (SE 2.8%) at 5 years and 14.2% (SE 5.2%) at 10 years, and for second non-lung cancers, it was 16.3% (SE 4.2%) at 5 years and 22.2% (SE, 5.7%) at 10 years. The rate of developing second cancer per patient per year was 4.3% (95% CI 2.7–5.9%), with the rates being 1.4% (CI 0.5–2.3%) for the second lung cancers and 2.8% (CI 1.5–4.1%) for second non-lung cancers. The rate of developing second cancers during the first and second 5-year period after RT (0–5 and 5–10 years) was 4.3% (CI 2.4–6.2%) and 4.2% (CI 0.6 to 7.8%), respectively, for all cancers. These rates were 1.0% (CI 0.1–1.9%) and 2.2% (CI 0–4.6%), respectively, for second lung cancers, and 3.2% (CI 1.6–4.8%) and 1.5% (CI 0–3.6%), respectively, for second non-lung cancers. It was, therefore, shown that the long-term survivors after RT alone for early stage NSCLC carry the same risk of developing second cancer, either lung or non-lung, as their counterparts treated surgically when the results of this study are compared with those of the published literature.

Avenues for an Improvement of RT Alone in Early NSCLC

To improve results obtained with RT alone, many attempts have been undertaken. Besides recent high-tech RT achievements such as IMRT/IGRT, Tomotherapy, CyberKnife, stereotactic RT was implemented with good success; protons and heavy ions as well. Only rarely, patients with early NSCLC were treated with combined radiochemotherapy. In one such attempt, Jeremic et al. [39] investigated the feasibility and activity of concurrent hyperfractionated radiotherapy (Hfx RT) and low-dose daily carboplatin and paclitaxel were investigated in patients with early-stage (I/II) non-small cell lung cancer in a phase II study. Fifty-six patients started their treatment on day 1 with 30 mg/m^2 of paclitaxel. Hfx RT using 1.3 Gy b.i.d. to a total dose of 67.6 Gy and concurrent low-dose daily carboplatin 25 mg/m^2 and paclitaxel 10 mg/m^2, both given Mondays through Fridays during the RT course, starting from the second day. There were 29 complete responses (52%) and 15 partial responses (27%), and 12 patients (21%), experienced stable disease. The median survival time was 35 months, and 3- and 5-year survival rates were 50 and 36%, respectively. The median time to local progression has not been achieved, but 3- and 5-year local progression-free survival rates were 56 and 54%, respectively. The median time to distant metastasis has not been achieved, but 3- and 5-year distant metastasis-free survival rates were 61 and 61%, respectively. The median and 5-year cause-specific survivals were 39 months and 43%, respectively. Acute high-grade (≥3) toxicity was hematological (22%), esophageal (7%), or bronchopulmonary (7%). No grade 5 toxicity was observed. Late high-grade toxicity was rarely observed (total 10%). Hfx RT and concurrent low-dose daily carboplatin/paclitaxel was feasible with low toxicity and effective in patients with stage I/II non-small cell lung cancer. It should continue to be investigated for this disease. What, however, should be clearly emphasized is the patient population which was very favorable. The majority of patients were in a good KPS, none had weight loss of >5 and 70% of patients enrolled into this study actually refused surgery.

Nevertheless, the results achieved showed an improvement over the results traditionally seen in an unselected and, therefore, unfavorable patient population of early NSCLC. They also showed that improvements in treatment outcome should also be sought by identifying subsets of patients within early NSCLC that may benefit from various approaches, a goal for future studies in this setting.

References

1 Jeremic B, Classen J, Bamberg M: Radiation therapy alone in technically operable, medically inoperable early stage (I/II) non-small-cell lung cancer. Int J Radiat Oncol Biol Phys 2002;54:119–130.

2 Zhang HX, Yin WB, Zhang LJ: Curative radiotherapy of early operable non-small cell lung cancer. Radiother Oncol 1989;14:89–94.

3 Morita K, Fuwa N, Suzuki Y: Radical radiotherapy for medically inoperable non-small cell lung cancer in clinical stage I: retrospective analysis of 149 patients. Radiother Oncol 1997;42:31–36.

4 Jeremic B, Shibamoto Y, Acimovic LJ, Milisavljevic S: Hyperfractionated radiotherapy alone for clinical stage I non-small cell lung cancer. Int J Radiat Oncol Biol Phys 1997;38:521–525.

5 Jeremic B, Shibamoto Y, Acimovic LJ, Milisavljevic S: Hyperfractionated radiotherapy for clinical stage II non-small cell lung cancer. Radiother Oncol 1999;51:141–145.

6 Cheung PCF, Mackillop WJ, Dixon P: Involved-field radiotherapy alone for early-stage non-small cell lung cancer. Int J Radiat Oncol Biol Phys 2000;48:703–710.

7 Sandler HM, Curran WJ Jr, Turrisi AT III: The influence of tumor size and pre-treatment staging on outcome following radiation therapy alone for stage I non-small cell lung cancer. Int J Radiat Oncol Biol Phys 1990;19:9–13.

8 Kaskowitz L, Graham MV, Emami B: Radiation therapy alone for stage I non-small cell lung cancer. Int J Radiat Oncol Biol Phys 1993;27:517–523.

9 Krol ADG, Aussems P, Noordijk EM: Local irradiation alone for peripheral stage I lung cancer: could we omit the elective regional nodal irradiation? Int J Radiat Oncol Biol Phys 1996;34:297–302.

10 Sibley GS, Jamieson TA, Marks LB: Radiotherapy alone for medically inoperable stage I non-small cell lung cancer: the Duke experience. Int J Radiat Oncol Biol Phys 1998;40:149–154.

11 Slotman BJ, Karim ABMF: Curative radiotherapy for technically operable stage I nonsmall cell lung cancer. Int JRadiat Oncol Biol Phys 1994;29:33–37.

12 Noordijk EM, van den Poest Clement E, Hermans J: Radiotherapy as an alternative to surgery in elderly patients with respectable lung cancer. Radiother Oncol 1988;13 :83– 89.

13 Slotman BJ, Antonisse IE, Njo KH: Limited field irradiation in early stage (T1–2 N0) non-small cell lung cancer. Radiother Oncol 1996;41:41–44.

14 Mountain CF: A new international staging system for lung cancer. Chest 1986;89:225S–233S.

15 Mountain CF: Revisions in the international system for staging lung cancer. Chest 1997;111:1710–1717.

16 Gauden S, Ramsay J, Tripcony L: The curative treatment by radiotherapy alone of stage I non-small cell carcinoma of the lung. Chest 1995;108: 1278–1282.

17 Dosoretz DE, Katin MJ, Blitzer PH: Radiation therapy in the management of medically inoperable carcinoma of the lung: results and implications for future treatment strategies. Int J Radiat Oncol Biol Phys 1992;25:3–9.

18 Hayakawa K, Mitsuhashi N, Nakajima N: Radiation therapy for stage III epidermoid carcinoma of the lung. Lung Cancer 1992;8:213–224.

19 Rosenthal SA, Curran WJ Jr, Herbert SH: Clinical stage II non-small cell lung cancer treated with radiation therapy alone: the significance of clinically staged ipsilateral hilar adenopathy (N1 disease). Cancer 1992;70:3410–3417.

20 Dosoretz DE, Galmarini D, Rubenstein JH: Local control in medically inoperable lung cancer: an analysis of its importance in outcome and factors determining the probability of tumor eradication. Int J Radiat Oncol Biol Phys 1993;27:507–516.

21 Ono R, Egawa S, Suemasu K: Radiotherapy in inoperable stage I lung cancer. Jpn J Clin Oncol 1991;21:125–128.

22 Jeremic B: Incidental irradiation of nodal regions at risk during limited-field radiotherapy (RT) in dose-escalation studies in non-small cell lung cancer (NSCLC): enough to convert no-elective into elective nodal irradiation (ENI)? Radiother Oncol 2004;71:123–125.
23 Jeremic B: Low incidence of isolated nodal failures after involved field radiation therapy (IFRT) for nonsmall cell lung cancer (NSCLC): blinded by the light? J Clin Oncol 2007;25:5543–5545.
24 Belderbos JSA, Kepka L, Kong FM, Martel MK, Videtic GMM, Jeremic B: Report from the International Atomic Energy Agency (IAEA) consultants' meeting on elective nodal irradiation in lung cancer. Non-Small Cell Lung Cancer (NSCLC). Int J Radiat Oncol Biol Phys 2008;72: 335–342.
25 Jeremic B, Shibamoto Y, Milicic B, Dagovic A, Nikolic N, Aleksandrovic J, Acimovic L, Milisavljevic S: Impact of treatment interruptions due to toxicity on outcome of patients with early stage (I/II) non-small-cell lung cancer (NSCLC) treated with hyperfractionated radiation therapy (Hfx RT) alone. Lung Cancer 2003;40:317–323.
26 Gauden SJ, Tripcony L: The curative treatment by radiation therapy alone of stage I non-small cell lung cancer in a geriatric population. Lung Cancer 2001;32:71–79.
27 Hayakawa K, Mitsuhashi N, Katano S: High-dose radiation therapy for elderly patients with inoperable or unresectable non-small cell lung cancer. Lung Cancer 2001;32:81–88.
28 Holsti LB, Vuorinen P: Radiation reaction in the lung after continuous and split-course megavoltage radiotherapy of bronchial carcinoma. Br J Radiol 1967;40:280–284.
29 Moss WT, Haddy FJ, Sweany SK: Some factors altering the severity of acute radiation pneumonitis: variation with cortisone, heparin, and antibiotics. Radiology 1960;75:50–54.
30 Rubin P, Casarett GW: Clinical Radiation Pathology. Philadelphia, Saunders, 1968, pp 423–470.
31 Mah K, Van Dyk J, Keane T: Acute radiation-induced pulmonary damage: a clinical study on the response to fractionated radiation therapy. Int J Radiat Oncol Biol Phys 1987;13:179–188.
32 McDonald S, Rubin P, Phillips TL: Injury to the lung from cancer therapy: clinical syndromes, measurable endpoints, and potential scoring systems. Int J Radiat Oncol Biol Phys 1995;31:1187–1203.
33 Braun SR, doPoco GA, Olson CE: Low-dose radiation pneumonitis. Cancer 1975;35:1322–1324.
34 Prasad SC: Relation between tolerance dose and treatment field size in radiation therapy. Med Phys 1978;5:430–433.
35 Garipagaoglu M, Munley MT, Hollis D: The effect of patient specific factors on radiation induced regional lung injury. Int J Radiat Oncol Biol Phys 1999;45:3331–3338.
36 Cox JD, Pajak TF, Asbell S: Interruptions of high-dose radiation therapy decrease long-term survival of favourable patients with unresectable non-small cell carcinoma of the lung: analysis of 1,244 cases from 3 Radiation Therapy Oncology Group (RTOG) trials. Int J Radiat Oncol Biol Phys 1993;27:493–498.
37 Chen M, Jiang G-L, Fu X-L: The impact of overall treatment time on outcomes in radiation therapy for nonsmall cell lung cancer. Lung Cancer 2000; 28:11–19.
38 Jeremic B, Shibamoto Y, Acimovic L, Nikolic N, Dagovic A, Aleksandrovic J, Radosavljevic-Asic G: Second cancers occurring in patients with early stage non-small cell lung cancer treated with chest radiation therapy alone. J Clin Oncol 2001; 19:1056–1063.
39 Jeremic B, Milicic B , Acimovic L, Milisavljevic S: Concurrent hyperfractionated radiotherapy and low-dose daily carboplatin/paclitaxel in patients with early stage (I/II) non-small cell lung cancer (NSCLC). Long -term results of a phase II study. J Clin Oncol 2005;23:6873–6880.

Branislav Jeremic, MD, PhD
Institute of Lung Disease
Institutski put 4
RS–21204 Sremska Kamenica (Serbia)
Tel. +381 65 4146663, E-Mail nebareje@gmail.com

Heide J, Schmittel A, Kaiser D, Hinkelbein W (eds): Controversies in the Treatment of Lung Cancer.
Front Radiat Ther Oncol. Basel, Karger, 2010, vol 42, pp 94–114

Stereotactic Body Radiation Therapy for Early Non-Small Cell Lung Cancer

Frank Zimmermann[b] · Jörn Wulf[a] · Ingmar Lax[d] · Yasushi Nagata[e] · Robert D. Timmerman[f] · Igor Stojkovski[c] · Branislav Jeremic[c]

[a]Institute of Radiation Oncology, Lindenhofspital, Bern, and [b]Department of Radiation Oncology, University Hospital, University Basel, Basel, Switzerland; [c]International Atomic Energy Agency (IAEA), Vienna, Austria; [d]Division of Oncology and Hospital Physics, Radiumhemmet, Karolinska University Hospital, Stockholm, Sweden; [e]Department of Radiation Oncology, Hiroshima University Hospital, Hiroshima, Japan; [f]Department of Radiation Oncology, The University of Texas Southwestern Medical Center, Dallas, Tex., USA

Abstract

For patients with early stage non-small cell lung cancer (NSCLC) unsuitable for resection local high-dose radiotherapy is the treatment of choice. In modern series even with escalated conformal radiotherapy local control rates of about 55% remain disappointing. Within the last years, stereotactic radiotherapy has been shown an effective treatment approach for early stage malignant lung tumors, combining the accurate focal dose delivery by stereotactic techniques with the biological advantages of dose escalated hypofractionated radiotherapy. Typical treatment regimens include three to five fractions over 1–2 weeks or 1 single fraction as radiosurgery. With adequate staging procedures including FDG-PET-CT scan and a low probability of subclinical involvement of unsuspicious locoregional lymph nodes, the concept is to irradiate the primary T1/2 tumor alone. Recent data report local control rates of up to 90%, with favorable results especially for patients in good general condition. Less than 10% of all patients develop isolated tumor recurrences in regional lymph nodes. Three-year survival is significantly improved to more than 80% when biological effective doses of more than 100 Gy are applied to patients in good conditions. Systemic tumor recurrence still is a major problem, making an additional systemic chemotherapy interesting for selected patients after hSRT, such as those younger than 75 years.

Cancer is one of the major health concerns worldwide. The burden of cancer is increasing globally, with an expected 20 million new cases per year in 2020, half of which will be in low and middle income countries [1].

In stage I non-small cell lung cancer (NSCLC) standard treatment is still surgery, in younger patients sometimes followed by systemic chemotherapy [2, 3]. At 3 years, mean overall survival rates of about 70% in stage IA and of less than 50% in stage IB were published [4–6]. Local tumor control is about 90% and depends on the type of resection. Lobectomy and pneumonectomy are superior to atypical resection [5]. It is reported that the worse outcome with atypical resection is not only influenced by an increased local failure rate but mainly by perioperative morbidity and mortality. For these patients in early NSCLC stages with pre-existing comorbidity, advanced age or refusal of operation, definitive local high dose radiotherapy alone may be the standard treatment option. Unfortunately, with conventionally fractionated and even moderately accelerated or hyperfractionated schedules, the results are still less favorable than those obtained with surgery alone. The reported 5-year survival rates are as low as 18% (5–42%), but it became obvious that the highest doses achieved a better local control than the standard 60 Gy in 30 fractions commonly used in practice. Furthermore, local failures continue to occur even at the highest dose levels, possibly owing to the very protracted overall treatment times [7–10].

Among many technologically advanced treatments that new informatic technologies brought to the field of radiation oncology, such as the use of sophisticated treatment planning systems and radiation therapy using three-dimensional software programs, stereotactic radiotherapy has been increasingly used in recent years [11, 12]. Combining the accurate focal dose delivery of stereotactic radiotherapy with the biological advantages of hypofractionated radiotherapy has been shown to be an effective treatment approach for both malignant and nonmalignant brain tumors. High biologically effective radiation doses are generally of advantage with regard to tumor cell kill and local tumor control. Patients with clinically T1–2 N0 tumors seem to be the ideal candidates for investigation of these new technologies of SBRT [11, 13–16]. This paper summarizes the current technique of SBRT and recent clinical data on local tumor control, overall survival and early and late toxicity of SBRT in early NSCLC.

Definitions of Stereotactic Body Radiation Therapy

SBRT evolved from the clinical experience of intracranial stereotactic radiosurgery and the technical development of radiotherapy in general. Today, SBRT is an accepted acronym for Stereotactic Body Radiation Therapy, which previously commonly was called extracranial stereotactic radiotherapy. The following essential components are collectively unique to SBRT [17–19]:

- The use of a well-defined reference system for localization of the target and for set-up at the accelerator. The reference (stereotactic) system is a 3D coordinate system as referenced to fiducials, which are 'markers' whose position can be confidently correlated both to the target and the treatment delivery device. A stereotactic treatment is one directed by such fiducial references.

- Direct geometrical verification of the target position in the reference system, as opposed to verification of surrogate markers in conventional radiotherapy.
- Secure immobilization and repositioning of the patient, as well as proper accounting for the internal organ motion.
- Small margins to PTV.
- Spatial dose distribution very conformal to and commonly intentionally heterogeneous within the PTV with a very rapid fall off to surrounding normal tissues.
- Treatment of solid tumors.
- Prescription of biologically very potent target doses, with a few fractions of very high dose delivered in a short time.

SBRT is thus used to treat well-demarcated visible gross tumors. It is not intended for prophylactic (adjuvant) treatment, independent of the technique used for SBRT (Linac, Protons, Cyberknife e.o.).

Different reference systems defined by fiducials in use in SBRT exist (fig. 1). The reference system relates both to the target (CTV) and to the treatment unit. *Set-up* is the alignment of the reference system used, to the coordinate system of the accelerator, according to what is determined during the dose planning, and the set-up margin is the margin used for the set-up error [20]. Characteristic for SBRT is a small set-up error, usually of less than 5 mm. To account for variations in position, shape and size of the CTV in the reference system used, a margin is added, an internal margin [20]. *PTV* is a geometrical concept used in treatment planning to ensure that the prescribed dose is delivered to the CTV, and includes both the set-up margin and an internal margin [20]. *Geometrical verification* aims at making confident that the volume of the CTV will be within the PTV during the treatment. This can be optimized by image guidance within the treatment room (IGRT) with conventional X-ray, CT scan or cone-beam CT as well, which is not necessarily obligat for SBRT. With a small set-up error (within 1 mm), the geometrical verification will be essential to make it confident that the volume of the CTV will be within PTV in the reference system used.

In some SBRT methods, set-up and geometrical verification are two separate steps in the process. However, when reference systems defined by tumor fiducials are used (for example, gold markers in the tumor and projection imaging or the tumor itself and cone-beam CT) the two steps are generally integrated to a single procedure, as the set-up also includes an on-line correction as a result of the geometrical verification.

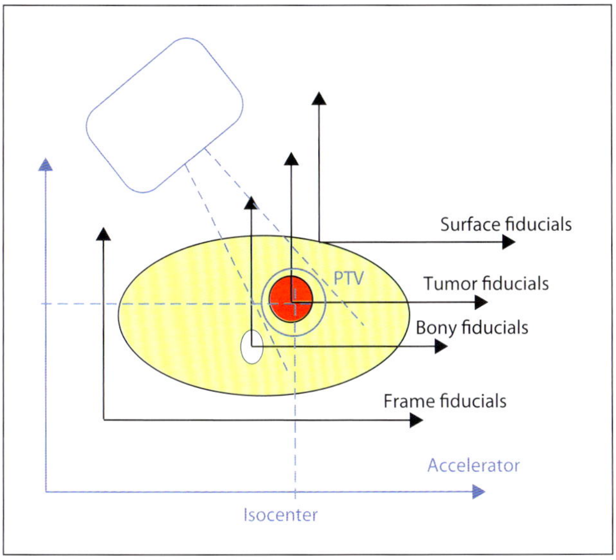

Fig. 1. Different reference systems defined by fiducials used in SBRT.

Staging Procedures before SBRT

Accurate clinical staging is critical in the evaluation of any patient with NSCLC. The clinical stage as determined by all available clinical, radiographic, and biopsy data, has to be performed as accurately and comprehensively as possible. Newer technologies such as autofluorescence bronchoscopy, narrow banding imaging, endoscopic ultrasound, endobronchial ultrasound and electromagnetic navigation are used to define the local tumor extension [21].

Mediastinoscopy remains the gold standard for regional nodal staging. Due to the fact that most patients presented for SBRT were not amenable for operative staging procedures due to poor functional status of lung and/or heart, CT scans have been used in principle to define both local and regional tumor extension. Invasive procedures can be omitted in patients with peripheral tumors and negative mediastinal positron emission tomography images [22]. Based on recent knowledge on the superiority of FDG-PET scan to CT scanning alone, with a 91% sensitivity and a 86% specificity for mediastinal staging and a negative predictive value of about 98%, nowadays, FDG-PET-CT scan is recommended in general [22, 23].

In SBRT, the concept to irradiate the primary tumor (T1 or T2) alone is based on the well-known observation that in these early T stages the probability of involvement of locoregional lymph nodes after adequate staging procedures, including a negative FDG-PET-CT scan for regional lymph nodes, is comparatively low, usually below 10% [24]. In all modern series, FDG-PET-CT is applied as the basic staging procedure and for radiation treatment planning to define target volume, especially in tumors causing subsequent atelectasis.

Unfortunately, data sets on overall survival with a longer follow-up after initial staging with FDG-PET-CT are still limited. In centrally located, undifferentiated carcinoma, MRI of the brain may be added to ascertain the staging of the brain [25, 26].

Implementation of Techniques in Clinical Routine

The clinical issue of SBRT is high local tumor control with low acute and late toxicity. Both goals are achieved by very high fraction doses applied to a small volume. Because the CTV is given, volume reduction can only be achieved by increased precision of treatment, which covers both – setup accuracy and target mobility. For this purpose two strategies are available: a frame-based stereotactic approach (external fiducials) and a frameless procedure, usually with internal markers (i.e. implanted in the tumor by CT punction or endoscopic techniques). In the latter, imaging is used for guidance, and in the previous situation, IGRT can be used additionally but is not needed in principle.

In both situations, patient fixation is required using a stereotactic body frame (SBF; ELEKTA, Inc.), BodyFix (Medical Intelligence/ELEKTA, Inc.) or comparable devices [13, 17, 27, 28]. In all devices, the patient is fixed by a tight vacuum pillow, which again can be related to an external (stereotactic) reference system. Breathing mobility can be easily decreased mechanically by abdominal pressure or – more advanced – controlled by gating techniques such as the active breathing control (ABC; ELEKTA, Inc.) or real-time positioning management (PRM, Varian, Inc.). Oxygen-assisted shallow breathing or JET ventilation are also in use, but its value is not yet proven.

In all scenarios setup accuracy and breathing mobility of the target have to be assessed for treatment planning and prior to irradiation. This can be performed by the use of fluoroscopy (if the target can be seen or is strongly related to bony structures) or by CT (if the target cannot be identified by conventional X-ray equipment). Recent advances in technology allow target verification and assessment of breathing mobility directly on the treatment couch using cone-beam CT. With the use of cone-beam CT prior to treatment stereotactic coordinates can be abandoned, because the isocenter position can be directly assigned to the appropriate position (image-guided radiotherapy).

Treatment planning is usually based on CT data. Further imaging modalities such as MRI or FDG-PET can be included, too. The scanned volume should not only cover the target but also the complete organs at risk, e.g. the lung and heart for pulmonary tumors. If non-coplanar irradiation techniques might be used, this should be regarded when determining the scanned volume. While slice thickness obviously depends on the size of the tumor, under normal conditions 3–5 mm will be appropriate in the majority of cases. Intravenous contrast will be helpful in central lung tumors. Prior to definite scanning potential breathing mobility has to be evaluated. Depending on the method used to decrease breathing mobility the amount of motion should be analyzed (it has to be regarded to determine appropriate margins for PTV definition). This can either be done by multislice CT, dynamic scans (repeated scans at the same couch position) or evaluation of the target position in maximum in- and expiration. While this approach is based on slices, which show the scanned tumor position in a very short (<1 s) period of time resulting in a 'sharp' image, the target also can be scanned by a slow CT. With this technique the tumor is scanned very slowly (e.g. scan time for a slice 3 s). The image shows a 'blurred' shape of the target including and depending on internal motion (ITV) [29], which represents the 'orbit' the target is moving in. This technique might have advantages especially when a cone-beam CT is used for target verification prior to irradiation, because due to the slow scan time (about 1 min) the shape of the target will also appear 'blurred' [30].

Ideally, both GTV and CTV should be geometrically defined in an unambiguous way in the reference system used. In clinical practice, however, there will always be more or less breathing motions during imaging (even with gating there will be a residual motion) as well as differences in tumor position during imaging and treatment. ICRU 62 [20] defines an internal margin (IM) and an internal target volume (ITV) for the physiologic movements and variations of the CTV during therapy (fig. 1). One way to get an estimate of the IM is to do the imaging during several breathing cycles (cf. Imaging for planning above). In clinical practice of SBRT, ITV is relatively seldom defined explicit, but PTV is usually drawn with standard margins to a CTV which has been defined by normal dose-planning imaging (table 1). Current clinical experience is basically based on this way of target definitions. The standard margins are determined from geometrical verification imaging of patient cohorts and basically only valid for the use of a particular set of conditions like methods for patient fixation, breathing reduction as well as choice of reference system and method for set-up and geometrical verification. However, due to similar geometrical requirement using different methodology for SBRT there is today a relatively narrow range of margins between CTV and PTV used in clinical practice. With the immobilization equipment and methods for reduction of the target motion described in this report, the longitudinal margin is generally 10 mm. In the transverse plane, margins are usually of the order of 5 mm up to 10 mm (table 1) [15, 30–40]. Even though the margins reported are relatively

Table 1. Margins for definition of planning target volume used in different recent trials of SBRT in early NSCLC

First author (year)	Margin trans mm	Margin long mm	Comment	Method for breathing reduction
Timmerman (2006) [19]	5	10		different methods
Baumann (2006) [31]	5, 10	10		Abd. Comp
Zimmermann (2006) [32]	individual	individual		Abd. Comp
Joyner (2006) [74]	5	10		
Okunieff (2006) [35]	7	10		Resp gating
Hoyer (2006) [34]	min 5	10	later ind. marg.	Abd. Comp
Wulf (2005) [33]	5	5, 10		Abd. Comp
Wurm (2006) [36]	5	5		adaptive gating
Hodge (2006) [37]	6	6	Marg. to ITV	Abd. Comp
Guckenberger (2007) [30]	5	5	Marg. to ITV	Abd. Comp
Nuyttens (2006) [38]	5	5		tracking
Nagata (2005) [39]	5	8–10	Marg. to ITV	Abd. Comp
Onishi (2007) [15]	0–5	0–5	Marg. to ITV	different methods
Hata (2007) [40]	5	5–10	Marg. to ITV	different methods

similar, it is important that the margins used should be based on experience from the particular methodology used at each center.

Treatment planning in SBRT is done on commercial treatment planning systems (TPS) used also for radiotherapy planning in general. Pencil beam algorithms have a limited accuracy, but acceptable to use [41]. Point kernel-based superposition/convolution algorithms give a more accurate estimate of the dose to the tumor and surrounding lung tissue [41]. The error in the dose calculation for tumors in the lungs is reduced if the photon energy is restricted to a maximum of 6 MV. Comparing different publications, these effects should be taken into account.

There are two different concepts of treatment planning for SBRT. One concept is to maintain dose homogeneity within the target derived from conventional radiotherapy. In this case, the homogeneity index (HI) is an important index and the dose is usually prescribed at the isocenter. The other concept is not to maintain

Table 2. Dose-volume constraints of various organs at risk, used in RTOG trial 0618 treating operable patients with early stage primary NSCLC

Organ	Volume	Dose, cGy
Spinal cord	any point	18 Gy (6 Gy per fraction)
Esophagus	any point	27 Gy (9 Gy per fraction)
Ipsilateral brachial plexus	any point	24 Gy (8 Gy per fraction)
Heart/Pericardium	any point	30 Gy (10 Gy per fraction)
Trachea and ipsilateral bronchus	any point	30 Gy (10 Gy per fraction)
Whole lung (right and left)	V-20	less than 5–10% of total lung volume
Skin	any point	24 Gy (8 Gy per fraction)

dose homogeneity derived from cranial stereotactic radiotherapy. In this case, the conformity index (CI) is an important index and the dose is prescribed at the PTV margin. To avoid serious complications, the most important issue for RTP of SBRT is to maintain the dose constraints of OAR, including the spinal cord, pulmonary artery, bronchus, and heart (table 2).

Biological Basis of Hypofractionated SBRT

Different to normofractionated radiotherapy, the biological purpose of stereotactic irradiation is lethal rather than sublethal cell damage in the high dose area without repair. Additionally due to short overall treatment time (single dose, hypofractionation within 1–3 weeks) avoidance of repopulation of tumor cells is another advantage. On the other hand the prescription of the amount of dose has to respect that re-oxygenation and re-distribution of cells in the cell cycle will not occur. Organs at risk are prevented from serious damage by sparing these tissues from high dose area. This is in accordance to the practice in intracranial stereotactic radiotherapy. The optimal amount of dose required to achieve local tumor control and the tolerance doses for normal tissue are a subject of evaluation [11, 16].

Besides dose escalation trials [13, 42, 43], a lot of prospective institutional-based reports on clinical results of SBRT have been published. Unfortunately, comparison of these results is difficult, because different dose fractionation schedules have been used and normalization and prescription of dose (PTV-enclosing isodose vs. isocenter, homogeneous vs. inhomogeneous dose distribution) is also very nonuniform. To overcome this problem, some authors used the biological effective dose (BED) based on the formula: BED (Gy) = dose/fraction × fraction number (1 + fraction dose/α/β) using an alpha/beta of 10 Gy for tumor tissue. Analyzing their data they found a BED of about 100 Gy to be appropriate to achieve a TCP of about 90% for lung tumors [15, 33]. Nevertheless, this approach can be criticized, because it is not proven that the LQ model will be reliable at such high fraction doses. Therefore eventually other radiobiological models might be better to predict the effect of ESRT including modifications of the multitarget model [44].

Historical Aspects and Early Clinical Experience in SBRT of Lung Cancer

The clinical experience from intracranial stereotactic radiosurgery introduced in the middle of the 20th century, together with the technical development in conventional radiotherapy, initiated the development of stereotactic radiotherapy with very high dose per fraction, delivered in a short time to targets in the body. This started at Karolinska University hospital, Sweden in 1991 with tumors in the liver and lungs [17]. In parallel, the method was developed in Japan and clinically introduced in 1994 for lung tumors [45]. During the last 5 years of the 1990s, SBRT was introduced at several centers in Europe, Japan and USA [28, 42, 46, 47]. Early reports already showed very promising results both with regard to local control and toxicity for the hypofractionation schedules adopted with 10–15 Gy/fraction given in a few fractions during a short time [27, 45]. However, due to the new aspects introduced in SBRT, clinical experience was gathered at a very slow rate at the beginning and it was not until the end of the 1990s and the first years of the 21st century that outcome data from several centers were at hand to confirm the initial promising results.

Clinical Experience

Considerable investigation of SBRT to treat both primary and metastatic cancers of the lungs has been carried out around the world. With the high prevalence of such tumors, the high rates of cancer-associated deaths, and the desire for more effective treatments, it is no wonder that lung tumors have been the most common site of SBRT treatment. In addition, the large volume and inherent functional redundancy of pulmonary tissue has allowed stereotactic treatments to be carried out effectively and with acceptable toxicity for many tumor presentations especially in the periphery of the lung.

So far, the experience in treating primary lung cancer using SBRT has mostly occurred in patients who were unfit for surgical resection (medically inoperable patients). Furthermore, nearly all reports describe outcomes in patients with stage I disease, particularly for peripheral tumor locations. As medically inoperable

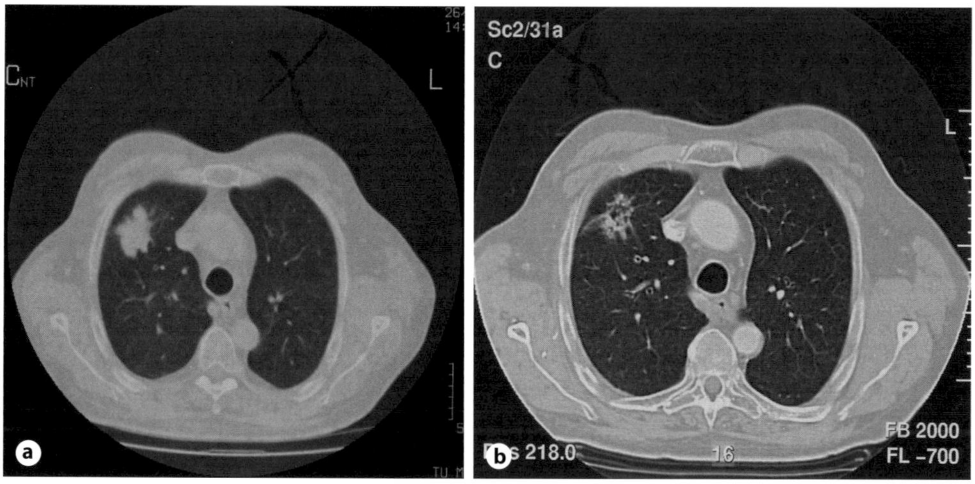

Fig. 2. NSCLC of the right upper lobe. T1 tumor. Before SBRT. 18 months after SBRT with 3 × 12.5 Gy (calculated on the 60%-isodose). Local lung fibrosis. Complete remission.

patients are at risk of dying from more causes than just their lung cancer, survival in these patients is ultimately compromised. On the other hand, initial data report on local control rates of up to 90%, with favorable results especially for patients in good general condition [15], asking for a further spread of this technique to new indications.

Local Tumor Response

Still the benefits of SBRT can be quantified by assessing local control (especially if reported as an actuarial rate). Numerous reports show dramatically improved rates of local control compared to results published using conventional radiotherapy methods and schedules. Historically, local control at 2 years from radiation treatment was only 30–45% with conventional schedules, yet with SBRT rates of 70–98% are reported in numerous phase II institutional protocols [15, 18, 27, 31, 32, 40, 42, 47–68] (fig. 2; table 3).

Unfortunately, a broad spectrum of fractionation schedules with different dose prescription resulting in various biologically effective doses have been used (tables 3, 4). The number of fractions have been 1 to more than 10, and the size of fractions 5–30 Gy at the PTV-surrounding isodose.

From the first clinical trials starting in the 1990s, local control rates of primary lung cancer with SBRT have been reported by to be 94% (47/50) for 50–60 Gy in 5 fractions with a median follow-up of 36 months [51], and 92% (22/24) for 60 Gy

Table 3. Local tumor control rates from different recent trials of SBRT in early NSCLC

First author (year)	Number of patients	Fraction	Total dose	Isodose	LC	CSS	OS	Comment
Ng (2008) [59]	20	3–4	45–54	85–90	94.7	77.6	73.3	
Salazar (2008) [62]	60	1–6	40	76	98	87	74	
						82	62	3 years data
Takeda (2009) [63]	63	5	50	80	95	92	79	
	38				93	100	90	3 years stage IA
	25				96	81	63	3 years stage IB
Onishi (2007) [15]	257	1–14	30–84	100	76.2	73.2	47.2	5 years data
Onimaru (2008) [60]	41	4	32–38.4	80	73	73	64	no consequent margins
Guckenberger (2007) [30]	38	1–8	26–56	65–80	89	n.g.	n.g.	
					83	59	37	3 years data
Timmerman (2007) [57]	70	3	60–66	80	95	n.g.	56	
Brown (2007) [64]	57	1–5	15–67.5	57–81	<75	~90	84	1.5 years data, indirect calculation
Fritz (2008) [58]	40	1	24	80	94	71	66	
					81	57	53	3 years data
Hof (2007) [47]	42	1	15.2–24	80	67.9	n.g.	65.4	
Baumann (2006) [31]	57	3	45	67	96	n.g.	n.g.	
Uematsu (2001) [51]	50	5–10	50–60	80	94	88	66	3 years data; 36% combined with CRT
Zimmermann (2006) [32]	68	3–5	24–40	60	88	82	71	
					88	73	53	3 years data
Wulf (2005) [33]	20	1–3	45–56.2	80	92	n.g.	32	
Nagata (2005) [39]	45	3	38.4	80	98	n.g.	83	stage IA
							72	stage IB
Hata (2007) [40]	21	10	50–60	90	96	86	74	proton therapy
Beitler (2006) [14]	75	5–40	30–90	70–95	n.g.	n.g.	45	some patients with prior chemotherapy

TD = Total dose, LC = local control, CSS = cause-specific survival, OS = overall survival. Isodose = PTV-encompassing isodose. n.g. = Not given.
All data are at 2 years of follow-up when not stated differently.

in 8 fractions with a median follow-up of 24 months [49]. This has prompted the initial investigation of using SBRT in operable patients [15]. In a multicentric approach, it could be demonstrated that patients in good condition have an even higher benefit than patients with severe comorbidity.

Within the following years, SBRT became more popular in areas besides the northern European countries and Japan. In all those clinical trials, the major focus was on local control. The authors report values of about 90%: 87% (30/37) for 60 Gy in 3 fractions with a median follow-up of 15 months [42], 85% for 48–60 Gy in 8 fractions with a median follow-up of 17 months [52], 95% for 45–56.2 Gy in 3 fractions with a median follow-up of 10 months [53], 90% for 30–40 Gy in 4 fractions with a median follow-up of 21 months [65], and 97% (44/45) for 48 Gy in 4 fractions with a median follow-up of 22–30 months [39]. In the most recent trials, with even higher BED of more than 150 Gy (with an α/β-relation of 3), local control reaches up to 98% [66, 63] (table 3).

A few publications exist on single fraction SBRT (radiosurgery), with doses between 15 and 40 Gy. Only two trials from Germany document the feasibility of this approach, whereas the other trials [64, 67, 68] lack both a good quality and long-term follow-up. In the trials from Hof et al. [47] and Fritz et al. [58], local control is at a similar level as with hypofractionated SBRT at 2 years when at least 26 Gy have been applied, but decreasing to 67.9 and 81% at 3 years. A comparison of the BED of all available concepts explains the difference, and is demanding for further dose escalation trials especially in radiosurgery.

However, the definition of local control after radiotherapy is difficult independent of the fractionation schedule, because local tumor failure and radiation-induced lung damage (RILD) cannot be clearly delineated. A so-called mass-like shadow which cannot be delineated from residual tumor has been reported by several authors [69–71]. To optimize follow-up, FDG-PET-CT scan may be introduced, but conclusive data are still lacking (fig. 3).

Even though the definition of local control is different between each trial, a BED larger than 100 Gy may be effective for SBRT of solitary lung cancer with a local control rate of more than 85% [15]. We recommend calculations for the PTV-including isodose, especially for calculation models using a dose prescription to less than the 80%-surrounding isodose.

Survival Data

The survival rates of stage IA (T1N0M0) and stage IB (T2N0M0) lung cancer have not been reported separately by several authors. In a series of stage IA cancer, the 1- and 5-year local relapse-free survival rates were 100 and 95%. The disease-free survival rates after 1, 3 and 5 years were 80, 72 and 72%, respectively, and the

Table 4. Side effects from different recent trials of SBRT in early NSCLC

First author (year)	BED	2 Gy equivalent dose	Lung toxicity >II° %	Pneumonitis I–II° %	Other toxicity
Ng (2008) [59]	270–297	162–178.2	0	n.g.	3 rib fractures
Takeda (2009) [63]	216.7	130	5	3	
Onishi (2007) [15]	252–330	151.2–198	5.4	5.5	0.8% esophagitis, 1.6% rib fracture
Onimaru (2008) [60]	117–161.3	70.4–96.8	~10		1 pleural effusion
Guckenberger (2007) [30]	186.7–251.3	112–150.8	0.6	12; >50% in CT scan	2 pneumothorax, 16% pleural effusion, 1 esophageal ulceration
Timmerman (2007) [57]	460–550	276–330	n.g.	n.g.	In total toxicity >II: peripheral tumors:17; central tumors:46
Brown (2007) [64]	90–371.3	54–222.8	~2	~5	3 esophagitis, 5 pneumothorax by fiducial implantation
Fritz (2008) [58]	216	129.6	0	75 (only on CT scan)	25% pleural effusion, 3 rib fractures
Hof (2007) [47]	92.2–216	55.3–129.6	0	64 (mostly on CT scan only)	
Baumann (2006) [31]	270	162	~5	16	21% toxicity III° in total, 2 pain, 1 rib fracture, 13 pleural effusion
Uematsu (2001) [51]	327.8–460	196.7–276	0	only on CT scan in most patients	
Zimmermann (2006) [32]	72–193.7	43.2–116.2	6.4	39.1 with symptoms	3.4% pleural effusion, 5.0% rib fractures
Wulf (2005) [33]	270–407	162–244.2	0	6	13% mild pain, fever, chills
Hata (2007) [40]	13–180	79.8–108	0	only in CT scan in most patients	3 mild hematologic, 2 chest wall pain
Salazar (2008) [62]	150.8–173.3	90.5–104	0	6	2 esophagitis, 1 pleural effusion

mBED = minimal biological effective dose (α/β = 3) in the PTV.

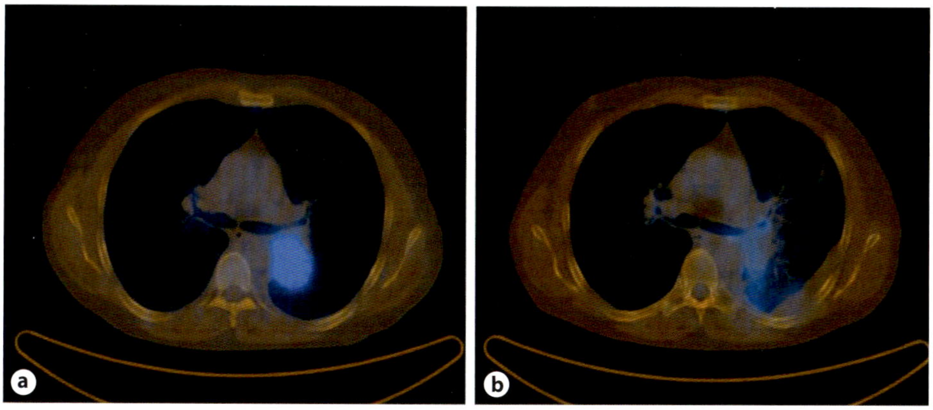

Fig. 3. NSCLC of the left lower lobe. T2/N1 tumor. FDG-PET-CT scan. **a** Before SBRT. **b** 12 months after SBRT with 5 × 7.0 Gy (calculated on the 60% isodose). Local lung fibrosis. Complete remission. SUV in PET scan <2. Courtesy of Institute of Nuclear Medicine, MRI, Munich.

overall survival rates were 93, 83 and 83%, respectively. In stage IB cancer, the local relapse-free survival rates were 100%. The disease-free survival after 1, 3 and 5 years were 92, 71 and 71%, respectively, and the overall survival rates were 82, 72 and 72%, respectively [39]. Onishi et al. [15] recently reported the results for 13 institutions in Japan, which summarized 245 patients: 155 with stage IA lung cancer and 90 with stage IB lung cancer. There were 87 operable and 158 inoperable patients, and their results showed that the intercurrent death rate was especially high in the inoperable patient group. Moreover, the 5-year survival rates of operable patients irradiated with more than BED = 100 Gy was 70.8% for the whole group, with 72.3% for stage IA and 65.9% for stage IB, and their clinical results were as good as those for surgery [15] (table 3).

These survival rates should be compared with the results of surgery; however, the results of SBRT may differ depending on how many patients of each groups are operable and inoperable, and how many of them have central and peripheral tumors. Additionally, the clinical staging is still less precise than the intraoperative one, mainly due to the detection of subclinical tumor spread around the primary and the higher detection rate of subclinical lymph node metastases by resection of N1 and N2 sites.

Side Effects

The great concern of pulmonary toxicity with this SBRT treatment was relieved by the very low rates of complications in early studies. Compared to conventional radiotherapy, lung toxicity occurs relatively late after SBRT (e.g. 9–12 months or more). The most serious toxicity after SBRT for lung tumors is predominantly related to the bronchi and bronchioles located in the vicinity of the treated tumor. Frequently, dramatic imaging changes can be seen on CT scans consisting of in-field and downstream consolidation and fibrosis. Nevertheless, symptomatic radiation pneumonitis which consists of inflammation and fluid extravasation within the terminal bronchioles and alveoli is seen less frequently after SBRT than with conventional radiotherapy. Drop in oxygen exchange parameters, including diffusing capacity and arterial oxygen tension can be seen soon after treatment, but are scarce. Most pulmonary complications are less than NCI-CTC version 2.0 grade 2 (table 4).

The effects of a hypofractionated dose on the main bronchus, pulmonary artery, heart and esophagus have not been followed up for a sufficiently long time. However, a few serious complications have recently been reported by several institutions in Japan [72]. These complications include grade 5 pulmonary complications, radiation pneumonitis, hemoptysis and radiation esophagitis. Lethal pulmonary bleeding and esophageal ulcer have been previously reported by several authors. Timmerman [43] recently reported a series of complications with SBRT. Most cases of grade 5 radiation pneumonitis were accompanied by interstitial pneumonitis. Cases of interstitial pneumonitis should be carefully considered. Thoracocutaneous fistula was reported in a patient with previous tuberculosis history. Acute cholecystis was reported in a patient with gallstones who had been pressed with an abdominal press board at the time of SBRT. Finally, it is not uncommon for patients to experience chest wall pain months after SBRT, especially if treating tumors adjacent to the pleura, as a sign of intercostal neuralgia. Some, but not all, of these patients will have pleural effusions associated with chest wall pain. The problem seems to be mostly self-limited and conservative management with over-the-counter analgesics or anti-inflammatory medicines is typically effective. Some of those patients later develop rib fractures, which should be strongly separated from local tumor progression, either by FDG-PET scan or biopsy. When the esophagus, trachea or main bronchus are near the target, there is a higher risk of early dysphagia, severe cough, and late strictures [43, 73]. Therefore, central hilar tumors adjacent to mediastinal organs should be carefully considered for SBRT, or only treated with lower single fraction doses [32, 74] (table 4).

Comparison of SBRT with Surgical Data

Less than 25% of all patients diagnosed with lung cancer will present with early stage disease (less than 10% in stage I). These patients have the greatest hope for cure following standard procedure of resection. Survival varies, with reports on

5-year overall survival of 36–84% for pathologically proven stage IA and IB diseases [5]. Mean values on overall survival at 5 years of 67% for postoperative pathological stage IA and of 57% in stage IB are reported, with a difference of 8–38% between stage IA and IB. The results decrease to 61 and 37% for preoperative clinically defined stage IA and IB, respectively [4]. Mean 3-year overall survival rates of about 70% in stage IA and of less than 50% for stage IB are published for surgical treatment. These figures are comparable to data after SBRT alone.

Unfortunately, data sets on overall survival with a longer follow-up after initial staging with FDG-PET-CT are still limited. This makes a direct comparison of recent data of SBRT with results after curative resection difficult [56]. Considering disease-specific survival data one has to be aware of the fact that these are even more scarce than results concerning overall survival. Onishi et al. [15] were able to demonstrate in a large multicenter trial that overall survival after SBRT is comparatively better when patients are operable but refuse resection. In this subgroup of patients 3-year survival was significantly improved to 88% when a biological effective dose of more than 100 Gy was applied. These results are even better than those usually achieved by surgical procedures.

We know from surgical data that even in patients with good general condition a difference of up to 20% between overall and disease-specific survival can be detected following resection, with a disease-specific survival of 72% for stage IA and of 32% for stage IB at 5 years [6]. For all stage I patients the disease-specific survival at 3 years was reported to be about 64%, which is even worse in comparison to data of SBRT [15, 32].

Comparable to surgical data, cancer relapse following SBRT is usually distant. Less than 10% of the patients die due to local recurrence, but more than 20% from distant metastases, predominately in brain and lung. This indicates that NSCLC is in part a systemic disease even in clinical stage I cancer patients. The use of additional systemic chemotherapy might be of benefit for selected patients after hSRT, such as those younger than 75 years. After resection the positive effect on survival has already been demonstrated in randomized clinical trials [3].

Follow-Up Recommendations

Follow-up of patients has a crucial aspect in quality assurance of the treatment. It should allow for assessment of efficacy of treatment in terms of local tumor control, patient condition in terms of clinically relevant side effects and patient selection in terms of survival and/or progression of disease.

Clinical anamnesis and focal physical examination are the basic diagnostic methods. For assessment of local tumor control and clinically not obvious side effects laboratory tests (differential blood account, tumor marker), CT, MRI, FDG-

PET and/or spirometry can be performed. The first examination is usually 6 weeks after irradiation followed by further examinations every 3–6 months. The results and especially the acquired images should be sent to and co-evaluated by the treating physician, because assessment of changes such as distinguishing scar tissue and inflammation from tumor (recurrence) might be difficult and requires a certain amount of experience [57] (fig. 2). Even with positive FDG-PET scan for months and years after SBRT, false-positive interpretation should be excluded by biopsy. Pneumonitis and pneumonia can pretend tumor progression, with SUV up to 7.

Future

While anatomical surgical resection has long been the standard treatment for stage I patients, SBRT could offer a less toxic, less costly, and more convenient alternative. With the promising preliminary results from single institutions, the maturing evaluation of late radiation toxicity, and the conduct of multicenter prospective trials in both operable and medically inoperable patients, SBRT shows considerable promise to be one of the most important recent innovations for effectively treating patients with primary and secondary lung cancer. However, prospective testing is required to insure that cure rates are not compromised. Clinical prospective phase II trials testing SBRT in operable patients is ongoing or planned in Japan (Japan Clinical Oncology Group, JCOG, protocol 0403) and the United States (Radiation Therapy Oncology Group, RTOG, protocol 0618), and a comparison of SBRT with surgery in the US. In medically inoperable patient groups, a Nordick multi-institutional consortium is comparing 3 fraction SBRT to conventional radiotherapy in an ongoing randomized phase II study. The RTOG has finished a phase II study of 3 fraction SBRT for peripheral tumors and is planning a phase I study with 5 fractions in patients with central tumors (RTOG 0633), and the JCOG is finishing a phase II study using a 4-fraction treatment for peripheral tumors and is planning a phase II study using a higher dose specifically for T2 tumors. Further trials in planning stages at the RTOG include the addition of targeted systemic therapies to SBRT (RTOG 0624) [12].

References

1 Kanavos P: The rising burden of cancer in the developing world. Ann Oncol 2006;17(suppl 8): viii15–viii23.

2 Alam N, Darling G, Shepherd FA, Mackay JA, Evans WK, Lung Cancer Disease Site Group of Cancer Care Ontario's Program in Evidence-Based Care: Postoperative chemotherapy in nonsmall cell lung cancer: a systematic review. Ann Thorac Surg 2006;81:1926–1936.

3 Bernstein ED, Herbert SM, Hanna NH: Chemotherapy and radiotherapy in the treatment of resectable non-small-cell lung cancer. Ann Surg Oncol 2006;13:291–301.
4 Mountain CF: The evolution of the surgical treatment of lung cancer. Chest Surg Clin N Am 2000;10:83–104.
5 Sugarbaker DJ, Strauss GM: Extent of surgery and survival in early lung carcinoma: implications for overdiagnosis in stage IA nonsmall cell lung carcinoma. Cancer 2000;89:S2432–S2437.
6 Reed MF, Molloy M, Dalton EL, Howington JA: Survival after resection for lung cancer is the outcome that matters. Am J Surg 2004;188:598–602.
7 Zimmermann FB, Bamberg M, Molls M, Jeremic B: Radiation Therapy Alone in Early Stage Non-small Cell Lung Cancer. Semin Surg Oncol 2003; 21:91–97.
8 Rosenzweig KE, Fox JL, Yorke E, Amols H, Jackson A, Rusch V, Kris MG, Ling CC, Leibel SA: Results of a phase I dose-escalation study using three-dimensional conformal radiotherapy in the treatment of inoperable nonsmall cell lung carcinoma. Cancer 2005;103:2118–2127.
9 Kong FM, Ten Haken RK, Schipper MJ, Sullivan MA, Chen M, Lopez C, Kalemkerian GP, Hayman JA: High-dose radiation improved local tumor control and overall survival in patients with inoperable/unresectable non-small-cell lung cancer: long-term results of a radiation dose escalation study. Int J Radiat Oncol Biol Phys 2005;63:324–333.
10 Bradley J, Graham MV, Winter K, Purdy JA Komaki R, Roa WH, Ryu JK, Bosch W, Emami B: Toxicity and outcome results of RTOG 9311:a phase I-II does-escalation study using three-dimensional conformal radiotherapy in patients with inoperable non-small-cell lung carcinoma. Int J Radiat Oncol Biol 2005;61:318–328.
11 Timmerman R, Abdulrahman R, Kavanagh BD, Meyer JL: Lung cancer: a model for implementing stereotactic body radiation therapy into practice; in Meyer JL (ed): IMRT, IGRT, SBRT – Advances in the Treatment Planning and Delivery of Radiotherapy. Front Radiat Ther Oncol. Basel, Karger, 2007, vol 40, pp 368–385.
12 Decker RH, Wilson LD: Advances in radiotherapy for lung cancer. Semin Respir Crit Care 2008;29:285–290.
13 Zimmermann FB, Geinitz H, Schill S, Grosu A, Schratzenstaller U, Molls M, Jeremic B: Stereotactic hypofractionated radiation therapy for stage I non-small cell lung cancer. Lung Cancer 2005;48: 107–114.
14 Beitler J, Badine EA, El-Sayah D, Makara D, Friscia P, Silverman P, Terjanian T: Stereotactic body radiation therapy for nonmetastatic lung cancer: an analysis of 75 patients treated over 5 years. Int J Radiat Oncol Biol Phys 2006;65:100–106.
15 Onishi H, Shirato H, Nagata Y, Hiraoka M, Fujino M, Gomi K, Niibe Y, Karasawa K, Hayakawa K, Takai Y, Kimura T, Takeda A, Ouchi A, Hareyama M, Kokubo M, Hara R, Itami J, Yamada K, Araki T: Hypofractionated stereotactic radiotherapy (HypoFXSRT) for stage I non-small cell lung cancer: updated results of 257 ptients in a Japanese multi-institutional study. J Thorac Oncol 2007;7: S94–S100.
16 Timmerman R, Bastasch M, Saha D, Abdulrahman R, Hittson W, Story M: Optimizing dose and fractionation for stereotactic body radiation therapy; in Meyer (ed): IMRT, IGRT, SBRT – Advances in the Treatment Planning and Delivery of Radiotherapy. Front Radiat Ther Oncol. Basel, Karger, 2007, vol 40, pp 352–365.
17 Lax I, Blomgren H, Naslund I, Svanstrom R: Stereotactic radiotherapy of malignancies in the abdomen: methodological aspects. Acta Oncol 1994;33:677–683.
18 Lax I, Blomgren H, Larson D, Näslund I: Extracranial stereotactic radiosurgery of localized targets. J Radiosurg 1998;1:135–148.
19 Timmerman R, Galvin J, Michalski J, Straube W, Ibbott G, Martin E, Abdulrahman R, Swann S, Fowler J, Choy H: Accreditation and quality assurance for Radiation Oncology Group: Multicenter clinical trials using stereotactic body radiation therapy in lung cancer. Acta Oncol 2006;45: 779–786.
20 ICRU 62: Prescription, Recording and Reporting Photon Beam Therapy. Bethesda, 1999.
21 El-Bayoumi E, Silvestri GA: Bronchoscopy for the diagnosis and staging of lung cancer. Semin Respir Crit Care Med 2008;29:261–270.
22 De Leyn P, Lardinois D, Van Schil PE, Rami-Porta R, Passlick B, Zielinski M, Waller DA, Lerut T, Weder W: ESTS guidelines for preoperative lymph node staging for non-small cell lung cancer. Eur J Cardio-Thorac Sur 2007;32:1–8.
23 Tanoue LT: Staging of non-small cell lung cancer. Semin Respir Crit Care Med 2008;29:248–260.

24 De Ruysscher D, Wanders S, van Haren E, Hochstenbag M, Geeraedts W, Utama I, Simons J, Dohmen J, Rhami A, Buell U, Thimister P, Snoep G, Boersma L, Verschueren T, van Baardwijk A, Minken A, Bentzen SM, Lambin P: Selective mediastinal node irradiation based on FDG-PET scan data in patients with non-small cell lung cancer: a prospective clinical study. Int J Radiat Oncol Biol Phys 2005;62:988–994.
25 Silvestri GA, Gould MK, Margolis ML, Tanoue LT, McCrory D, Toloza E, Detterbeck F: Noninvasive staging of non-small cell lung cancer. Chest 2007;132:S178–S201.
26 Yi CA, Shin KM, Lee KS, Kim H, Kim H, Kwon OJ, Choi JY, Chung MJ: Non-small cell lung cancer staging: efficacy comparison of integrated PET/CT versus 3.0-T whole-body MR imaging. Radiology 2008;248:632–642.
27 Blomgren H, Lax I, Naslund I, Svanstrom R: Stereotactic high dose fraction radiation therapy of extracranial tumors using an accelerator: clinical experience of the first thirty-one patients. Acta Oncol 1995;34:861–870.
28 Wulf J, Haedinger U, Oppitz U, Thiele W, Ness-Dourdoumas R, Flentje M: Stereotactic radiotherapy of targets in the lung and liver. Strahlenther Onkol 2001;177:645–655.
29 Lagerwaard F, Van Sornsen de Koste J, Nijssen-Visser M, Schuchard-Schippeer RH, Oei SS, Munne A, Senan S: Multiple 'slow' CT scans for incorporating lung tumor mobility in radiotherapy planning. Int J Radiat Oncol Biol Phys 2001; 51:932–937.
30 Guckenberger M, Meyer J, Wilbert J, Richter A, Baier K, Mueller G, Flentje M: Pulmonary injury and tumor response after stereotactic body radiotherapy (SBRT): Results of a serial follow-up CT study. Radiother Oncol 2007;85:435–442.
31 Baumann P, Nyman J, Lax I, Friesland S, Hoyer M, Rehn Ericsson S, Johansson KA, Ekberg , Morhed E, Paludan M, Wittgren L, Blomgren H, Lewensohn R: Factors important for efficacy of stereotactic body radiotherapy of medically inoperable stage I lung cancer: a retrospective analysis of patients treated in the Nordic countries. Acta Oncol 2006;45:787–795.
32 Zimmermann FB, Geinitz H, Schill S, Thamm R, Nieder C, Schratzenstaller U, Molls M: Stereotactic hypofractionated radiotherapy in stage I (T1–2 N0 M0) non-small cell lung cancer (NSCLC). Acta Oncol 2006;45:796–801.
33 Wulf J, Baier K, Mueller G, Flentje MP: Dose-response in stereotactic irradiation of lung tumors. Radiother Oncol 2005;77:83–87.
34 Hoyer M, Roed H, Traberg Hansen A, Ohlhuis L, Petersen J, Nellemann H, Kiil Berthelsen A, Grau C, Aage Engelholm S, von der Maase H: Phase II study on stereotactic body radiotherapy of colorectal metastases. Acta Oncol 2006;45:823–830.
35 Okunieff P, Petersen AL, Philip A, Milano MT, Katz AW, Boros L, Schell MC: Stereotactic body radiation therapy (SBRT) for lung metastases. Acta Oncol 2006;45:808–817.
36 Wurm RE, Gum F, Erbel S, Schlenger L, Scheffler D, Agaoglu D, Schild R, Gebauer B, Rogalla P, Plotkin M, Ocran K, Budach V: Image guided respiratory gated hypofractionated stereotactic body radiation therapy (H-SBRT) for liver and lung tumors: initial experience. Acta Oncol 2006; 45:881–889.
37 Hodge W, Tomê W, Jaradat HA, Orton NP, Khuntia D, Traynor A, Weigel T, Mehta MP: Feasibility report of image guided stereotactic body radiotherapy (IG-SBRT) with tomotherapy for early stage medically inoperable lung cancer using extreme hypofractionation. Acta Oncol 2006;45: 890–896.
38 Nuyttens JJ, Prevost JB, Praag J, Hoogeman M, van Klaveren RJ, Levendag PC, Pattynama PM: Lung tumor tracking during stereotactic radiotherapy treatment with the Cyberknife: marker placement and early results. Acta Oncol 2006;45:961–965.
39 Nagata Y, Takayama K, Matsuo Y, Norihisa Y, Mizowaki T, Sakamoto T; Sakamoto M, Mitsumori M, Shibuya K, Araki N, Yano S, Hiraoka M: Clinical outcomes of a phase I/II study of 48Gy of stereotactic body radiation therapy in 4 fractions using a stereotactic body frame. Int J Radiat Oncol Biol Phys 2005;63:1427–1431.
40 Hata M, Tokuuye K, Kagel K, Sugahara S, Nakayama H, Fukumitsu N, Hashimoto T, Mizumoto M, Ohara K, Akine Y: Hypofractionated high-dose proton beam therapy for stage I non-small cell lung cancer: preliminary results of a phase I/II clinical study. Int J Radiat Oncol Biol Phys 2007;68:786–793.
41 Panettieri V, Wennberg B, Gagliardi G, Duch MA; Ginjaume M, Lax I: SBRT of lung tumours: Monte Carlo simulation with PENELOPE of dose distributions including resiratory motion and comparison with different treatment planning systems. Phys Med Biol 2007;52:4265–4281.
42 Timmerman R, Papiez L, McGarry R, Likes L, DesRosiers C, Bank M, Frost S, Randall M, Williams M: Extracranial stereotactic radioablation: results of a phase I study in medically inoperable stage I non-small cell lung cancer. Chest 2003;124: 1946–1955.

43 Timmerman R, McGarry R, Yiannoutsos C, Papiez L, Tudor K, DeLuca J, Ewing M, Abdulrahman R, DeRosiers C, Williams M, Fletcher J: Excessive toxicity when treating central tumors in a phase II study of stereotactic body radiation therapy for medically inoperable early-stage lung cancer. J Clin Oncol 2006;24:4833–4839.

44 Park C, Papiez L, Zhang S, Story M, Timmerman RD: Universal survival curve and single fraction equivalent dose: useful tools in understanding potency of ablative radiotherapy. Int J Radiat Oncol Biol Phys 2008;70:847–852.

45 Uematsu M, Yamamoto F, Takai K, Ozeki Y, Tsumadori G, Aoki T, Tahara K, Shioda A, Fukui S, Kusano S: Stereotactic radiation therapy for primary or metastatic lung cancer: Preliminary experience with a linear accelerator-based treatment unit. Int J Radiat Oncol Biol Phys 1996; 36(suppl):352.

46 Nagata Y, Negoro Y, Aoki T, Mizowaki T, Takayama K, Kokubo M, Araki N, Mitsumori M, Sasai K, Shibamoto Y, Koga S, Yano S, Hiraoka M: Clinical outcomes of 3D conformal hypofractionated single high-dose radiotherapy for one or two lung tumors using a stereotactic body frame. Int J Radiat Oncol Biol Phys 2002;52:1041–1046.

47 Hof H, Muenter M, Oetzel D, Hoess A, Debus J, Herfarth K: Stereotactic single-dose radiotherapy (radiosurgery) of early stage nonsmall-cell lung cancer. Cancer 2007;110:148–155.

48 Uematsu M, Shioda A, Tahara K, Fukui T, Yamamoto F, Tsumatori G, Ozeki Y, Aoki T, Watanabe M, Kusano S: Focal, high dose, and fractionated modified stereotactic radiation therapy for lung carcinoma patients: a preliminary experience. Cancer. 1998;82:1062–1070.

49 Arimoto T, Usubuchi H, Matsuzawa T, Yonesaka A, Shimizu S; Shirato H, Miyasaka K: Small volume multiple non-coplanar arc radiotherapy for tumors of the lung, head and neck and the abdominopelvic region; in Lemke H, Vannier MW, Inamura K, Garman AG (eds): Computer Assisted Radiology and Surgery. Proc 12th Int Symp and Exhibition on Computer Assisted Radiology and Surgery. CARS ´98 Tokyo, 1998. Elsevier Press, Amsterdam, 1998, pp 257–261.

50 Shirato H, Shimizu S, Tadashi S, Nishioka T, Miyasaka K: Real time tumour tracking radiotherapy. Lancet 1999;353:1331–1332.

51 Uematsu M, Shioda A, Suda A, Fukui T, Ozeki Y, Hama Y, Wong JR, Kusang S. computed tomography-guided frameless stereotactic radiotherapy for stage I non-small-cell lung cancer: a 5-year experience. Int J Radiat Oncol Biol Phys 2001;51:666–670.

52 Onimaru R, Shirato H, Shimizu S, Kitamura K, Xu B, Fukumoto S, Chang TC, Fujita K, Oita M, Miyasaka K, Nishimura M, Dosaka-Akita H: Tolerance of organs at risk in small-volume, hypofractionated, image-guided radiotherapy for primary and metastatic lung cancers. Int J Radiat Oncol Biol Phys 2003;56:126–135.

53 Wulf J, Haedinger U, Oppitz U, Thiele W, Mueller G, Flentje M: Stereotactic radiotherapy for primary lung cancer and pulmonary metastases: a noninvasive treatment approach in medically inoperable patients. Int J Radiat Oncol Biol Phys 2004;60:186–196.

54 Nyman J, Johansson KA, Hulten U: Stereotactic hypofractionated radiotherapy for stage I non-small cell lung cancer: mature results for medically inoperable patients. Lung Cancer 2006;51: 97–103.

55 Xia T, Li H, Sun Q, Wang Y, Fan N, Yu Y, Li P, Chang JY: Promising clinical outcome of stereotactic body radiation therapy for patients with inoperable Stage I/II non-small-cell lung cancer. Int J Radiat Oncol Biol Phys 2006;66:117–125.

56 Hara R, Itami J, Kondo T, Aruga T, Uno T, Sasano N, Onishi K, Kiyozuka M, Fuse M, Ito M, Naoi K, Kohno Y: Clinical outcomes of single-fraction stereotactic radiation therapy of lung tumors. Cancer 2006;106:1347–1352.

57 Timmerman RD, Park C, Kavanagh BD: The North American experience with stereotactic body radiation therapy in non-small cell lung cancer. J Thorac Oncol 2007;2:S101–S112.

58 Fritz P, Kraus HJ, Blaschke T, Mühlnickel W, Strauch K, Engel-Riedel W, Chemaissani A, Stoelben E: Stereotactic, high single-dose irradiation of stage I non-small cell lung cancer (NSCLC) using four-dimensional CT scans for treatment planning. Lung Cancer 2008;60:193–199.

59 Ng AW, Tung SY, Wong VY. Hypofractionated stereotactic radiotherapy for medically inoperable stage I non-small cell lung cancer: report on clinical outcome and dose to critical organs. Radiother Oncol 2008;87:24–28.

60 Onimaru R, Fujino M, Yamazaki K, Onodera Y, Taguchi H, Katoh N, Hommura F; Oizumi S, Nishimura M, Shirato H: Steep-dose-response relationship for stage I non-small-cell lung cancer using hypofractionated high-dose irradiation by real-time tumor-tracking radiotherapy. Int J Radiat Oncol Biol Phys 2008;70:374–381.

61 McCammon R, Schefter TE, Gaspar LE, Zaemisch R, Gravdahl D, Kavanagh B: Observation of a dose-control relationship for lung and liver tumors after stereotactic body radiation therapy. Int J Radiat Oncol Biol Phys 2009;73:112–118.

62 Salazar OM, Sandhu TS, Lattin PB, Chang JH, Lee CK, Groshko GA, Lattin CJ: Once-weekly, high-dose stereotactic body radiotherapy for lung cancer: 6-year analysis of 60 early-stage, 42 locally advanced, and 7 metastatic lung cancers. Int J Radiat Oncol Biol Phys 2008;72:707–715.

63 Takeda A, Sanuki N, Kunieda E, Ohashi T, Oku Y, Takeda T, Shigematsu N, Kubo A: Stereotactic body radiotherapy for primary lung cancer at a dose of 50 Gy total in five fractions to the periphery of the planning target volume calculated using a superposition algorithm. Int J Radiat Oncol Biol Phys 2009;73:442–448.

64 Brown WT, Wu X, Wen BC, Fowler JF, Fayad F, Amendola BE, Garcia S, De La Zerda A, Huang Z, Schwade JG: Early results of CaberKnife image-guided robotic stereotactic radiosurgery for treatment of lung tumors. Comp Aided Surg 2007;12:253–261.

65 Lee S, Choi EK, Park HJ, Ahan SD, Kim JH, Kim KJ, Yoon SM, Kim YS, Yi BY: Stereotactic body frame based fractionated radiosurgery in the consecutive days for primary and metastatic tumor in the lung. Lung Cancer 2003;40:309–315.

66 Timmerman RD, Park C, Kavanagh BD: The North American experience with stereotactic body radiation therapy in non-small cell lung cancer (appendix). J Thorac Oncol 2007;2:S101–S112.

67 Collins BT, Vahdat S, Erickson K, Collins SP, Suy S, Yu X, Zhang Y, Subramaniam D, Reichner CA, Sarikaya I, Esposito G, Yousefi S, Jamis-Dow C, Banovac F, Anderson ED: Radical cyberknife radiosurgery with tumor tracking: an effective treatment for inoperable small peripheral stage I non-small cell lung cancer. J Hematol Oncol 2009;2:1–9.

68 Pennathur A, Luketich JD, Heron DE, Abbas G, Burton S, Chen M, Gooding WE, Ozhasoglu C, Landreneau RJ, Christie NA: Stereotactic radiosurgery for the treatment of stage I non-small cell lung cancer in high-risk patients. J Thorac Cardiovasc Surg 2009;137:597–604.

69 Koenig TR, Kunden RF, Erasmus JJ, Sabloff BS, Gladish GW, Komaki R, Stevens CW: Radiation injury of the lung after three-dimensional conformal radiotherapy. AJR 2002;178:1383–1388.

70 Aoki T, Nagata Y, Negoro Y, Takayama K, Mizowaki T, Kokubo M, Oya N, Mitsumori M, Hiraoka M: Evaluation of lung injury after three-dimensional conformal stereotactic radiotherapy for solitary lung tumors. Radiology 2004;230:101–108.

71 Takeda T, Takeda A, Kunieda E, Ishizaka A, Takemasa K, Shimado j, Yamamoto S, Shigematsu N, Kawaguchi O, Fukada J, Ohashi T, Kuribayashi S, Kubo A: Radiation injury after hypofractionated stereotactic radiotherapy for peripheral small lung tumors: serial changes on CT. AJR 2004;182:1123–1128.

72 Inoue T, Shimizu S, Onimaru RE, Takeda A, Onishi H, Nagata Y, Kimura T, Karasawa K, Arimoto T, Hareyama M, Kikuchi E, Shirato H: Clinical outcomes of stereotactic body radiotherapy for small lung lesions clinically diagnosed as primary lung cancer on radiologic examination. Int J Radiat Oncol Biol Phys 2009;in press.

73 McGarry RC, Papiez L, Williams M, Whitford T, Timmerman RD: Stereotactic body radiation therapy of early stage non-small cell lung cancer: phase I study. Int J Radiat Oncol Biol Phys 2005;63:1010–1015.

74 Joyner M, Salter BJ, Papanikolaou N, Fuss M: Stereotactic body radiation therapy for centrally located lung lesions. Acta Oncol 2006;45:802–807.

Prof. Dr. Frank Zimmermann
Department of Radiation Oncology, University Hospital, University Basel
Petersgraben 4
CH–4031 Basel (Switzerland)
Tel. +41 61 265 49 54, Fax +41 61 265 45 89, E-Mail fzimmermann@uhbs.ch

Heide J, Schmittel A, Kaiser D, Hinkelbein W (eds): Controversies in the Treatment of Lung Cancer.
Front Radiat Ther Oncol. Basel, Karger, 2010, vol 42, pp 115–121

Extended Surgical Resection in Stage III Non-Small Cell Lung Cancer

Sven Hillinger · Walter Weder

Division of Thoracic Surgery, University Hospital, Zürich, Switzerland

Abstract

Stage III includes a large variety of clinical situations from chest wall invasion together with intralobar lymph node metastasis to any size of a lung cancer in combination with mediastinal lymph node involvement (N2/N3). Furthermore, the prognosis of patients with lymph node metastasis depends largely on the extent of the disease, which may range from micro-metastasis occasionally found during surgery to bulky and/or multilevel involvement of the mediastinum or extracapsular infiltration. Not surprising the optimal treatment including the role of surgery for stage IIIA (N2) and stage IIIB (T4/N3) non-small cell lung cancer is discussed controversially. Adequate analysis of the clinical stage is key to select the best treatment. In general, patients benefit from surgery, when a radical resection can be achieved with a low morbidity and mortality. A multidisciplinary approach is indicated in most patients, which present with stage III disease at diagnosis. Preferentially patients should be treated in study protocols whenever they are available. Radical surgery including chest wall resection may result in a 5-year survival rate of up to 50% in T3N1 disease. Adjuvant chemotherapy is recommended and radiotherapy is reserved for cases with unclear resection margins. Clinical trials of preoperatively proven N2 patients could show a better outcome when downstaging is achieved after neoadjuvant chemo- or chemoradiotherapy prior to surgery. Patients who may need a pneumonectomy should be selected with caution since some centers experience a high perioperative mortality rate. If unforeseen N2 disease is found during surgery, an adjuvant therapy is recommended. Patients with T4 tumors (infiltration of great vessels, trachea, esophagus, vertebral bodies, etc.) show an increasing 5-year survival from 15 to 35% after radical resection with acceptable perioperative mortality if treated in experienced centers. In stage III non-small cell lung cancer, surgery should be performed within a multimodality approach. Surgery should be recommended when resection is radical including systematic lymph node dissection and mortality and morbidity are low.

Stage III non-small cell lung cancer (NSCLC) is a very heterogeneous group, harboring up to 30% of all TNM classified patients. It includes a large variety of clinical situations, which have to be approached individually [1].

Stage IIIA includes T3N1M0 tumors, centrally located or peripheral tumors infiltrating either the chest wall, diaphragm, mediastinal pleura or parietal pericardium in addition to intrapulmonary lymph node metastasis. Special entities are tumors infiltrating the superior sulcus. On the other side of the spectrum are locally less advanced tumors within the lungs of any size with ipsilateral and mediastinal lymph node involvement (T2N2M0). Lymph node involvement itself may already be clinically recognizable as bulk on one or several levels or microscopically recognized only on histology or cytology. All these factors have to be included in the individual decision process on treatment since they are relevant for the prognosis.

Stage IIIB consists of tumors of any size with contralateral mediastinal lymph node metastasis (N3) or tumors with mediastinal organ infiltration (great vessels, carina, left atrium, superior vena cava, esophagus and vertebral bodies), malignant effusions or satellite tumor nodule(s) within the ipsilateral primary tumor lobe of the lung (T4). N3 disease is usually no indication for surgery, except in rare palliative situations. However some promising results have been achieved in the recent past in selected patients with successful response to induction therapy and surgery (Swiss Group for Clinical Cancer Research (SAKK), publication is currently under review).

Locally advanced tumors with infiltration into neighboring organs (T4) have to be evaluated separately since treatment goals relate more towards local radicality in contrast to N3 disease where control of the systemic disease is of predominant importance.

The role of optimal treatment including the role of surgery is discussed controversially in these advanced stages and depends beside proper patient selection and individual staging also on the local expertise of the treatment teams and their possibilities.

Discussion of Stage-Related Treatment

Various centers worldwide have investigated the surgical treatment in these advanced stages of lung cancer mostly in multimodality approaches.

Stage IIIA

The Mayo Clinic group summarized 95 en bloc lung and chest wall resections in locally advanced tumors and reported an operative mortality 6.3% [2]. Overall 5-year survival was 38.7%. Long-term survival was strongly dependent on nodal involvement and complete resection. Adjuvant chemotherapy in patients with positive lobar lymph nodes was not used at that time when the study was conducted.

A special entity of stage IIIA tumors are the superior sulcus or pancoast tumors because of the limitations to resection due to their anatomic location. It has been shown that preoperative radiation therapy increases the 5-year survival rates. Complete resection and nodal involvement are again major prognostic factors.

With additional chemotherapy (induction chemoradiotherapy) a complete resection rate of 76% and a 5-year survival rate of 54% with complete resection can be achieved [3]. Similar results have been achieved by the Stamatis group with a complete resection rate of even 94% and a 5-year survival of 46% [4].

Of high importance is the sub-classification of N2 disease. Andre et al. [5] defined subgroups of single and multiple level minimal (detected at the time of surgery) N2 disease and those with single and multiple level clinical N2 disease. Their 5-year survival rates have been 34, 11, 8 and 3%, respectively. Therefore, in occult N2 disease, complete resection of the primary tumor as well as the lymph nodes is recommended, followed by an adjuvant platinum-based chemotherapy. Adjuvant radiotherapy after chemotherapy for local recurrence control should be considered [6].

For clinically diagnosed N2 preoperatively, surgical resection is not recommended as a single treatment. Those patients should be referred for a multidisciplinary evaluation (including a thoracic surgeon) before embarking on definitive treatment. In most of the cases with a good performance status, surgical resection might be a valuable option after induction chemo- or chemoradiotherapy [6].

Some studies in the past suggested missing benefits as well as inacceptable high morbidity and mortality rates when advanced lung cancers have been surgically resected following neoadjuvant therapy. For instance, the EORTC trial published by van Meerbeck et al. [7] could not show an improved overall and progression-free survival in 154 proven and primarily unresectable stage IIIA N2 patients. After induction and surgery more than 50% remained incompletely resected. Not surprisingly, the overall survival in this subgroup of patients with N2 disease did not differ compared to the same number who had received radiation therapy. Nevertheless, patients with complete resection reached a 27% 5-year survival compared to an overall 5-year survival rate of 15.7% in the surgery arm and 14% in the radiation arm.

The interim analysis of the RTOG 9309 trial in a total of 396 included proven stage IIIA N2 patients also could not show an overall survival benefit between the surgery and radiation arm following neoadjuvant chemotherapy [8].

A closer insight into these studies, however, shows that the mortality rate for patients after pneumonectomy has been as high as 26%, and that 79% were right-sided pneumonectomies. Patients, who only received a lobectomy after chemoradiotherapy and without this exceedingly high perioperative mortality rate showed a clear survival benefit after 60 months of follow-up compared to the radiotherapy treatment.

This high mortality rate of pneumonectomies after induction chemo- and/or radiotherapy has not been observed in other centers. Between 2003 and 2006, we reviewed 59 sleeve resections, 30% thereof have been performed after induction therapy, and 74 pneumonectomies (25% after induction therapy) at the division of thoracic surgery at the University Hospital in Zürich. In-hospital mortality was 1.2 and 1.3%, respectively.

The MD Anderson cancer center group evaluated a series of 76 patients who underwent induction chemotherapy followed by surgery compared to 259 patients who had only surgical treatment [9]. Chemotherapy followed by surgery did not significantly affect overall morbidity or mortality based on clinical or postoperative stage, or the extent of resection.

A Swiss multicenter phase II trial with cisplatin/docetaxel chemoinduction summarized 75 resections (37 pneumonectomies, 38 bi- or lobectomies) reported a 30-day mortality of 3% [10]. Successful downstaging of the mediastinal lymph nodes was the most important prognostic factor and 3-year survival after surgery in this subgroup was 61% compared to 11% in the nonresponders.

The Columbia group reviewed 40 of their patients from 1994 to 2000 (follow-up closing interval until 2003) with locally advanced lung cancer, which had been surgically resected following curative intent radiotherapy and concurrent chemotherapy with 0% mortality and highly favorable survival rates (5-year overall survival 46.2% and 5-year progression-free survival 56.4%) [11].

Kaya et al. [12] evaluated 54 stage III patients (75.9% stage IIIB and 24.1% stage IIIA) after concomitant chemoradiotherapy with cisplatin and doxetaxel. Downstaging was possible in 32 (59.3%) of the patients. In the 26 (48.1%) surgically resected patients, median progression-free survival and overall survival (in the entire cohort 14 months and 22 months, respectively) has not been reached with a median follow-up duration of 24 months.

Cerfolio et al. [13] reviewed a series of 216 advanced lung cancer patients over a decade (1998–2008), which had been surgically resected after concurrent chemotherapy and high-dose (60 Gy) radiation with a major morbidity of 17% and a mortality of only 2.3%. They reported an overall 5-year survival of 34%. It was 42% for R0 resections, 38% for those with initial N2 disease and 45% for the 71 complete responders.

Evolving advanced surgical techniques such as sleeve resections allow performing lung volume saving procedures in functionally impaired patients and at the same time a complete resection. A meta-analysis (13 studies) by Ma et al. [14] compared sleeve lobectomies (SL) and pneumonectomies (PN) including more than 1,000 stage III patients for morbidity and survivals. They summarized that SL is effective and can be accomplished safely in selected patients without increasing the morbidity and mortality as compared to PN, that SL offers better long-term survival than does PN, and that a more radical operation such as PN is not a more appropriate procedure, even in higher stage tumors.

Stage IIIB

Progress has also been made for stage IIIB patients over the past decades including surgical therapy in selected patients.

Grunenwald [15] proposed that selected patients in IIIB subgroups, of which the groups A ('nodal' stage IIIB) and B ('mediastinal' T4) should be differently analyzed, may profit from radical surgery, whereas T4/N3 and pleural effusions offer rare indications for curative surgical intents.

Farjah et al. [16] analyzed 13,077 T4 tumors in a cohort study between 1992 and 2002, from which 1,177 (9%) underwent surgical resection. The 5-year survival rate increased from 15% in 1992 to 35% in 2002 with still high 30-day mortality of 10%. Over time mediastinal lymphadenectomy has increased (from 10 to 29%) as well as the use of neoadjuvant therapy (from 4 to 8%). Adjuvant radiation therapy is used for local control of incompletely resected tumors and adjacent lymph nodes, whereas adjuvant chemotherapy is used to treat suspected occult systemic disease.

A meta-analysis of 26 series including 675 patients with T4 involvement of trachea, carina, heart, great vessels and vertebral bodies shows a median survival of 19 months and a 5-year survival of up to 31% [17].

After radical resection of the distal trachea or carina 312 patients of this series showed a median survival of 23 months [17].

The Paris group summarized their 8-year experience in 19 patients with vertebral body involvement who underwent radical en bloc resection with no postoperative mortality and an acceptably low morbidity. They could present a median overall survival of 26 months with 1- and 5-year survivals of 59 and 14%, respectively [18].

One and a half decades ago Naruke [19] already stated that within the stage IIIB patients N3 does have a worse prognosis than T4, but several studies show remarkable results after resection with 5-year survivals of 10%. Meanwhile, surgery plays an increasingly important role, especially in combination with induction chemotherapy or chemoradiotherapy.

The importance of surgery in selected stage IIIB patients has been reviewed by Albain [20], as 2-year survival rates with N3 and T4N2 tumors have been similar; however, in T4N0/1 patients induction chemoradiotherapy and additional surgery resulted in 64% 2-year survival versus 33% with chemoradiotherapy alone.

In a phase II study of 40 stage IIIB (T4 and/or N3) patients, to whom surgery was offered after clinical response to chemoradiotherapy, the overall 5-year survival was 19% and as high as 42% for patients having no mediastinal lymph node involvement at the time of complete resection surgery. Patients who had persistent viable tumor cells at surgery (chemoradiotherapy failed to control disease) had a remarkable 28% 5-year survival after complete resection [21].

Conclusions

Surgical resection remains the single most consistent and successful option for cure for patients diagnosed with NSCLC. For this option to be successful, the cancer must be completely resectable, and the patient must be able to tolerate the proposed surgical intervention well with low mortality [22].

However, these goals can be achieved in early stages only and in the more advanced stage III, a multimodality approach is needed in most cases to achieve a successful radical therapy. Since stage III disease includes a large variety of different stages, which have to be treated with different approaches these patients should be evaluated for best treatment by an interdisciplinary tumor board after clinical evaluation.

References

1 Lababede O, Meziane MA, Rice TW: TNM staging of lung cancer: a quick reference chart. Chest 1999;115:233–235.

2 Burkhart HM, Allen MS, Nichols FC 3rd, Deschamps C, Miller DL, Trastek VF, Pairolero PC: Results of en bloc resection for bronchogenic carcinoma with chest wall invasion. J Thorac Cardiovasc Surg 2002;123:670–675.

3 Rusch VW, Giroux DJ, Kraut MJ, Crowley J, Hazuka M, Winton T, Johnson DH, Shulman L, Shepherd F, Deschamps C, Livingston RB, Gandara D: Induction chemoradiation and surgical resection for superior sulcus non-small-cell lung carcinomas: long-term results of Southwest Oncology Group Trial 9416 (Intergroup Trial 0160). J Clin Oncol 2007;25:313–318.

4 Marra A, Eberhardt W, Pöttgen C, Theegarten D, Korfee S, Gauler T, Stuschke M, Stamatis G: Induction chemotherapy, concurrent chemoradiation and surgery for Pancoast tumour. Eur Respir J 2007;29:117–126.

5 Andre F, Grunenwald D, Pignon JP, Dujon A, Pujol JL, Brichon PY, Brouchet L, Quoix E, Westeel V, Le Chevalier T: Survival of patients with resected N2 non-small-cell lung cancer: evidence for a subclassification and implications. J Clin Oncol 2000;18:2981–2989.

6 Robinson LA, Ruckdeschel JC, Wagner H Jr, Stevens CW, American College of Chest Physicians: Treatment of non-small cell lung cancer-stage IIIA: ACCP evidence-based clinical practice guidelines, ed 2. Chest 2007;132(3 suppl):243S–265S.

7 van Meerbeeck JP, Kramer GW, Van Schil PE, Legrand C, Smit EF, Schramel F, Tjan-Heijnen VC, Biesma B, Debruyne C, van Zandwijk N, Splinter TA, Giaccone G, European Organisation for Research and Treatment of Cancer-Lung Cancer Group: Randomized controlled trial of resection versus radiotherapy after induction chemotherapy in stage IIIA-N2 non-small-cell lung cancer. J Natl Cancer Inst 2007;99:442–450.

8 Albain KS, Swann RS, Rusch VR, Turrisi AT, Shepherd FA, Smith CJ, Gandara DR, Johnson DH, Green MR, Miller RC, North American Lung Cancer Intergroup: Phase III study of concurrent chemotherapy and radiotherapy (CT/RT) vs. CT/RT followed by surgical resection for stage IIIA(pN2) non-small cell lung cancer (NSCLC): outcomes update of North American Intergroup 0139 (RTOG 9309). J Clin Oncol 2005;23:624s.

9 Siegenthaler MP, Pisters KM, Merriman KW, Roth JA, Swisher SG, Walsh GL, Vaporciyan AA, Smythe WR, Putnam JB Jr: Preoperative chemotherapy for lung cancer does not increase surgical morbidity. Ann Thorac Surg 2001;71:1105–1111.

10 Betticher DC, Hsu Schmitz SF, Tötsch M, Hansen E, Joss C, von Briel C, Schmid RA, Pless M, Habicht J, Roth AD, Spiliopoulos A, Stahel R, Weder W, Stupp R, Egli F, Furrer M, Honegger H, Wernli M, Cerny T, Ris HB: Mediastinal lymph node clearance after docetaxel-cisplatin neoadjuvant chemotherapy is prognostic of survival in patients with stage IIIA pN2 non-small-cell lung cancer: a multicenter phase II trial. J Clin Oncol 2003;21:1752–1759.

11 Sonett JR, Suntharalingam M, Edelman MJ, Patel AB, Gamliel Z, Doyle A, Hausner P, Krasna M: Pulmonary resection after curative intent radiotherapy (>59 Gy) and concurrent chemotherapy in non-small-cell lung cancer. Ann Thorac Surg 2004;78:1200–1205; discussion 1206.

12 Kaya AO, Buyukberber S, Benekli M, Coskun U, Sevinc A, Akmansu M, Yildiz R, Ozturk B, Yaman E, Kalender ME, Orhan O, Yamac D, Uner A, Anatolian Society of Medical Oncology (ASMO): Concomitant chemoradiotherapy with cisplatin and docetaxel followed by surgery and consolidation chemotherapy in patients with unresectable locally advanced non-small cell lung cancer. Med Oncol 2009. [Epub ahead of print]

13 Cerfolio RJ, Bryant AS, Jones VL, Cerfolio RM: Pulmonary resection after concurrent chemotherapy and high dose (60 Gy) radiation for non-small cell lung cancer is safe and may provide increased survival. Eur J Cardiothorac Surg 2009;35:718–723.

14 Ma Z, Dong A, Fan J, Cheng H: Does sleeve lobectomy concomitant with or without pulmonary artery reconstruction (double sleeve) have favorable results for non-small cell lung cancer compared with pneumonectomy? A meta-analysis. Eur J Cardiothorac Surg 2007;32:20–28.

15 Grunenwald DH: Surgery for advanced stage lung cancer. Semin Surg Oncol 2000;18:137–142.

16 Farjah F, Wood DE, Varghese TK Jr, Symons RG, Flum DR: Trends in the operative management and outcomes of T4 lung cancer. Ann Thorac Surg 2008;86:368–374.

17 Rice TW, Blackstone EH: Radical resections for T4 lung cancer. Surg Clin North Am 2002;82:573–587.

18 Grunenwald DH, Mazel C, Girard P, Veronesi G, Spaggiari L, Gossot D, Debrosse D, Caliandro R, Le Guillou JL, Le Chevalier T: Radical en bloc resection for lung cancer invading the spine. J Thorac Cardiovasc Surg 2002;123:271–279.

19 Naruke T: Significance of lymph node metastases in lung cancer. Semin Thorac Cardiovasc Surg 1993;5:210–218.

20 Albain KS: Induction chemotherapy with/without radiation followed by surgery in stage III non-small-cell lung cancer. Oncology (Williston Park). 1997;11(9 suppl 9):51–57.

21 Grunenwald DH, André F, Le Péchoux C, Girard P, Lamer C, Laplanche A, Tarayre M, Arriagada R, Le Chevalier T: Benefit of surgery after chemoradiotherapy in stage IIIB (T4 and/or N3) non-small cell lung cancer. J Thorac Cardiovasc Surg 2001;122:796–802.

22 Molina JR, Yang P, Cassivi SD, Schild SE, Adjei AA: Non-small cell lung cancer: epidemiology, risk factors, treatment, and survivorship. Mayo Clin Proc 2008;83:584–594.

Sven Hillinger, MD
Division of Thoracic Surgery, University Hospital
Rämistrase 100
CH–8091 Zürich (Switzerland)
Tel. +41 44 255 8802, Fax +41 44 255 8805, E-Mail sven.hillinger@usz.ch

Heide J, Schmittel A, Kaiser D, Hinkelbein W (eds): Controversies in the Treatment of Lung Cancer.
Front Radiat Ther Oncol. Basel, Karger, 2010, vol 42, pp 122–134

Stage III: Definitive Chemoradiotherapy

Rainer Fietkau · Sabine Semrau

Department of Radiotherapy, University of Erlangen-Nürnberg, Erlangen, Germany

Abstract

Concurrent chemoradiotherapy is presently the standard treatment for stage III inoperable non-small cell lung cancer. Within this treatment framework, conventionally fractionated radiotherapy to a total dose of 60–66 Gy has proven effective. The chemotherapy should be performed using a cisplatin-based regimen or, if contraindicated, carboplatin. The base drug can be combined with another cytostatic, such as etoposide, vinorelbine, paclitaxel or gemcitabine. There is no evidence from randomized clinical trials suggesting that addition of induction chemotherapy or adjuvant chemotherapy to the concurrent chemotherapy regimen improves the prognosis of these patients. Therefore, induction or adjuvant chemotherapy should not be used outside the framework of clinical trials. Age over 70 years and concomitant diseases are not contraindications for concurrent radiochemotherapy per se, but an increased rate of side effects can be expected in such elderly patients or patients with comorbidities. Consequently, these patients require intensive supportive care. Presumably, advanced age is not an adverse prognostic factor per se, but reduced heart and lung function are. Conclusive evidence confirming this assumption is lacking.

Until the mid-1990s, treatment of technically or functionally inoperable stage III non-small cell lung cancer (NSCLC) consisted of radiotherapy alone, which achieved median survival times of 9–11 months. Few patients survived more than 5 years (fig. 1). The introduction of combined radiotherapy and chemotherapy significantly improved the survival of these patients, as was initially shown in randomized clinical trials and later in meta-analyses. A recent meta-analysis by Rolland et al. [1] showed that sequential chemoradiotherapy (chemotherapy followed by radiotherapy) results in significant improvement of survival rates (hazard ratio (HR) 0.88, p = 0.001; absolute survival gain 2.6% at 3 years; increase from 8.7 to 11.3%). Concurrent chemoradiotherapy was compared to radiotherapy alone in the same study. The investigators found that concurrent radiochemotherapy resulted in a significant improvement of prognosis (HR 0.88, 0.81–0.95;

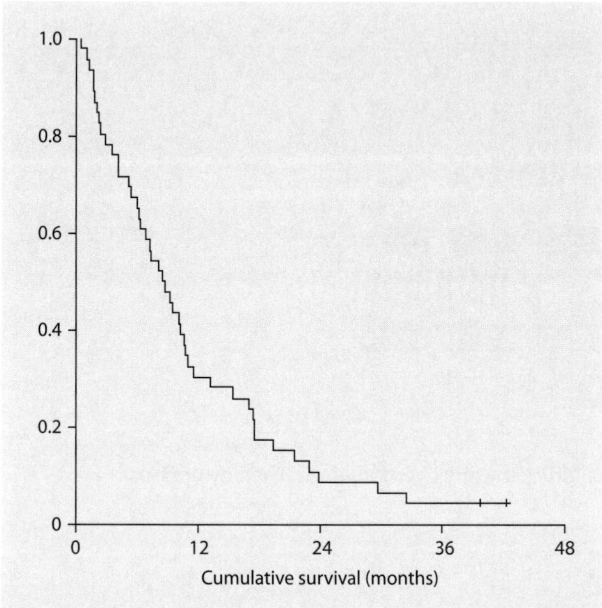

Fig. 1. Survival following radiotherapy alone of inoperable advanced NSCLC without distant metastases (n = 46). Median survival was 8.4 months: 1-year survival 30%, 2-year survival 9%, and 5-year survival 0%. Data from the Radiation Department of Rostock; radiotherapy between 01.01.1994 and 31.12.1997.

p = 0.0008; absolute survival gain 3.2% at 3 years; increase from 13.4 to 16.6%) in a population of 2,910 patients with inoperable stage III NSCLC.

Based on these data, the present review will answer the following questions:

- Which combination of chemotherapy and radiotherapy is currently the most promising?
- How should optimal chemoradiotherapy be performed?
- How do comorbidities influence the performance of concurrent chemoradiotherapy?

Optimization of Combined Radiotherapy and Chemotherapy

Concurrent and sequential chemotherapy (fig. 2) regimens have been compared in four large-scale randomized clinical trials to date [2–5] (table 1). These studies differ with regard to the radiation doses used. Total radiation doses of 60 Gy were used in two studies (Czech study and RTOG 9410-Trial), 56 Gy in the third study (Japanese), and 66 Gy in the fourth (French). All four studies used a

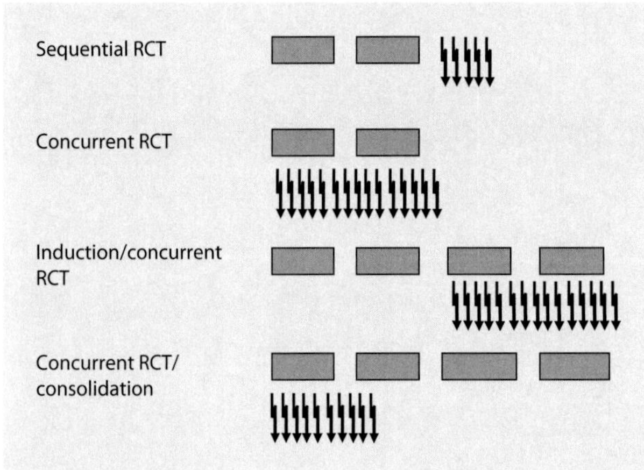

Fig. 2. Principle combination of radiotherapy and chemotherapy. Therapy options.

cisplatin-based regimen combined with either vinorelbine, vincristine or, in the case of the Japanese study, mitomycin C. These RCTs also differed with regard to the number of cycles of sequential chemotherapy completed, which ranged from 2 to 4.

Different from these studies was the trial by the European Organization for Research and Treatment of Cancer (EORTC 08972–22973), where low dose of platinum cytostatic was used in the concurrent chemoradiotherapy arm of the study [6]. While in the four studies with significantly higher cytostatic doses a more or less significant survival benefit of concurrent chemoradiotherapy was observed, the EORTC study detected no difference in survival rates. This equated to a median survival gain of up to 3 months. The benefit was more pronounced in the 2- to 3-year survival statistics: the differences in survival rates at this time were about 10% higher following concurrent radiotherapy than after sequential chemoradiotherapy (table 2). This was confirmed by a recent meta-analysis by Auperin et al. [7]. Their meta-analysis of seven randomized clinical trials showed a survival benefit of concurrent chemoradiotherapy over sequential chemoradiotherapy (HR 0.83 (0.73–0.94); p = 0.0026; absolute gain 6.6%, increase from 18.2 to 24.8%). In particular, concurrent chemoradiotherapy was superior in terms of local control (HR 0.76, p = 0.011). There was no significant difference in the incidence of distant metastases in the two treatment arms (HR 1.04, p = 0.669). This finding is important because a main point of criticism of concurrent chemoradiotherapy has been the assumption that simultaneous administration of radiotherapy and chemotherapy decreases the dose density of chemotherapy and thus reduces the control of distant metastases.

Table 1. Design of studies comparing sequential and concurrent chemoradiotherapy

Study	Stage	Arm		
Furuse, 1999 WJLCG [2]	III A/B	$4 \times M_8V_3P_{80}$	→	56 Gy
		56 Gy (split course)	+	$4\ M_8V_3P_{80}$
Curran, 2003 RTOG 9410 [3]	II/III	$2 \times V_5P_{100}$	→	60 Gy
		60 Gy	+	$2 \times V_5P_{100}$
Fournel, 2005 GLOT-GFPC NPC 95-01 [4]	III A/B	$3 \times P_{120}/Vinor_{30}$	→	66 Gy
		$2 \times Cis_{20}/Eto_{50}$ + 66 Gy	→	2 Cis/Vinor.
Zatloukal, 2004 [5]	III A/B	$4 \times P_{80}/Vinor._{25}$	→	60 Gy
		60 Gy	+	$2 \times P_{80}$, q28 $Vinor._{12,5./d1,8,15}$ + $2 \times P_{80}/Vinor._{25}$

Table 2. Survival results of trials comparing sequential and concurrent chemo-radiotherapy randomized studies

	Median survival, months		2-year survival, %		
	concurrent RCT	sequential RCT	concurrent RCT	sequential RCT	
Furuse et al. [2], 1999	16.5	13.3	22,3	14.7	$p < 0.05$
Curran et al. [3], 2003	17.0	14.6	21*	12*	$p = 0.04$
Fournel et al. [4], 2005	16.3	14.5	21*	14*	$p = 0.24$
Zatlukal et al. [5], 2004	16.6	12.9	42	15	$p = 0.02$

* 4-year data.

All of the studies indicated that concurrent chemoradiotherapy results in higher rates of acute toxicity than sequential chemoradiotherapy (table 3). This was particularly true of acute esophagitis (grade III/IV) (HR 5.7, $p < 0.0001$). The rate of hematologic toxicity was also higher in the concurrent arm of most studies. Specifically, the rate of grade 3–4 hematologic toxicity was about 20% higher

Table 3. Toxicity results of trials comparing sequential and concurrent chemo-radiotherapy: acute toxicity – grade III/IV

	Neutropenia, %		Esophagitis, %		Pneumonitis, %	
	sequential	concurrent	sequential	concurrent	sequential	concurrent
Furuse et al. [2], 1999	73	94	2	3	1	1
Fournel et al. [4], 2005	88	77	3	32	11	5
Zatloukal et al. [5], 2004	40	65	4	18	2	4

after concurrent chemoradiotherapy that after sequential chemoradiotherapy. In the EROTC study, the reverse was true due to the use of low-dose cisplatin. The rate of neutropenia in the concurrent arm was only 3%.

Closer analysis of the data reveals that, in the majority of studies, the feasibility of radiotherapy was decidedly unsatisfactory, especially in the sequential arm. Only 60% of patients in the sequential arms of the Czech and French studies received an adequate irradiation dose of more than 50–60 Gy. In contrast, radiotherapy was completed as planned in 80–90% of patients in the concurrent arms. The Japanese trial suggests that the intensity of chemotherapy was higher in the concurrent arm. The difference was not as great in the Czech study, but the percentage of patients completing four or more cycles of chemotherapy tended to be higher in the concurrent chemoradiotherapy arm than in the sequential arm (83 vs. 58%).

Overall, these data show that concurrent chemoradiotherapy can achieve a significantly higher treatment intensity than sequential chemoradiotherapy. The reason why only 60% of patients in the sequential arm received radiotherapy could be that the patients were so debilitated after two to four cycles of chemotherapy that they had little motivation to continue with further treatment.

Which Chemotherapy and Radiotherapy Regimens Are Optimal for Concurrent Chemoradiotherapy?

Most radiotherapy regimens employed for concurrent chemoradiotherapy use conventionally fractionated doses, e.g. 2 Gy once daily. The total dose is set based on previous experience with radiotherapy alone and should be at least 60 Gy or, ideally, 66 Gy. Relevant randomized clinical trial data on accelerated radiotherapy are not available. Curran et al. [8] compared hyperfractionated radiotherapy to a total dose of 69.6 Gy to conventionally fractionated radiotherapy in a study of different chemoradiotherapy regimens. Hyperfractionated radiotherapy not only failed to improve median survival, but also resulted in higher rates of grade 3–4 toxicity; however, there was no significant difference between the two groups with regard to the long-term toxicity statistics. As dose-limiting toxicities, particularly esophagitis, are a frequent impediment to concurrent chemoradiotherapy, these results suggest that conventionally fractionated radiotherapy should always be used if possible.

The standard chemotherapy regimens most commonly used by different working groups in the scope of concurrent chemoradiotherapy are:

- Cisplatin/etoposide
- Cisplatin/vinorelbine
- Cisplatin/paclitaxel
- Cisplatin/gemcitabine

If cisplatin is contraindicated, carboplatin can be used, but studies on the use of carboplatin in chemoradiotherapy are scarce. The CALGB phase II randomized clinical trial (CALGB 9431) compared the efficacy and toxicity of the drug combinations cisplatin/vinorelbine, cisplatin/gemcitabine and cisplatin/paclitaxel [9], but these regimens were administered in the scope of induction chemotherapy followed by concurrent chemoradiotherapy. The investigators found no significant differences between the groups in terms of the efficacy of treatment, as determined based on the rates of remission, median survival, and 1-year survival. It must be noted that no P values were provided because this was a phase II trial. However, concurrent chemoradiotherapy resulted in considerable differences in the rates of toxicity. The rates of neutropenia and thrombopenia were lowest in the cisplatin/vinorelbine group. The highest rates of grade 3–4 toxicity were observed in the cisplatin/gemcitabine group, with figures ranging from 51% for neutropenia, 51% for esophagitis, and 56% for thrombocytopenia. Again, no definitive conclusions are possible because of the lack of P values.

Our group at the University of Rostock can confirm the comparatively good experiences with the combination of cisplatin/carboplatin and vinorelbine (fig. 3). We treated 94 patients with this combination from 1998 to 2007 [10, 11]. The rates of the grade 3–4 toxicity were 25.3% for thrombocytopenia, 48.9% for neutropenia, and 13.2% for esophagitis. The median survival rate of 13 months in our patients was similar to the rates reported in other publications (fig. 4). The 5-year survival rate of 7.6% was the first occurrence of long-term survival, which is particularly remarkable considering that, based on the historical data, no patients survive five years after radiotherapy alone (fig. 1).

Findings from the first phase I/II studies on novel cytostatic drugs are now available, e.g. on the novel antifolate permetrexed [12–15] and the monoclonal

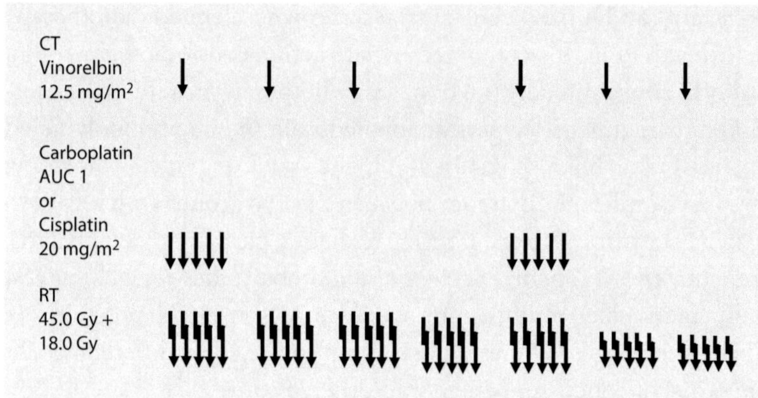

Fig. 3. Treatment schedule of concurrent chemoradiotherapy with cisplatin/carboplatin and vinorelbin [10, 11].

antibody cetuximab [15, 16]. Combination of cisplatin/carboplatin with pemetrexed resulted in grade 3–4 neutropenia rates of 21–35%; feasibility rates ranged from 72 to 90%. Cetuximab was studied in combination with carboplatin/pemetrexed (CALGB 30407) and carboplatin/paclitaxel (RTOG 0324). The grade 3–4 toxicity rates for these combinations also ranged between 20 and 34%; the RTOG study reported a median survival time of about 23 months. As far as can be determined at this time, these regimens seem to be feasible, but no clear advantages can be discerned at first glance.

The administration of additional chemotherapy before or after concurrent chemoradiotherapy has not resulted in any significant improvement of survival in the randomized clinical trials performed so far. In the two randomized clinical trials on the usefulness of performing induction chemotherapy before concurrent chemoradiotherapy [17, 18], induction chemotherapy did not result in any significant difference in median survival (median survival: 12 vs. 14 months in Vokes et al. [17] and 18 vs. 12 months in Kim et al. [18]). Furthermore, there was no significant difference in the 2-year survival rates (29 vs. 31% in Vokes et al. [17] and 43 vs. 25% in Kim et al. [18]). In fact, the study by Kim et al. [18] detected a significant reduction of progression-free survival in the patients receiving additional induction chemotherapy (median progression-free survival following concurrent chemoradiotherapy with and without induction chemotherapy; 7.5 vs. 11.6 months; $p = 0.04$). Vokes et al. [17] concluded that the administration of additional induction chemotherapy prior to concurrent chemoradiotherapy increases the rates of grade 4 toxicities significantly, from 24 to 41% ($p = 0.001$).

The preliminary results on consolidation chemotherapy after completion of chemoradiotherapy are also disappointing. The retrospective analysis of the

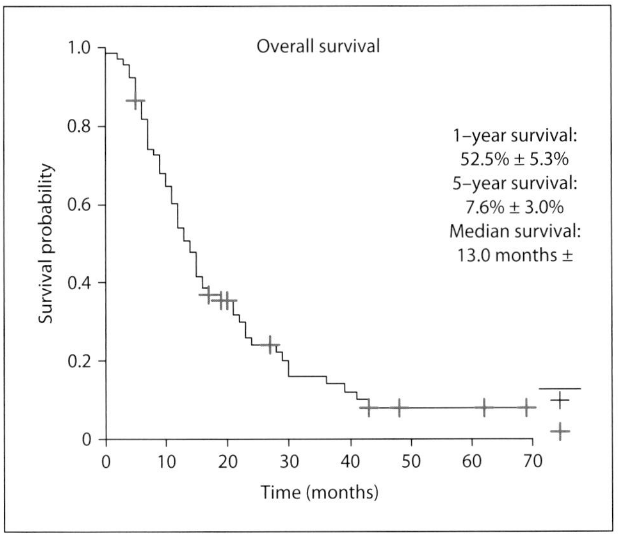

Fig. 4. Survival following concurrent chemoradiotherapy of inoperable advanced NSCLC without distant metastases (n = 94). Data from the Radiation Department of Rostock; chemoradiotherapy between 01.01.1998 and 31.12.2007.

Southwest Oncology Group (SWOG) study 9504 [19] initially indicated that consolidation chemotherapy with docetaxel after definitive chemoradiotherapy significantly improved 3-year survival (26 vs. 37%), but the randomized data from the Hoosier Oncology Group study HOG LUN 01–24 [20] later showed that there was no significant improvement of either median survival (22 vs. 24 months) or 3-year survival (26.1 vs. 24.2%). Another especially critical point is that 5.5% of patients died on consolidation docetaxel. The administration of maintenance gefitinib after concurrent chemoradiotherapy also did not improve the survival of patients with stage III inoperable NSCLC [21]. In fact, the median survival of patients receiving gefitinib after concurrent chemoradiotherapy was only 23 months compared to 35 months in patients receiving concurrent chemoradiotherapy alone (p = 0.013). This difference cannot be explained by higher rates of toxicity in the gefitinib arm.

Based on the current state of knowledge, concurrent chemoradiotherapy can be classified as the current standard of care in patients with inoperable stage III non-small cell lung cancer. The administration of additional chemotherapy before or after chemoradiation does not improve survival. The reader is referred to the German Intergroup Lung Cancer Trial (GILT-1 study), which also analyzed the available data on additional chemotherapy after completion of definitive chemoradiation in this context.

How Do Comorbidities Influence the Performance of Concurrent Chemoradiotherapy?

Several limitations make it difficult to translate the findings of randomized clinical trials into general treatment recommendations. For example, the patients included in the randomized clinical trials described above had a median age of 59 years, whereas that of the general population of patients with stage III inoperable non-small cell lung cancer is 67 years (table 4). Furthermore, the inclusion and exclusion criteria of the randomized clinical trials generally ensure that patients with significant comorbidities are not included in the studies. A Dutch research group showed that only 59% of all patients with stage III non-small cell or small cell lung cancer met the inclusion criteria for concurrent chemoradiation [22]. A statistical analysis by our group of the data at the University of Rostock showed that about one-third of these patients have significant comorbidities. Ten to twenty percent of the patients have renal failure and secondary cancer, and the percentage with a left ventricular ejection fraction of less than 50% of the age-related normal value is at least twice as high as that in the normal population [23].

Our research group has studied the potential effects of age and dysfunction of various organ systems on the toxicity and feasibility of concurrent chemoradiotherapy using a platinum derivative and vinorelbine in 66 patients with inoperable lung cancer to date [24]. Compared to the younger patients, patients over 70 years of age have significantly higher rates of WHO grade 3–4 leukopenia (33 vs. 58%) and thrombopenia (17 vs. 46%) at the same dose intensities of radiochemotherapy (table 5). Many investigators assume that old age (>70 years) alone implies an inability to tolerate chemoradiation; consequently, these patients receive concurrent chemoradiotherapy less often than other cancer patients, even though age was not identified as an independent factor for survival in multivariate analyses [25]. Schild et al. [26] showed that patients aged 70 years and older achieve comparable median survival rates after concurrent radiation and chemotherapy with etoposide and cisplatin versus hyperfractionated radiation therapy. This is in agreement with Atagi et al. [27], who found that concurrent radiation and daily low-dose carboplatin could be successfully administered to over-75-year-olds, with the predominant dose-limiting factor being hematologic toxicity. In contrast, the multivariate analysis of the randomized trial by Vokes et al. [17] showed that age was an independent prognostic factor. However, considering that the hazard ratio was 1.02, the survival rate in the older patient population was only 2% worse than that of younger patients. Thus, age has very little effect on the prognosis.

Further analysis showed that the effect of cardiopulmonary factors on prognosis is at least as great as that of the tumor stage itself. Survival of patients with an ejection fraction below 50% or significantly reduced lung function was significantly worse than that of those with good heart or lung function.

Table 4. Comparison of the median age of patients with NSCLC recruited in clinical phase III trial and in the general population of different regions

	Median age, years
Trials	
Furuse et al. [2], 1999	63–64
Zatlaukal et al. [5], 2004	61–62
Fournel et al. [4], 2005	56–57
General population	
Rostock [pers. commun.]	68
Australia [32], 2006	68

Reduced left ventricular ejection fraction (LVEF ≤50%; p = 0.043; HR 1.74), decreased lung function (p = 0.001; HR: 1.70/5.05), and tumor stage (p = 0.026; HR: 1.3) were identified as independent prognostic factors in multivariate analyses [23]. The median survival time of patients with normal age-related lung function was twice as long (16 months) as that of patients in whom lung function was impaired (p = 0.001) [23]. The median survival times of 8–10 months in the group with unfavorable prognostic factors are essentially identical with those obtained with radiotherapy alone (fig. 1). A priori, one must consider that patients with reduced heart and lung function have a worse prognosis. A LVEF of less than 50% following myocardial infarction is an unfavorable prognostic factor in non-cancer patients. Six-month mortality rates of 16% have been observed in patients with a recurrent cardiac decompensation [28]. With a slightly lower mortality, this applies in the scope of chronic obstructive pulmonary disease too [29].

Using common rating scales, such as the Cumulative Illness Rating Scale for Geriatrics (CIRSG), investigators demonstrated that concurrent chemoradiotherapy resulted in a worse survival more than radiotherapy alone in patients with high CIRSG scores [30]. Other scoring systems, such as the Charlson Index, did not show any reproducible correlation [25].

Our data suggest that concurrent chemoradiotherapy is feasible, even in patients with reduced general health and comorbidities. However, the long-term prognosis of these patients is influenced by common comorbidities, especially cardiac and pulmonary dysfunction, in addition to the known tumor-related factors. This was confirmed by the results of a Spanish research group, which found that, in high-risk patients, concurrent chemoradiotherapy (60 Gy plus carboplatin/vinorelbine)

Table 5. Acute toxicity of patients with NSCLC treated with concurrent chemoradiotherapy in different age groups

	Age 18–59 years	Age 60–69 years	Age 70–77 years
Leukopenia 3 and 4	36	43	51
Thrombocytopenia 3 and 4	8	29	31
Transfusions needed	30	37	50
Esophagitis 3 and 4	15	20	17
Infection 3 and 4	36	29	23

Data (%) from the Radiation Department of Rostock; chemoradiotherapy between 01.01.1998 and 31.12.2007 with cisplatin/carboplatin and vinorelbin [10, 11] (courtesy of Sabine Semrau).

is more feasible than sequential chemoradiotherapy and results in higher remission rates than sequential chemoradiotherapy [31].

Our review of the data indicates that comorbidity and old age are not exclusion criteria for concurrent chemoradiotherapy per se. However, these patients require more intensive supportive care. Presumably, the prognosis of these patients is also influenced by the comorbidities as well as the classical prognostic factors.

References

1 Rolland E, Le Chevalier T, Auperin A, et al: Sequential radio-chemotherapy (RT-CT) versus radiotherapy alone (RT) and concomitant RT-CT versus RT alone in locally advanced non-small cell lung cancer (NSCLC): Two meta-analyses using individual patient data (IPD) from randomised clinical trials (RCTs): A1–04. J Thor Oncol 2007;2(suppl 4):S309–S310.

2 Furuse K, Fukuoka M, Kawahara M, et al: Phase III study of concurrent versus sequential thoracic radiotherapy in combination with mitomycin, vindesine, and cisplatin in unresectable stage III non-small-cell lung cancer. J Clin Oncol 1999;17: 2692–699.

3 Curran W, Scott C, Langer C, et al: Long-term benefit is observed in a phase III comparison of sequential vs. concurrent chemo-radiation for patients with unresected stage III nsclc: RTOG 9410. Proc Am Soc Clin Onc 2003;22:abstr 2499.

4 Fournel P, Robinet G, Thomas P, et al: Randomized phase III trial of sequential chemoradiotherapy compared with concurrent chemoradiotherapy in locally advanced non-small-cell lung cancer: Groupe Lyon-Saint-Etienne d'Oncologie Thoracique-Groupe Français de Pneumo-Cancerologie NPC 95–01 Study. J Clin Oncol 2005;23:5910–5917.

5 Zatloukal P, Petruzelka L, Zemanova M, et al: Concurrent versus sequential chemoradiotherapy with cisplatin and vinorelbine in locally advanced non-small cell lung cancer: a randomized study. Lung Cancer 2004;46:87–98.

6 Belderbos J, Uitterhoeve L, van Zandwijk N, et al: Randomised trial of sequential versus concurrent chemo-radiotherapy in patients with inoperable non-small cell lung cancer (EORTC 08972–22973). Eur J Cancer 2007;43:114–121.

7 Auperin A, Rolland E; Curran W, et al: Concomitant radio-chemotherapy (RT-CT) versus sequential RT-CT in locally advanced non-small cell lung cancer (NSCLC): a meta-analysis using individual patient data (IPD) from randomised clinical trials (RCTs): A1–05. J Thorac Oncol 2007; 28(suppl 4):S310.
8 Curran W, Scott C, Langer C, et al: Phase III comparison of sequential vs. concurrent chemoradiation for patients with unresected stage III non-small cell lung cancer (NSCLC): initial report of Radiation Therapy Oncology Group (RTOG) 9410. Proc Am Soc Clin Oncol 2000;19:abstr 1891.
9 Vokes EE, Herdon JE, Crawford J, et al: Randomized phase II study with gemicitabine or paclitaxel or vinorelbine as induction chemotherpy followed by concomitant chemoradiotherapy for stage IIIB non-small-cell lung cancer: cancer and Leukemia Group B study 9431. J Clin Oncol. 2002; 20:4191–4198
10 Semrau S, Bier A, Thierbach U, Virchow C, Ketterer P, Klautke G, Fietkau R. 6-year experience of concurrent radiochemotherapy with vinorelbine plus a platinum compound in multimorbid or aged patients with inoperable non-small cell lung cancer. Strahlenther Onkol 2007;183:30–35.
11 Semrau S, Bier A, Thierbach U, Virchow C, Ketterer P, Fietkau R: Concurrent radiochemotherapy with vinorelbine plus cisplatin or carboplatin in patients with locally advanced non-small-cell lung cancer (NSCLC) and an increased risk of treatment complications: preliminary results. Strahlenther Onkol 2003;179:823–831.
12 Gadgeel SM, Ruckdeschel JC, Wozniak A, et al: Pemetrexed and cisplatin with concurrent thoracic radiation therapy (TRT) followed by docetaxel in stage III non-small cell lung cancer (NSCLC) patients (pts). Proc Am Soc Clin Oncol 2008;26:abstr 7569.
13 Machtay M, Werner-Wasik M, DeNittis A, et al: Pilot study of carboplatin/radiotherapy plus 'dose-dense' pemetrexed for locally advanced non-small cell lung carcinoma. Proc Am Soc Clin Oncol 2008;26:abstr 7571.
14 Brade AM, Bezjak A, MacRae R, et al: A phase I study of concurrent pemetrexed (P)/cisplatin (C)/radiation (RT) for unresectable stage IIIA/B non-small cell lung cancer (NSCLC). Proc Am Soc Clin Oncol 2008;26:abstr 7550.
15 Govindan R, Bogart J, Wang X, Liu D, Kratzke RA, Vokes EE: A phase II study of pemetrexed, carboplatin and thoracic radiation with or without cetuximab in patients with locally advanced unresectable non-small cell lung cancer: CALGB 30407 – Early evaluation of feasibility and toxicity. Proc Am Soc Clin Oncol 2008;26:abstr 7518.
16 Blumenschein GR, Paulus R, Curran WJ, et al: A phase II study of cetuximab (C225) in combination with chemoradiation (CRT) in patients (PTS) with stage IIIA/B non-small cell lung cancer (NSCLC): a report of the 2 year and median survival (MS) for the RTOG 0324 trial. Proc Am Soc Clin Oncol 2008;26:abstr 7516.
17 Vokes EE, Herndon JE, Kelley MJ, et al: Induction chemotherapy followed by chemoradiotherapy compared with chemoradiotherapy alone for regionally advanced unresectable stage III Non-small-cell lung cancer: cancer and leukemia group B. J Clin Oncol 2007;25:1698–704.
18 Kim S, Kim M, Choi E, et al: Induction chemotherapy followed by concurrent chemoradiotherapy (CCRT) versus CCRT alone for unresectable stage III non-small cell lung cancer (NSCLC): randomized phase III trial. Proc Am Soc Clin Oncol 2007;25:abstr 7528.
19 Gandara DR, Chansky K, Albain KS, et al: Consolidation docetaxel after concurrent chemoradiotherapy in stage IIIB non-small cell lung cancer: phase II Southwest Oncology Group Study S9504. J Clin Oncol 2003;21:2004–2010.
20 Mina LA, Neubauer MA, Ansari RH, et al: Phase III trial of cisplatin (P) plus etoposide (E) plus concurrent chest radiation (XRT) with or without consolidation docetaxel (D) in patients (pts) with inoperable stage III non-small cell lung cancer (NSCLC): HOG LUN 01–24/USO-023 – Updated results. Proc Am Soc Clin Oncol 2008;26:abstr 7519.
21 Kelly K, Chansky K, Gaspar LE, et al: Phase III trial of maintenance gefitinib or placebo after concurrent chemoradiotherapy and docetaxel consolidation in inoperable stage III non-small cell lung cancer: SWOG S0023. J Clin Oncol 2008; 26:2450–456.
22 De Ruysscher D, Botterweck A, Dirx M, et al: Eligibility for concurrent chemotherapy and radiotherapy of locally advanced lung cancer patients: a prospective, population-based study. Ann Oncol 2009;20:98–102.

23 Semrau S, Klautke G, Fietkau R: Baseline cardiopulmonary function as an independent prognostic factor for survival of inoperable non-small-cell lung cancer following concurrent chemoradiotherapy: a single-center analysis of 161 cases. Submitted.
24 Semrau S, Klautke G, Virchow JC, Kundt G, Fietkau R. Impact of comorbidity and age on the outcome of patients with inoperable NSCLC treated with concurrent chemoradiotherapy. Respir Med 2008;102:210–218.
25 Firat S, Byhardt RW, Gore E: Comorbidity and Karnofksy performance score are independent prognostic factors in stage III non-small-cell lung cancer: an institutional analysis of patients treated on four RTOG studies. Radiation Therapy Oncology Group. Int J Radiat Oncol Biol Phys 2002;54:357–364.
26 Schild SE, Stella PJ, Geyer SM, et al: North Central Cancer Treatment Group. The outcome of combined-modality therapy for stage III non-small-cell lung cancer in the elderly. J Clin Oncol 2003;21:3201–3206.
27 Atagi S, Kawahara M, Ogawara M, et al: Phase II trial of daily low-dose carboplatin and thoracic radiotherapy in elderly patients with locally advanced non-small cell lung cancer. Jpn J Clin Oncol 2000;30:59–64.
28 Bursi F, Weston SA, Redfield MM, et al: Systolic and diastolic heart failure in the community. JAMA 2006;296:2209–2216.
29 Pelkonen M, Notkola IL, Nissinen A, et al: Thirty-year cumulative incidence of chronic bronchitis and COPD in relation to 30-year pulmonary function and 40-year mortality: a follow-up in middle-aged rural men. Chest 2006;130:1129–1137.
30 Firat S, Pleister A, Byhardt RW, Gore E: Age is independent of comorbidity influencing patient selection for combined modality therapy for treatment of stage III nonsmall cell lung cancer (NSCLC). Am J Clin Oncol 2006;29:252–257.
31 Cardenal F, Arnaiz MD, Isla D, et al: Randomized phase II study of sequential versus concurrent chemoradiotherapy (CRT) in poor-risk patients with inoperable stage III non-small cell lung cancer (NSCLC): Interim analysis. Proc Am Soc Clin Oncol 2004;22:abstr 7255.
32 Jennens RR, Giles GG, Fox RM: Increasing under-representation of elderly patients with advanced colorectal or non-small-cell lung cancer in chemotherapy trials. Intern Med J 2006;36:216–220.

Rainer Fietkau
Department of Radiotherapy, University of Erlangen-Nürnberg
Universitätsstrasse 27
DE–91054 Erlangen (Germany)
Tel. +49 9131 85 33405, Fax +49 9131 85 39335, E-Mail rainer.fietkau@uk-erlangen.de

Heide J, Schmittel A, Kaiser D, Hinkelbein W (eds): Controversies in the Treatment of Lung Cancer.
Front Radiat Ther Oncol. Basel, Karger, 2010, vol 42, pp 135–144

Adjuvant Therapy in Early-Stage Non-Small Cell Lung Cancer

Monika Serke

CÄ Pneumologie III, Lungenklinik Hemer, Hemer, Germany

Abstract

Evidence clearly supports adjuvant chemotherapy following resection in patients with stage II or III non-small cell lung cancer (NSCLC). Based on 3 landmark studies, adjuvant chemotherapy has become standard in completely resected NSCLC stage II and IIIA. Survival benefit from adjuvant chemotherapy is estimated to be between 3% and 15%, depending on stage. Treatment should include 4 cycles of platinum-based combination chemotherapy. There is uncertainty about chemotherapy prescription in those patients with resected stage IB NSCLC, as the risk of recurrence is lower in early NSCLC and the magnitude of benefit of adjuvant therapy is proportional to the risk of relapse according to stage. Postoperative radiotherapy (PORT) should not be used for stage I or II NSCLC, and remains controversial in resected stage IIIA (N2) disease. All positive adjuvant trials have utilized a cisplatin-based regimen, usually in combination with vinorelbine, and this should be considered the standard approach. Prognostic factors to select patients who will benefit from adjuvant therapy in general or from platinum-based chemotherapy are under discussion, but not yet established. In future we hope to optimize treatment convenience for the patients by using other combinations with the hope of better efficacy results. Work is currently under way to identify prognostic factors which in future may help to identify patients who are most likely to benefit from chemotherapy.

Treatment of choice for early non-small cell lung cancer (NSCLC) is surgical resection, however only 50% of all patients will be cured. The survival rates range from 67% for stage IA disease (T1 N0) to 23% for stage IIIA patients (T1–3N2). Relapse may occur local (in about 30%) or, more often at distant sites, indicating that NSCLC may be a systemic disease [1]. One of the most significant advances in the treatment of lung cancer has been the identification of benefit associated with the use of adjuvant chemotherapy in completely resected early stage disease.

A meta-analysis in 1995 [2] suggested that adjuvant chemotherapy could yield an overall survival advantage of 5% at 5 years and this caused several

Table 1. Landmark studies adjuvant

Trial	Chemotherapy	Number of patients	% 5-year survival	Hazard ratio (all stages)	Radiotherapy
IALT [6], 2004	cisplatin + etoposide or vinca	1,867	40 vs. 44.5	0.86*	+
JBR.10 [7], 2005	cisplatin + vinorelbine	482	54 vs. 69	0.69*	–
ANITA [8], 2006	cisplatin + vinorelbine	840	43 vs. 51	0.80*	+

* Significant.

large randomized studies on adjuvant chemotherapy with results in the years 2003–2006.

Concomitant adjuvant chemoradiotherapy failed to improve the results [3] and the PORT meta-analysis 1998, updated 2005 [4, 5], indicated a deleterious effect of postoperative radiotherapy on long-term survival in stage I and II patients and a small positive effect in NSCLC IIIA N2-patients.

Landmark Studies Concerning Adjuvant Platinum-Based Chemotherapy

Three landmark studies (see table 1), published between 2003 and 2005, established the role of adjuvant platinum-based chemotherapy: the IALT [6], JBR.10 [7] and the ANITA studies [8].

In 2003, the IALT trial [6], the first large positive adjuvant NSCLC trial, was presented. Nearly 2,000 patients with resected stage I-IIIA NSCLC were randomized to observation or to 4 cycles of adjuvant cisplatin-based doublet chemotherapy (with the free choice of vindesine, vinblastine, vinorelbine, or etoposide as the second drug). The 5-year overall survival improved (44.5 vs. 40.4%) with a survival hazard ratio (HR) of 0.86 ($p = 0.03$) in favor of chemotherapy. However, an IALT update 2008 found no survival benefit at 7 years with an updated survival HR of 0.91. Patients with adjuvant therapy had fewer local recurrences and fewer distant metastases but had a higher non-lung cancer death rate (3 and 4% compared to 1 and 5%). Radiotherapy was optional according to pN status and given after chemotherapy.

The National Cancer Institute of Canada (NCIC) with the JBR.10 [7] trial included only stage IB and II patients and was positive again with a 15% 5-year survival advantage in the adjuvant therapy group (69% compared with 54%, p =

0.04, HR 0.69). Patients were randomized between observation or 4 cycles of cisplatin (50 mg/m^2 days 1 and 8, every 4 weeks) and vinorelbine (25 mg/m^2 weekly for 16 weeks). Radiotherapy was not allowed.

The ANITA [8] (Adjuvant Navelbine International Trialist's Association) trial, published 2005 was the third positive study. 840 patients were included with stage I, II and IIIA NSCLC and half of them were treated with 4 cycles cisplatin (100 mg/m^2 on day 1 every 4 weeks) and vinorelbine (30 mg/m^2 per week). This study demonstrated an 8.6% 5-year overall survival benefit (51% compared with 43%, survival HR: 0.80, p = 0.017). This survival advantage did not diminish over time and was 8.4% at 7 years of follow-up.

IALT, JBR.10 and ANITA established the role of routine adjuvant treatment in early NSCLC.

Negative Studies

The Cancer and Leukaemia Group B (CALGB) 9633 [9] study was negative. Exclusively stage IB patients were enrolled and the carboplatin/paclitaxel regimen was used. Though chemotherapy was well tolerated, the study failed to reach statistical significance for survival benefit with a survival HR of 0.80 (p = 0.10), despite a highly positive result at an interim analysis in 2004. A subgroup analysis in patients with larger tumors (4 cm or larger in size) showed a statistically significant survival benefit with the addition of adjuvant chemotherapy.

This study, combined with the result of the meta-analysis of the cisplatin-based trials, argues against the use of a carboplatin-based combination and against adjuvant chemotherapy in general in stage IB patients.

The ALPI trial [10] included 1,088 stage I–IIIA patients treated with 3 cycles MVP (mitomycin, vindesine, cisplatin) and showed a nonsignificant survival improvement under chemotherapy. The Big Lung Trial [11] investigated a subgroup of 307 stage I–III patients under 3 cycles platinum-based chemotherapy and showed a nonsignificant survival improvement under chemotherapy and optional radiotherapy.

The LACE (Lung Adjuvant Cisplatin Evaluation) Meta-Analysis (table 2)

Survival

In 2006, the LACE meta-analysis [12] evaluated the results of 5 adjuvant studies (IALT, JBR.10, ANITA, ALPI and Big Lung Trial) including 4,510 patients and confirmed the positive results with an 5.4% 5-year overall survival improvement (from 43.5 to 48.8%). The survival benefit was statistically significant (HR: 0.89) with an 11% reduction in the risk of death. Furthermore, the disease-free survival improved for 5, 8% at 3 and 5 years, respectively. Only patients in performance status 2 did not benefit from adjuvant chemotherapy.

Toxicity
Treatment-related deaths were rare but may be considered. In the LACE meta-analysis 19 chemotherapy-related deaths (0.9%) were reported and one third of adjuvant- treated patients experienced grade 3/4 toxicities with neutropenia being most frequent (9% grade III, 28% grade IV). The rate of overall grade IV toxicity was 32%. A small excess of deaths not related to lung cancer was seen in the treatment group with cardiovascular and pulmonary deaths, possibly related to the detrimental cardiovascular effect of cisplatin.

Compliance to Therapy
59% of all patients received at least 240 mg of cisplatin, 14% received only one chemotherapy cycle and 10% received only two cycles. In comparison, the effect of cisplatin plus vinorelbine was marginally better than the effect of other drug combinations. Comparing two doses levels of cisplatin (<300 or >300 mg/m^2), a trend in favor of higher dose was seen.

Postoperative Radiotherapy (PORT)
The effect of chemotherapy in the LACE meta-analysis was independent of the use of postoperative radiotherapy (PORT). Most of the patients, who received postoperative radiotherapy had stage III (N2) tumors.

Stages
Benefit varied considerably by stage of disease, with potential harm seen in patients with stage IA NSCLC, a trend towards benefit in stage IB patients and clear benefit in patients with stage II and IIIA NSCLC (HR 0.83; for patients with nodal involvement). This result supports the use of adjuvant chemotherapy for patients with resected stage II and IIIA NSCLC but leaves questions about therapy for those with stage I disease.

Adjuvant Chemotherapy and Stage (table 3)

- *Stage IA:* Adjuvant chemotherapy is not recommended in completely resected stage IA NSCLC patients. Studies included only a minority of patients in stage IA and survival analysis indicated that the prognosis of those patients did not improve with adjuvant chemotherapy.
- *Stage IB:* LACE showed a nonsignificant 3% improvement in stage IB (5-year survival improved from 64 to 67%). The IALT stage IB subgroup did not ben-

Table 2. LACE meta-analysis

Study	Result	Hazard ratio
ALPI [10], 2003	negative	0.95
ANITA [8], 2006	positive	0.82
BLT [11], 2004	negative	1.0
IALT [6], 2004	positive	0.91
JBR.10 [7], 2005	positive	0.71

Hazard ratio total: 0.89.
5-year overall survival: 43.5% (observation) vs. 48.8% (chemotherapy) = 5.3%.

Table 3. Adjuvant therapy: stages

Trial	Stage IA	Stage IB	Stage II	Stage IIIA
ALPI [10], 2003	negative	negative	negative	negative
IALT [6], 2004	negative	negative	negative	positive
JBR.10 [7], 2005	not tested	negative	positive	not tested
CALGB [9], 2008	not tested	positive ?	not tested	not tested
ANITA [8], 2006	not tested	negative	positive	positive

efit from chemotherapy and the JBR.10 study was only positive for stage II, not for IB patients (with the exception of IB tumors, larger than 4 cm in diameter). Subset analysis of the ANITA trial demonstrated that significant improvement in survival was restricted to stage II and IIIA patients and no benefit was observed in stage IB disease.

- *Conclusion:* Adjuvant chemotherapy is not recommended for routine use in IB patients.
- *Stage II:* Adjuvant cisplatin-based chemotherapy improves the overall survival in completely resected stage II NSCLC for 17% with a hazard ration of 0.83. All studies in stage II patients were clearly positive. Most patients (NCIC, ANITA, and IALT) were treated with a cisplatin/vinorelbine combination for 4 cycles.
- *Stage IIIA:* Adjuvant chemotherapy improved survival in stage IIIA completely resected patients, as shown in the IALT and ANITA trial. In the ANITA trial

(cisplatin/vinorelbine) the hazard ratio was 0.69 and in the IALT trial (n = 728, cisplatin and any combination partner, including second-generation NSCLC regimens) the hazard ratio was 0.79.

Which Chemotherapy Combination?

Most studies used a cisplatin-based combination. The only study using a carboplatin-based combination (carboplatin/paclitaxel) (9 CALB) in stage IB patients was negative. Data do not support the routine use of carboplatin in the adjuvant setting. Most patients were treated with cisplatin/vinorelbine, in conclusion cisplatin/vinorelbine is the best tested combination in adjuvant chemotherapy.

Adjuvant Radiotherapy

The PORT meta-analysis [4, 5] demonstrated adverse effects of postoperative radiotherapy in stage I and II patients on survival (HR: 1.21), mostly due to long-term detrimental effects on pulmonary and cardiac function. Of note is that radiotherapy techniques used in the PORT studies are considered suboptimal today.

In stage IIIA patients, the role of postoperative radiotherapy is controversial. Modern radiotherapy may reduce local recurrences and hopefully improves survival, but at the moment no modern prospective trials support this hypothesis. A large retrospective analysis of SEER data indicates superior survival rates for N2 patients under postoperative radiotherapy [13]. Simultaneous postoperative chemo- and radiotherapy in stage II and III was not superior to postoperative radiotherapy alone [3]. Survival did not differ between the two randomized treatment groups and even a trend towards better survival was seen in the only radiotherapy group (median survival 39 months only radiotherapy versus 38 months combination group with radiotherapy and 3 cycles cisplatin/etoposide). An unplanned analysis of the influence of postoperative radiotherapy in the ANITA study demonstrated a survival benefit under sequential chemo- and radiotherapy in a small subgroup of N2 patients [8].

Patient Selection and Predictive or Prognostic Factors

Age

Patients in the LACE meta-analysis [14] were divided into three age groups: 3,269 young (71%; <65 years), 901 mid-category (20%; 65–69 years), and 414 elderly patients (9%; >70 years) to study the effect of chemotherapy on survival according to age. More elderly patients died from non-lung cancer-related causes (12% young, 19% mid-category, 22% elderly; $p < 0.0001$). The analysis demonstrated that elderly patients who met the eligibility criteria for trial enrolment had a survival benefit from chemotherapy that was similar to that of their younger counterparts. These findings are consistent with those of the elderly analysis of JBR.10, which did not find any significant difference in survival benefit for patients older than 65 years of age [15]. Adjuvant cisplatin-based chemotherapy should not be withheld from elderly patients with NSCLC purely on the basis of age.

Performance Score 2

The LACE meta-analysis showed a significant interaction between chemotherapy effect and stage and performance score. Chemotherapy effect increased with better performance score and higher stage and may be detrimental in performance score 2.

ERCC1 (Excision Repair Cross-Complementation Group 1)

A retrospective analysis based on tumor specimens from patients included in the IALT trial indicated a better survival in patients with ERCC1-negative tumors and cisplatin treatment, indicating that ERCC1 analysis may be predictive for the response to cisplatin-based adjuvant chemotherapy [16]. Expression of RRM1, a regulatory subunit of ribonucleotide reductase, appears to be a good predictor for response to gemcitabine [17]. Future studies will investigate tumor expression of ERCC1 and RRM1 and will use these levels to assign patients to adjuvant therapy. Genomic tumor analysis is under investigation. Analysing tumor samples using the 'lung metagene' [18] protocol using the 'lung metagene score' has been shown to be a prognostic factor.

Other Biomarker Studies

No biomarker has been fully validated as a method to identify subgroups of patients. Published adjuvant trials have failed to show that biomarkers such as p53 mutations, p53 protein expression, and KRAS mutations have any prognostic or predictive value [19]. Class III beta-tubulin expression is under investigation as well as p27Kip1 expression.

Future studies will investigate the role of antivascular agents as bevacizumab and of 'small molecules' tyrosine kinase inhibitors in the adjuvant treatment (e.g. the RADIANT study). An ongoing study examines a vaccine to MAGE-A3, a tumor antigen found in up to 50% of early-stage NSCLC.

Neoadjuvant Chemotherapy

The use of preoperative (neoadjuvant) chemotherapy is under investigation. Recently, a meta-analysis of nearly 500 patients found a survival HR of 0.82 (95% CI 0.69–0.97), which is very close to the HR seen in the LACE meta-analysis of adjuvant therapy [20]. Until results of ongoing studies are known, adjuvant therapy will remain the standard. The NATCH trial, presented at ASCO and WCLC 2009, showed that preoperative chemotherapy had a nonsignificant trend towards improved 5-year DFS when compared to surgery alone.

Conclusion

The recommendation of 4 cycles of adjuvant platinum-based combination chemotherapy in patients with fully resected stage II and IIIA NSCLC is generally established. For example, the current ESMO clinical recommendation (2008) [22] is: 'Cisplatin-based adjuvant combination chemotherapy is recommended in stage II and IIIA [I, A], and can be considered in selected stage IB patients (T >4 cm).'

There is uncertainty about its prescription in those with resected stage IB NSCLC. The magnitude of benefit of adjuvant therapy is proportional and dependent on the risk of relapse according to stage. However, those high-risk factors that might support selection for adjuvant chemotherapy have not been defined with certainty.

The magnitude of survival benefit from adjuvant therapy based on the LACE meta-analysis therapy is estimated to be between 3% and 15%, depending on stage. The LACE analysis clearly confirms the benefits of adjuvant cisplatin-based chemotherapy in resected NSCLC patients in stage II and IIIA and further supports its use in routine clinical practice.

Both the National Comprehensive Cancer Network and the American Society of Clinical Oncology [21] recommend a cisplatin-based doublet as adjuvant therapy for patients with resected stage II and IIIA NSCLC; the role of adjuvant therapy for stage IB disease remains unknown. 15–20 patients must be treated for 1 patient to benefit.

PORT should not be used for stage I or II NSCLC, and it remains highly controversial in resected stage IIIA (N2) disease.

All of the positive adjuvant trials have utilized a cisplatin-based regimen, usually in combination with vinorelbine, and this should be considered the standard approach. Substitution with other platinum doublets can be considered, but cisplatin may be slightly superior to carboplatin and should remain the platinum drug of choice.

In future, it should be one of the treatment goals to optimize treatment convenience for the patients by using other combinations, with the hope of better efficacy results because of better patient's adherence to chemotherapy.

References

1 Mountain CF: Revisions in the international system for staging lung cancer. Chest 1997;111:1710–1717.

2 Non-Small Cell Lung Cancer Collaborative Group: Chemotherapy in non-small cell lung cancer: a meta-analysis using updated data on individual patients from 52 randomised clinical trials. Br Med J 1995;311:899–909.

3 Keller SM, Adak S, Wagner H, et al: A randomized trial of postoperative adjuvant therapy in patients with completely resected stage II or IIA non-small cell lung cancer. N Engl J Med 2000;343: 1217–1222.

4 PORT Meta-Analysis Trialists Group: Postoperative radiotherapy in non-small cell lung cancer: systematic review and meta-analysis of individual patient data from nine randomized controlled trials. Lancet 1998;352:257–263.

5 PORT Meta-Analysis Group, Burdett S, Stewart L: Postoperative radiotherapy in non-small-cell lung cancer: update of an individual patient data meta-analysis. Lung Cancer 2005;47:81–83.

6 Arriagada R, Bergman B, Dunant A, et al, The International Adjuvant Lung Cancer Trial Collaborative Group: Cisplatin-based adjuvant chemotherapy in patients with completely resected non-small cell lung cancer. N Engl J Med 2004; 350:351–360.

7 Winton T, Livingston R, Johnson D, et al: Vinorelbine plus cisplatin vs. observation in resected non-small-cell lung cancer. N Engl J Med 2005;352: 2589–2597.

8 Douillard JY, Rosell R, De Lena M, et al: Adjuvant vinorelbine plus cisplatin versus observation in patients with completely resected stage IB-IIIA non-small cell lung cancer (Adjuvant Navelbine International Trialist Association [ANITA]): a randomised controlled trial. Lancet Oncol 2006;7: 719–727.

9 Strauss GM, Herndon JE, Maddaus MA, Johnstone DW, Johnson EA, Harpole DH, Gillenwater HH, Watson DM, Sugarbaker DJ, Schilsky RL, Vokes EE, Green MR : Adjuvant paclitaxel plus carboplatin compared with observation in stage IB non–small-cell lung cancer: CALGB 9633 with the Cancer and Leukemia Group B, Radiation Therapy Oncology Group, and North Central Cancer Treatment Group Study Groups. J Clin Oncol 2008;26:5043–5051.

10 Scagliotti GV, Fossati R, Torri V, et al. Randomized study of adjuvant chemotherapy for completely resected stage I, II, or IIIA non-small-cell lung cancer. J Natl Cancer Inst 2003;95:1453–1461.

11 Waller D, Peake MD, Stephens RJ, et al: Chemotherapy for patients with non-small cell lung cancer: the surgical setting of the Big Lung Trial. Eur J Cardiothorac Surg 2004;26:173–182.

12 Pignon J-P, Tribodet H, Scagliotti GV, et al: Lung adjuvant cisplatin evaluation: a pooled analysis by the LACE Collaborative Group. J Clin Oncol 2008; 26:3552–3559.

13 Lally BE, Zelterman D, Colasanto JM, et al: Postoperative radiotherapy for stage II and III non–small-cell lung cancer using the Surveillance, Epidemiology, and End Results database. J Clin Oncol 2006;24:2998–3006.

14 Früh Martin, Rolland E, Pignon JP, Seymour L, Ding K, Tribodet H, Winton T, Le Chevalier T, Scagliotti GV, Douillard JY, Spiro S, Shepherd FA: Pooled analysis of the effect of age on adjuvant cisplatin-based chemotherapy for completely resected non–small-cell lung cancer. J Clin Oncol 2008;26:3573–3581.

15 Pepe C, Hasan B, Winton T, et al: Adjuvant vinorelbine and cisplatin in elderly patients: National Cancer Institute of Canada and Intergroup Study JBR.10. J Clin Oncol 2007;25:1553–1561.

16 Olaussen KA, Dunant A, Fouret P, et al: DNA repair by ERCC1 in non-small-cell lung cancer and cisplatin-based adjuvant chemotherapy. N Engl J Med 2006;355:983–991.

17 Zheng Z, Chen T, Li X, Haura E, Sharma A, Bepler G. DNA synthesis and repair genes RRM1 and ERCC1 in lung cancer. N Engl J Med. 2007;356: 800–808.
18 Potti A, Mukherjee S, Petersen R, et al: A genomic strategy to refine prognosis in early-stage non-small-cell lung cancer. N Engl J Med 2006;355: 570–580.
19 Schiller JH, Adak S, Feins RH, et al: Lack of prognostic significance of p53 and K-ras mutations in primary resected non-small-cell lung cancer on E4592: a laboratory ancillary study on an Eastern Cooperative Oncology Group prospective randomized trial of postoperative adjuvant therapy. J Clin Oncol 2001;19:448–457.
20 Gilligan D, Nicolson M, Smith I, et al: Preoperative chemotherapy in patients with respectable non-small cell lung cancer: results of the MRC LU22/NVALT 2/EORTC 08012 multicentre randomised trial and update of systematic review. Lancet 2007;369:1929–1937.
21 Pisters KM, Evans WK, Azzoli CG, et al: Cancer Care Ontario and American Society of Clinical Oncology Adjuvant Chemotherapy and Adjuvant Radiation Therapy for Stages I-IIIA Resectable Non Small-Cell Lung Cancer Guideline. J Clin Oncol 2007;25:5506–5518.
22 D'Addario G, Felip E, on behalf of the ESMO Guidelines Working Group: Non-small-cell lung cancer: ESMO Clinical Recommendations for diagnosis, treatment and follow-up. Ann Oncol 2009;20(suppl 4):iv68–iv70.

Dr. med. Monika Serke
CÄ Pneumologie III, Lungenklinik Hemer
Theo-Funccius-Strasse 1
DE–58675 Hemer (Germany)
Tel. +49 2372 9082201, Fax +49 2372 9089201, E-Mail monika.serke@lkhemer.de

Heide J, Schmittel A, Kaiser D, Hinkelbein W (eds): Controversies in the Treatment of Lung Cancer.
Front Radiat Ther Oncol. Basel, Karger, 2010, vol 42, pp 145–149

Postoperative Irradiation in Non-Small Cell Lung Cancer

Stefan Höcht[a,b] · Jürgen Heide[a] · Ronald Bischoff[b] · Olaf Gründel[b] · Detlef Carstens[b]

[a]Klinik für Radioonkologie und Strahlentherapie, Charité Universitätsmedizin Berlin, Campus Benjamin Franklin, Berlin, und [b]Gemeinschaftspraxis für Strahlentherapie an der Asklepios-Klinik St. Georg, Hamburg, Deutschland

Abstract

Adjuvant radiotherapy following radical surgery in NSCLC has long been a matter of debate. The pros and cons have all been discussed thoroughly and the data existing due to their partial outdated nature in respect of the diagnostic and therapeutic maneuvers used make it difficult to rely on them. Based on the existing level of evidence from randomized studies, the decision to irradiate a NSCLC patient postoperatively does not seem to be prudent, as several meta-analyses in fact have rather shown a detrimental effect than any benefit. As the majority of the randomized trials that are the bases of the meta-analyses are neither of good quality nor include those patients that are nowadays regarded as those for whom adjuvant irradiation should be discussed, other sources of information are of relevance. Subanalyses of randomized phase III trials and recently published SEER data are indicative that there is a benefit from adjuvant irradiation not only in terms of freedom from local failure but of overall survival as well. Notably, this is not at the expense of unacceptably high rates of long-term side effects.

Radiotherapy as an adjunct to surgery after potentially curative resection of non-small cell lung cancer (NSCLC) has since long been discussed as being controversial. The main argument in the debate is the uncontradicted ability of postoperative radiotherapy to reduce the probability of a recurrent intrathoracic tumor, which besides being lethal in many cases may also be a source of considerable morbidity and certainly has a tremendous impact on the quality of life in the remaining time span especially if not accompanied by distant metastasis.

On the other hand, side effects of radiotherapy can have a negative effect on several outcome parameters and due to potential worsening of pulmonary and cardiac functioning even be lethal. Given the high rates of metastasis, especially in locally advanced stages of NSCLC, the potential impact of adjuvant irradiation on survival by reducing the risk of locoregionally recurrent disease can only be marginal. From this point of view, a strategy of delayed palliative radiotherapy only for those patients who are symptomatic for intrathoracic tumor recurrence would be an acceptable option.

On the basis of the published meta-analysis of phase III trials on postoperative irradiation in NSCLC, early termination of this article would be possible, as the plain language summary of the latest version of the PORT-MATG [1] seems to leave no room for further debate: 'Radiotherapy given after surgery increases the risk of death for patients with early stage completely resected non-small cell lung cancer' due to an 18% increase of the relative risk of death for the irradiated patients [1].

Evidence-based medicine – nowadays sometimes regarded the utmost scientific recognition that obviates any further need to scrutinize the underlying data – cannot improve the quality of the original data nor the trial design. Although 10 randomized trials including 2,232 patients at first glance seem to be a robust basis for such a meta-analysis, the majority of the trials are very outdated and given the incidence of lung cancer worldwide the paucity of data from recently treated patients is astonishing [2–12]. In 1966, when the first studies started, staging and therapy were obviously dramatically different as neither computed tomography nor modern radiotherapy facilities existed and even since termination of the trial that ended patient accrual as the last one in 1997, huge developments in diagnostic and therapeutic maneuvers such as PET-CT and endoscopic ultrasound-guided fine-needle aspiration have taken place and have in part been validated [13–15].

This is not the only detail that makes it difficult to rely on the results. From today's point of view, adjuvant irradiation should be limited to patients with stage IIIA N2 disease or to the rare situation of stage IIIB N3 disease that was not realized preoperatively; on the other hand, the benefit of resection over concurrent chemoradiation in N2 disease is nowadays under debate. Single doses of 1.8–2.0 Gy and total doses of 50 Gy in the absence of residual disease are recommended [16]. If these criteria are applied, none of the 10 phase III studies would be regarded as state of the art, limiting any conclusions that can be drawn from them [2–12]. Even if less stringent criteria would be applied, only two of the studies, where stage II and III patients were treated with single and total doses in the range cited above, would seem acceptable [4, 9].

Limiting the meta-analysis to patients treated for stage III or N2 disease completely abandoned the negative effect of radiotherapy, although none of the criticisms on inadequate technique or dosing are resolved by that limitation. In these patients the meta-analysis showed a nonsignificant relative survival advantage of 3–4% [1].

We have to admit that inadequate irradiation, be it by outdated technique, obsolete single or total doses or improper patient selection, therefore has a proven detrimental effect on survival. Whether this still holds true for patients treated more recently and with adequate therapeutic regimens is of considerable interest. Two studies examined these issues by looking at DID data (dead of intercurrent disease) in comparison to a population adopted for age, sex and smoking habits, and both did not find a significant difference [17, 18]. Interestingly, the study by Machtay et al. [17] showed a strong negative effect of total doses above 54 Gy on the DID rate.

The potential survival benefit by an additive local therapy is not easy to detect and it is probably not unrelated to the benefits of systemic therapy. In breast cancer, for example, it took some 42,000 patients and 78 randomized phase III trials to elucidate the relationship of improved locoregional control and a survival benefit that became detectable later on [19]. As a benefit of a local therapy will only be detectable and of clinical relevance quo ad vitam, it is not unlikely that the now widespread use of adjuvant chemotherapy in NSCLC patients enhances the chance of a survival benefit by achieving a higher probability of local control due to adjuvant irradiation [20–22].

The analysis of the ANITA trial on adjuvant chemotherapy showed some hints of such an interaction, as in the initial publication of that study the results seemed to favor adjuvant irradiation added to adjuvant chemotherapy in NSCLC patients with N2 disease [23]. Additional information provided recently on that study makes these clues more likely to be artifacts and caused by chance, as the huge differences detected in different subgroups are unlikely to be attributable to the respective therapeutic interventions [24].

In the absence of other data with validity generated recently, the SEER analysis on the outcome of 7,465 stage II and IIIA NSCLC patients may be regarded a rather strong argument for adjuvant irradiation as in the subgroup of 1,987 N2 disease patients the use of adjuvant irradiation was associated with an improved survival hazard ratio of 0.85, i.e. a solid 15% benefit in overall survival. Given the retrospective nature of these data, it is not unlikely that the decision to administer irradiation in the presence of conflicting data on the general benefit of adjuvant irradiation was based on negative selection criteria in the patients treated and hence the real benefit of radiotherapy may even be greater [25]. Hopefully, the planned EORTC protocol 22055–08053 on adjuvant irradiation in resected N2 NSCLC will be able to solve many of the problems discussed above and will present a realistic view of the status of postoperative radiotherapy.

The target for adjuvant radiotherapy is a topic that has to be assessed separately. The benefit of local control is achieved by the eradication of microscopic or low volume macroscopic disease in the mediastinum. The likelihood of residual disease after surgery is probably not unrelated to the ability to detect metastatic spread preoperatively. PET-CT, EUS-FNA and innovative surgical techniques as VAMLA might therefore have the potential to reduce residual tumor burden and by doing so reduce the probability that the addition of radiotherapy may be beneficial [26–28]. The relatively low rates of elective nodal failure in involved-field radiation therapy in NSCLC point in the same direction, thus increasing the need for data generated in the third millennium [29].

References

1 PORT Meta-Analysis Trialists Group: Postoperative radiotherapy for non-small cell lung cancer. Cochrane Database of Systematic Reviews 2005, Issue 2. Art. No.: CD002142. DOI: 10.1002/14651858.CD002142.pub2.

2 van Houtte P, Rocmans P, Smets P, et al: Postoperative radiation therapy in lung cancer: a controlled trial after resection of curative design. Int J Radiat Oncol Biol Phys 1980;6:983–986.

3 Feng QF, Wang M, Wang LJ, et al: A study of postoperative radiotherapy in patients with non-small cell lung cancer: a randomized trial. Int J Radiat Oncol Biol Phys 2000;47:925–929.

4 van Zandwijk N, Gregor A, Rocmans P: EORTC 08861 – phase III randomised trial of adjuvant radiotherapy vs. no adjuvant therapy with completely resected non-small cell lung cancer. Data reported in PORT Meta-analysis Trialists Group [1].

5 Dautzenberg B, Arriagada R, Chammard AB, et al: A controlled study of postoperative radiotherapy for patients with completely resected non-small cell lung carcinoma: Groupe d'Etude et de Traitement des Cancers Bronchiques. Cancer 1999;86: 265–273.

6 Dautzenberg B, Arriagada R, Chammard AB, et al: A randomised trial evaluating post-op RT in NSCLC after complete surgical resection. Additional data reported in PORT Meta-analysis Trialists Group [1].

7 Dautzenberg B, Arriagada R, Chammard AB, et al: A randomised trial evaluating post-op RT in NSCLC after complete surgical resection. Additional data reported in: PORT Meta-analysis Trialists Group [1].

8 Trodella L, Granone P, Valente S, et al: Adjuvant radiotherapy in non-small cell lung cancer with pathological stage I: definitive results of a phase III randomised trial. Radiother Oncol 2002;62:11–19.

9 Lung Cancer Study Group: Effects of postoperative mediastinal radiation on completely resected stage II and stage III epidermoid cancer of the lung. N Engl J Med 1986;315:1377–1381.

10 Lafitte JJ, Ribet ME, Prévost BM, Gosselin BH, Copin M-C, Brichet AH: Post-irradiation for T2 N0 M0 non-small cell carcinoma: a prospective randomized study. Ann Thorac Surg 1996;62:830–834.

11 Stephens RJ, Girling DJ, Bleehen NM, Moghissi K, Yosef HMA, Machin D: The role of post-operative radiotherapy in non-small cell lung cancer: a multicentre randomised trial in patients with pathologically staged T1–2, N1–2, M0 disease. Br J Cancer 1996;74:632–639.

12 Debevec M, Bitenc M, Vidmar S, et al: Post-operative radiotherapy for radically resected N2 non-small cell lung cancer: randomised clinical study 1988–92. Lung Cancer 1996;14:99–107.

13 Eloubeidi MA: Endoscopic ultrasound-guided fine-needle aspiration in the staging and diagnosis of patients with lung cancer. Semin Thorac Cardiovasc Surg 2007;19:206–211.

14 de Geus-Oei LF, van der Heijden HF, Corstens FH, Oyen WJ: Predictive and prognostic value of FDG-PET in nonsmall-cell lung cancer: a systematic review. Cancer 2007;110:1654–1664.

15 de Langen AJ, Raijmakers P, Riphagen I, Paul MA, Hoekstra OS: The size of mediastinal lymph nodes and its relation with metastatic involvement: a meta-analysis. Eur J Cardiothorac Surg 2006; 29:26–29.

16 National Comprehensive Cancer Network: NCCN Practice Guidelines in Oncology: Non-small cell lung cancer: v2.2009:http://www.nccn.org/professionals/physician_gls/PDF/nscl.pdf (accessed November 9th, 2008).

17 Machtay M, Lee JH, Shrager JB, Kaiser LR, Glatstein E: Risk of death from intercurrent disease is not excessively increased by modern postoperative radiotherapy for high-risk resected non-small-cell lung carcinoma. J Clin Oncol 2001;19: 3912–3917.

18 Wakelee HA, Stephenson P, Keller SM, et al: Eastern Cooperative Oncology Group: Post-operative radiotherapy (PORT) or chemoradiotherapy (CPORT) following resection of stages II and IIIA non-small cell lung cancer (NSCLC) does not increase the expected risk of death from intercurrent disease (DID) in Eastern Cooperative Oncology Group (ECOG) trial E3590. Lung Cancer 2005; 48:389–397.

19 Early Breast Cancer Trialists' Collaborative Group (EBCTCG): Effects of radiotherapy and of differences in the extent of surgery for early breast cancer on local recurrence and 15-year survival: an overview of the randomised trials. Lancet 2005; 366:2087–2106.

20 Punglia RS, Morrow M, Winer EP, Harris JR: Local therapy and survival in breast cancer. N Engl J Med 2007;356:2399–2405.

21 Le Chevalier T, Arriagada R, Pignon JP, Scagliotti GV: Should adjuvant chemotherapy become standard treatment in all patients with resected non-small-cell lung cancer? Lancet Oncol 2005;6: 182–184.

22 Pignon JP, Tribodet H, Scagliotti GV, et al: Lung adjuvant cisplatin evaluation: a pooled analysis by the LACE Collaborative Group. J Clin Oncol 2008; 26:3552–3559.

23 Douillard JY, Rosell R, De Lena M, et al: Adjuvant vinorelbine plus cisplatin versus observation in patients with completely resected stage IB-IIIA non-small-cell lung cancer (Adjuvant Navelbine International Trialist Association ANITA): a randomised controlled trial. Lancet Oncol 2006;7: 719–727.

24 Douillard JY, Rosell R, De Lena M, Riggi M, Hurteloup P, Mahe MA, Adjuvant Navelbine International Trialist Association: Impact of postoperative radiation therapy on survival in patients with complete resection and stage I, II, or IIIA non-small-cell lung cancer treated with adjuvant chemotherapy: the Adjuvant Navelbine International Trialist Association (ANITA) Randomized Trial. Int J Radiat Oncol Biol Phys 2008;72:695–701.

25 Lally BE, Detterbeck FC, Geiger AM, et al: The risk of death from heart disease in patients with nonsmall cell lung cancer who receive postoperative radiotherapy: analysis of the Surveillance, Epidemiology, and End Results database. Cancer 2007;110:911–917.

26 Craanen ME, Comans EF, Paul MA, Smit EF: Endoscopic ultrasound guided fine-needle aspiration and 18FDG-positron emission tomography in the evaluation of patients with non-small cell lung cancer. Interact Cardiovasc Thorac Surg 2007;6:433–436.

27 Kramer H, Sanders J, Post WJ, Groen HJ, Suurmeijer AJ: Analysis of cytological specimens from mediastinal lesions obtained by endoscopic ultrasound-guided fine-needle aspiration. Cancer 2006; 108:206–211.

28 Witte B, Hürtgen M: Video-assisted mediastinoscopic lymphadenectomy (VAMLA). J Thorac Oncol 2007;2:367–369.

29 Rosenzweig KE, Sura S, Jackson A, Yorke E: Involved-field radiation therapy for inoperable non small-cell lung cancer. J Clin Oncol 2007; 25:5557–5561.

Prof. Dr. Stefan Höcht
Gemeinschaftspraxis für Strahlentherapie an der Asklepios-Klinik St. Georg
Lohmühlenstrasse 5
DE–20099 Hamburg
Tel. +49 40 18 18 85 25 76, Fax +49 40 18 18 85 31 29, E-Mail stefan.hoecht@alice-dsl.net

Heide J, Schmittel A, Kaiser D, Hinkelbein W (eds): Controversies in the Treatment of Lung Cancer.
Front Radiat Ther Oncol. Basel, Karger, 2010, vol 42, pp 150–156

Altered Fractionation Schemes in Radiotherapy

Martin Stuschke · Christoph Pöttgen

Department of Radiotherapy, University of Duisburg-Essen, Essen, Germany

Abstract

Hyperfractionation and hypofractionation combined with acceleration have been investigated in stage I-III NSCLC patients. In stage I tumors, hypofractionated radiation schedules given with highly conformal stereotactic body radiotherapy (SBRT) techniques have been proven safe and effective with local control rates >85% and meanwhile have been accepted as the standard treatment in stage I patients who are medically unfit for surgery or who refuse resection. When comparing the dose-effect relationship derived from local control data of various clinical studies using conventional fractionation (CF) with that obtained from SBRT trials using doses per fraction from 7.5 to 30 Gy based on the linear quadratic model without parameters considering repopulation or hypoxia, the α/β ratio for biological equivalent doses with the different fractionation schedules was found to be 8.2 (7.0–9.4) Gy for stage I NSCLC. From this, it can be concluded that using an α/β value of 10 Gy for tumors is conservative, underestimating the BED of SBRT schedules relative to CF schedules with regard to tumor control. If repopulation is the dominant resistance-promoting factor for CF schedules and hypoxia for hypofractionated SBRT schedules, and the true α/β value of tumors is assumed to be 10 Gy, then the observed α/β value of 8.2 Gy can imply that the effect of repopulation during CF is higher than the effect of hypoxia during SBRT. Patients with locally advanced NSCLC in whom contraindications preclude the use of concurrent chemotherapy with CF radiotherapy may be treated outside clinical trials with CHART. Combinations of hyperfractionated-accelerated RT schedules with concurrent platinum-based chemotherapy have been proven safe and effective in stage III NSCLC patients.

External-beam radiotherapy in conventional fractionation (CF; 2 Gy/fraction, 5 daily fractions per week) up to total doses of 60–74 Gy in combination with concurrent platinum-based chemotherapy represents a standard treatment option in stage III NSCLC [1]. Similarly, CF radiotherapy has been considered standard for a long time in stage I patients who do not qualify for surgery [2]. Meanwhile, altered fractionation schedules have gained an accepted role in radiation oncology concepts for stage I–III NSCLC which will be reviewed in the following sections.

Hypofractionated Stereotactic Body Radiotherapy for NSCLC (Stage I)

Fractionation represents a method for improving the therapeutic ratio between the effects of ionizing irradiation on tumor cells on the one hand and on normal tissues on the other. Especially, when sensitive dose-limiting normal tissues are included in the PTV or a considerable dose-volume exposure of sensitive organs around the PTV exists, the often assumed lower fractionation sensitivity of tumor cells offers the possibility to reduce normal tissue toxicity to a greater extent than tumor control by fractionated irradiation in comparison with single-session high-dose radiotherapy. However, the amount of normal tissue at risk might be rather low, especially in peripheral stage I tumors. Furthermore, highly conformal radiotherapy plans with multiple (usually ≥7) fields and additional maneuvers to reduce tumor motion due to breathing (gating, tracking, breath hold) will produce sufficiently steep dose gradients around the PTV. Consequently, the integral lung dose will remain within tolerable limits and even the critical amount of normal tissue receiving high doses per fraction (>2 Gy) when using a hypofractionated treatment regime will remain low.

Several studies have shown mature results with regard to effectiveness and tolerability of SBRT with 1–8 fractions of 7.5–30 Gy in stage I NSCLC.

For the present analysis, we used the minimum dose values within the PTV for comparison of the effectiveness of the different fractionation schedules given in published SBRT studies. The results of these studies demonstrate that the PTV can be treated with SBRT as a means of hypofractionated high-precision radiotherapy with sufficiently high doses within normal tissue constraints achieving local control rates >85%. The group from Amsterdam has shown that the application of 8 × 7.5 Gy in stage I tumors adjacent to central structures (heart, hilum, mediastinum) remain safe and effective with a local control rate >90% [3], whereas Timmerman et al. [4] observed an increased (grade 3–5) toxicity following irradiation of perihilar/centrally located tumors with 3 × 20 Gy. However, stage I tumors in peripheral location have been treated effectively with 3 × 20 Gy (within 2 weeks) resulting in local control rates >90% at 2 years with excellent acute and chronic toxicity profiles [3, 4].

In order to compare the dose-effect relation of hypofractionated SBRT in stage I NSCLC with doses per fraction ≥7.5 Gy and total treatment times ≤14 days with CF or hyperfractionated RT and total treatment times of 6–8 weeks, we analyzed published SBRT series which included ≥25 patients with stage I tumors. Studies were selected for this analysis when the amount of patients with T1 tumors was

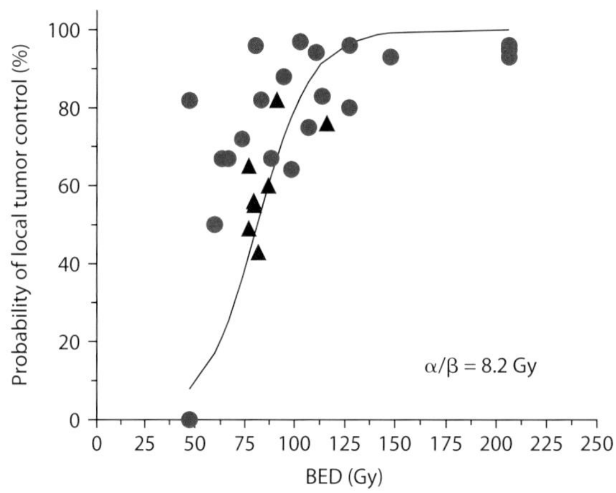

Fig. 1. Logistic dose-effect relation fitted to the data from clinical studies using hypofractionated SBRT (●) [3–11, 28–33] or CF (▲) schedules [14–20]. The curves for SBRT and CF schedules were not significantly different using α/β values for BED calculation of 8.2 Gy (7.0–9.4).

similar to the amount of T2 tumors, accounting for 35–65% of the treated lesions. Especially, phase I studies with dose-finding phases were included. A large variety of doses per fraction and total doses were given within the selected SBRT series [4–11]. Figure 1 shows the relation between local control rates and biologic effective doses (BED) of the different SBRT series. The dose response relation fitted to the data was a logistic model assuming 0% tumor control at 0 Gy BED (SAS statistical software: proc probit). The BED according to the linear-quadratic (LQ) model depends on the dose per fraction dose d, the total dose D, and the fractionation sensitivity of the tumor α/β: $BED = D*(1+d/(\alpha/\beta))$. When repopulation or hypoxia are not effective during RT, α/β represents a parameter for recovery from the sublethal radiation damage. Some extensions of this model exist in order to account for the influence of repopulation and reoxygenation [12, 13]. However, in the present analysis, the basic version of the LQ model was chosen for the description of the SBRT data as it is common practice. Furthermore, the clinical data are not sufficient to estimate multiple parameters of more complex models. In addition, figure 1 shows the local tumor control-BED data pairs from clinical series using doses per fraction of ≤2.5 Gy, labeled as 'CF' schedules [14–20]. The α/β value obtained was optimized so that SBRT and CF series follow the same BED-response relation. The resulting α/β ratio was 8.2 (7.0–9.4) Gy. This value allows calculation of an isoeffective CF schedule for a given SBRT schedule. Usually, an α/β of 10 Gy has been assumed for tumors [3, 7]. The here obtained α/β ratio of 8.2 (7.0–9.4) Gy which is significantly lower, indicates that the assumption $\alpha/\beta = 10$

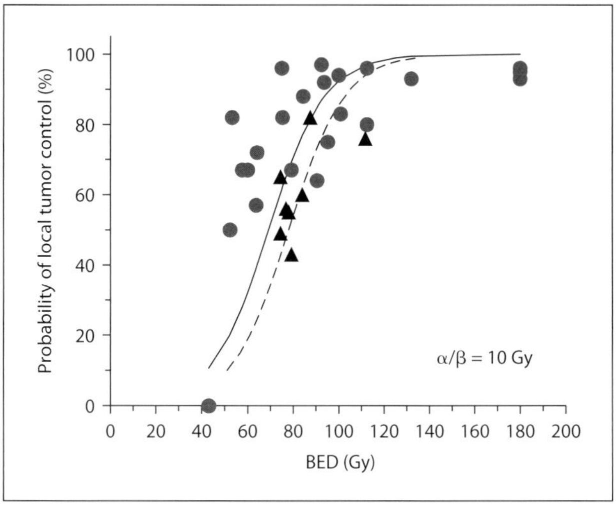

Fig. 2. Logistic dose-effect curves of the data from SBRT (●) [3–11, 28–33] and CF schedules (▲) [14–20] assuming an α/β value of 10 Gy for BED calculation. The BED needed to control 50% of the tumors was 69 Gy (67–71) for SBRT schedules. The dose-response curve for CF schedules was shifted to higher BED in comparison to SBRT schedules, the difference was 8.8 Gy (5.8–11.9).

Gy is conservative in that the efficacy of an SBRT in comparison to CF will be underestimated.

Due to the increasing log-linear tumor cell kill beyond the shoulder and the confounding effects of repopulation and hypoxia, deviations from the basic LQ model might exist for schedules with doses per fraction ≥7.5 Gy. Since the available clinical data are not sufficient for a multiparameter estimation, the obtained overall α/β value can be influenced by these confounding factors. For the SBRT series hypoxia due to less reoxygenation between the limited number fractions might be considered as the prevailing factor parameter modifying radiation response of the tumors whereas repopulation might be considered the major factor for CF schedules. The obtained α/β of 8.2 (7.0–9.4) Gy underscores that SBRT schedules might have higher efficacy than has been expected with the traditional α/β value of 10 Gy without considering repopulation and hypoxia. The other way round, it can be concluded that the influence of repopulation on the effect of CF is larger than that of hypoxia on the effect of SBRT under the assumption that the traditional α/β value of 10 Gy correctly describes the fractionation sensitivity of tumors over the range of doses per fractions used for stage I NSCLC in the clinic.

Figure 2 shows the separate dose-effect relations of SBRT and CF schedules under the assumption of α/β = 10 Gy. A statistically significant difference between both curves exists, characterized by a BED difference of 8.8 Gy (5.8–11.9) which is less than the calculated BED difference of 15 Gy obtained from the CHART trial for differences in repopulation between CHART and CF irradiation [12].

In summary, high BED can be applied by hypofractionated SBRT regimes within normal tissue constraints so that local control rates >90% are achievable. Based on the obtained dose-effect curves, a BED of >110 Gy is necessary assuming an α/β ratio of 8.2 Gy (fig. 1). An α/β ratio of 8.2 Gy was found to be the best α/β estimate for the comparison of the different fractionation schemes for stage I NSCLC. From the high tumor control rates after SBRT, it can be concluded that hypoxia is of less importance for SBRT regimes than repopulation for CF schedules.

Hyperfractionated Accelerated Radiotherapy for Stage III NSCLC

Randomized trials were performed using pure hyperfractionation (i.e. smaller doses per fraction than CF, same overall treatment time, 10–20% higher total dose than CF [21]) or pure acceleration (i.e. same dose per fraction and total dose than CF, shorter overall treatment time [22]) in comparison to CF for patients with inoperable NSCLC without distant metastases, most in stage III. Both of these trials did not demonstrate a significant increase in effectiveness of these schedules though their power to detect reasonable fractionation effects was low due to the limited number of patients treated. Before simultaneous chemotherapy became the standard in combination with definitive radiotherapy, the CHART (continuous hyperfractionated accelerated radiotherapy) trial was conducted [23]. A dose of 1.5 Gy per fraction, given three times a day at intervals of at least 6 h to a limited target volume over 12 consecutive days up to a total dose of 54 Gy was found to be more effective than CF up to 60 Gy. The majority of patients in the CHART trial had stage III disease. CHART is a recognized trial in European guidelines and can be given for patients with locally advanced disease not suited for surgery or definitive radio-chemotherapy (NICE guideline [24]). Hyperfractionated accelerated radiotherapy (HART) and concomitant chemotherapy has also been successfully combined with concurrent cisplatin-containing chemotherapy. Especially, a schedule of 2 × 1.5 Gy per fraction with at least 6 h interval at 5 days per week to total doses of 45 Gy has been employed. In limited-disease small-cell lung cancer, Turrisi et al. [25] have shown a gain of HART of up to 45 Gy over CF to 45 Gy given early together with 4 cycles of cisplatin/etoposide chemotherapy. The Essen Group uses HART up to 45 Gy followed by CF up to a total dose of 71 Gy for NSCLC in stage III in the running ESPATÜ trial with promising toxicity data [26]. However, the superiority of concurrent chemo-radiotherapy with hyperfractionated accelerated schedules in comparison with conventional fractionation parallel to chemotherapy has not yet been proven by randomized trials despite theoretical advantages and documented safety [26, 27].

References

1 NCCN Guideline: Assessed March 2009: Non-small cell lung cancer V.2.2009; in Network NCC (ed): Clinical Practice Guidelines in Oncology, vol 2008. NCCN, 2009.

2 Rowell NP, Williams CJ: Radical radiotherapy for stage I/II non-small cell lung cancer in patients not sufficiently fit for or declining surgery (medically inoperable): a systematic review. Thorax 2001;56:628–638.

3 Lagerwaard FJ, Haasbeek CJA, Smit EF, Slotman BJ, Senan S: Outcomes of risk-adapted fractionated stereotactic radiotherapy for stage I non-small cell lung cancer. Int J Radiat Oncol Biol Phys 2008;70:685–692.

4 Timmerman R, McGarry R, Yiannoutsos C, Papiez L, Tudor K, DeLuca J, Ewing M, Abdulrahman R, DesRosiers C, Williams M, Fletcher J: Excessive toxicity when treating central tumors in a phase II study of stereotactic body radiation therapy for medically inoperable early-stage lung dancer. J Clin Oncol 2006;24:4833–4839.

5 Nagata Y, Takayama K, Matsuo Y, Norihisa Y, Mizowaki T, Sakamoto T, Sakamoto M, Mitsumori M, Shibuya K, Araki N, Yano S, Hiraoka M: Clinical outcomes of a phase I/II study of 48 Gy of stereotactic body radiotherapy in 4 fractions for primary lung cancer using a stereotactic body frame. Int J Radiat Oncol Biol Phys 2005;63:1427–1431.

6 Onimaru R, Fujino M, Yamazaki K, Onodera Y, Taguchi H, Katoh N, Homura F, Oizumi S, Nishimura M, Shirato H: Steep dose-response relationship for stage I non-small cell lung cancer using hypofractionated high-dose irradiation by real-time tumor-tracking radiotherapy. Int J Radiat Oncol Biol Phys 2008;70:374–381.

7 Onishi H, Shirato H, Nagata Y, Hiraoka M, Fujino M, Gomi K, Niibe Y, Karasawa K, Hayakawa K, Takai Y, Kimura T, Takeda A, Ouchi A, Hareyama M, Kokubo M, Hara R: Hypofractionated stereotactic radiotherapy (HypoFXSRT) for stage I non-small cell lung cancer: updated results of 257 patients in a Japanese multi-institutional study. J Thorac Oncol 2007;2(suppl 3):S94–S100.

8 Takeda A, Sanuki N, Kunieda E, Ohashi T, Oku Y, Takeda T, Shigematsu N, Kubo A: Stereotactic body radiotherapy for primary lung cancer at a dose of 50 Gy total in five fractions to the periphery of the planning target volume calculated using a superposition algorithm. Int J Radiat Oncol Biol Phys 2009;73:442–448.

9 Xia T, Li H, Sun Q, Wang Y, Fan N, Yu Y, Li P, Chang JY: Promising clinical outcome of stereotactic body radiation therapy for patients with inoperable stage I/II non-small cell lung cancer. Int J Radiat Oncol Biol Phys 2006;66:117–125.

10 Zimmermann FB, Geinitz H, Schill S, Thamm R, Nieder C, Schratzenstaller U, Molls M: Stereotactic hypofractionated radiotherapy in stage I (T1–2 N0 M0) non-small-cell lung cancer (NSCLC). Acta Oncol 2006;45:796–801.

11 Nymann J, Johansson KA, Hultén U: Stereotactic hypofractionated radiotherapy for stage I non-small cell lung cancer: mature results for medically inoperable patients. Lung Cancer 2006;51: 97–103.

12 Bentzen SM, Saunders MI, Dische S: From CHART to CHARTWEL in non-small cell lung cancer: clinical radiobiological modeling of the expected change in outcome. Clin Oncol 2002;14: 372–381.

13 Nahum AE, Movsas B, Horwitz EM, Stobbe CC, Chapman JD: Incorporating clinical measurements of hypoxia into tumor local control modeling of prostate cancer: implications for the a/b ratio. Int J Radiat Oncol Biol Phys 2003;57:391–401.

14 Jeremic B, Shibamoto Y, Acimovic L, Milisavljevic S: Hyperfractionated radiotherapy alone for clinical stage I non-small cell lung cancer. Int J Radiat Oncol Biol Phys 1997;38:521–525.

15 Lagerwaard FJ, Senan S, van Meerbeeck JP, Graveland WJ, on behalf of the Rotterdam Oncological Thoracic Study Group: Has 3-D conformal radiotherapy improved the local tumour control for stage I non-small cell lung cancer. Radiother Oncol 2002;63:151–157.

16 Morita K, Fuwa N, Suzuki Y, Nishio M, Sakai K, Tamaki Y, Niibe H, Chujo M, Wada S, Sugrawara T, Kita M: Radical radiotherapy for medically inoperable non-small cell lung cancer in clinical stage I: a retrospective analysis of 149 patients. Radiother Oncol 1997;42:31–36.

17 Bogart JA, Alpert TE, Kilpatrick MC, Keshler BL, Pohar SS, Shah H, Dexter E, Aronowitz JN: Dose-intensive thoracic radiation therapy for patients with early-stage non-small-cell lung cancer. Clin Lung Cancer 2005;6:350–354.

18 Henning GT, Littles JF, Martel ML, Ten Haken R, Lichter AS, Hayman JA: Preliminary results of 92.4 Gy or more for non-small cell lung cancer (abstract). Int J Radiat Oncol Biol Phys 2000; 48(suppl 1):233.

19 Kupelian PA, Komaki R, Allen P: Prognostic factors in the treatment of node-negative nonsmall cell lung carcinoma with radiotherapy alone. Int J Radiat Oncol Biol Phys 1996;36:607–613.

20 Dosoretz DE, Katin MJ, Blitzer PH: Radiation therapy in the management of medically inoperable carcinoma of the lung: results and implications for future treatment strategies. Int J Radiat Oncol Biol Phys 1992;24:3–9.

21 Sause W, Kolesar P, Taylor S, Johnson D, Livingston R, Komaki R, Emami B, Curran W, Byhardt R, Dar AR, Turrisi A: Final results of phase III trial in regionally advanced unresectable non-small cell lung cancer. Chest 2000;117:358–364.

22 Ball D, Bishop J, Smith J, O'Brien P, Davis S, Ryan G, Olver I, Toner G, Walker Q, Joseph D: A randomised phase III study of accelerated or standard fraction radiotherapy with or without concurrent carboplatin in inoperable nonsmall cell lung cancer: final report of an Australian multi-centre trial. Radiother Oncol 1999;52:129–136.

23 Saunders M, Dische S, Barrett A, Harvey A, Gibson D, Parmar M, on behalf of the CHART Steering Committee: Continuous hyperfractionated accelerated radiotherapy (CHART) versus conventional radiotherapy in non-small-cell lung cancer: a randomised multicentre trial. Lancet 1997; 350:161–165.

24 National Institute for Clinical Excellence: Clinical Guideline 24; Lung cancer: the diagnosis and treatment of lung cancer: February 2005. www.nice.org.uk/CG024NICEguideline.

25 Turrisi AT, Kim K, Blum R, Sause WT, Livingston RB, Komaki R, Wagner H, Aisner S, Johnson DH: Twice-daily compared with once-daily thoracic radiotherapy in limited small-cell lung cancer treated concurrently with cisplatin and etoposide. N Engl J Med 1999;340:265–271.

26 Pöttgen C, Eberhardt W, Gauler T, Krbek T, Berkovic K, Abu Jawad J, Korfee S, Teschler H, Stamatis G, Stuschke M: Intensified high-dose chemoradiotherapy with induction chemotherapy in patients with locally advanced non-small-cell lung cancer – safety and toxicity results within a prospective trial. Int J Radiat Onol Biol Phys 2009 May 7 [epub ahead of print, PMID 19427744].

27 Van Baardwijk A, Bosmans G, Bentzen SM, Boersma L, Decker A, Wanders R, Wouters BG, Lambin P, De Ruysscher D: Radiation dose prescription for non-small-cell lung cancer according to normal tissue dose constraints: an in silico clinical trial. Int J Radiat Oncol Biol Phys 2008; 71:1103–1110.

28 Baumann P, Nyman J, Lax I, Friesland S, Hoyer M, Ericsson SR, Johansson KA, Ekberg L, Morhed E, Paludan M, Wittgren L, Blomgren H, Lewensohn R: Factors important for efficacy of stereotactic body radiotherapy of medically inoperable stage I lung cancer: a retrospective analysis of patients treated in the Nordic countries. Acta Oncol 2006;45:787–795.

29 Baumann P, Nyman J, Hoyer M, Gagliardi G, Lax I, Wennberg B, Drugge N, Ekberg L, Friesland S, Johansson KA, Lund JS, Morhed E, Nilsson K, Levin N, Paludan M, Sederholm C, Traberg A, Wittgren L, Lewensohn R: Stereotactic body radiotherapy for medically inoperable patients with stage I non-small cell lung cancer: a first report of toxicity related to COPD/CVD in a non-randomized prospective phase II study. Radiother Oncol 2008;88:359–367.

30 Fritz P, Kraus HJ, Mühlnickel W, Hammer U, Dölken W, Engel-Riedel W, Chemaissani A, Stoelben E: Stereotactic, single-dose irradiation of stage I non-small cell lung cancer and lung metastases. Radiat Oncol 2006;1:30–39

31 Hof H, Muenter M, Oetzel D, Hoess A, Debus J, Herfarth K: Stereotactic single-dose radiotherapy (radiosurgery) of early stage nonsmall-cell lung cancer (NSCLC). Cancer 2007;110:148–155.

32 Koto M, Takai Y, Ogawa Y, Matsushita H, Takeda K, Takahashi C, Britton KR, Jingu K, Takai K, Mitsuya M, Nemoto K, Yamada S: A phase II study on stereotactic body radiotherapy for stage I non-small cell lung cancer. Radiother Oncol 2007;85:429–434.

33 McGarry RC, Papiez L, Williams M, Whitford T, Timmerman RD: Stereotactic body radiation therapy of early-stage non-small-cell lung carcinoma: phase II study. Int J Radiat Oncol Biol Phys 2005;63:1010–1015.

Prof. Dr. med. Martin Stuschke
Department of Radiotherapy, University of Duisburg-Essen
Hufelandstrasse 55
DE–45122 Essen (Germany)
Tel. +49 201 723 2321, Fax +49 201 723 5960, E-Mail martin.stuschke@uk-essen.de

Heide J, Schmittel A, Kaiser D, Hinkelbein W (eds): Controversies in the Treatment of Lung Cancer.
Front Radiat Ther Oncol. Basel, Karger, 2010, vol 42, pp 157–163

Chemotherapy of Advanced Non-Small Cell Lung Cancer

Robert Pirker · Wilma Minar

Department of Medicine I, Medical University of Vienna, Vienna, Austria

Abstract

Patients with advanced NSCLC receive palliative chemotherapy with platinum-based doublets. Cisplatin-based doublets are preferred in patients with good performance status, whereas carboplatin-based protocols are preferred in patients with impaired organ functions (kidney, heart). Customized chemotherapy appears promising but still remains experimental. Improvements of the outcome of first-line chemotherapy have been achieved by the addition of cetuximab in patients with EGFR-positive NSCLC and of bevacizumab in selected patients with non-squamous cell NSCLC. The optimal combination of chemotherapy with targeted therapies remains a challenge. Maintenance therapy and early second-line chemotherapy might improve outcome but are not yet considered as standard treatments. Patients progressing after first-line chemotherapy are treated with docetaxel, pemetrexed or erlotinib. Finally, the efficacy of new anticancer treatments should be assessed by several clinical endpoints with overall survival remaining the most important endpoint in patients with advanced NSCLC.

Palliative chemotherapy of advanced non-small cell lung cancer (NSCLC) is well established. Chemo-naïve patients are treated with up to 6 cycles of platinum-based doublets containing third-generation anticancer drugs [1]. Chemotherapy improves cancer-related symptoms and increases survival compared to best supportive care alone. Patients progressing after first-line chemotherapy are currently treated with either docetaxel, pemetrexed or erlotinib.

Open issues including controversies are the role of pemetrexed, the preferential platin, the possibility of customized chemotherapy, the optimal integration of targeted therapies, the impact of maintenance therapy, the optimal time for initiation as well as the type of second-line therapy, and the most appropriate endpoint in clinical trials.

Pemetrexed

Pemetrexed is a multitargeted antifolate and has been established as a second-line therapy in patients with advanced NSCLC [2]. Cisplatin plus pemetrexed was recently compared to cisplatin/gemcitabine in chemo-naive patients with advanced NSCLC [3]. The primary goal to demonstrate noninferiority of cisplatin/pemetrexed compared to cisplatin/gemcitabine was achieved with a median survival of 10.3 months in both arms. In a pre-planned subgroup analysis, however, cisplatin/pemetrexed was shown to be superior to cisplatin/gemcitabine in patients with nonsquamous NSCLC with median survival times of 12.6 and 10.9 months, respectively. In patients with squamous cell carcinomas, survival was better for cisplatin/gemcitabine than for cisplatin/pemetrexed (median 10.8 vs. 9.4 months). Thus, this is the first prospective trial to demonstrate the predictive value of histology for the outcome of palliative chemotherapy in patients with advanced NSCLC. Based on these findings, cisplatin plus pemetrexed is increasingly used as a first-line treatment in patients with nonsquamous NSCLC. However, some doctors are still reluctant to consider it as a standard option due to its high costs and the fact that its superiority has been shown only in a subgroup analysis.

Cisplatin- vs. Carboplatin-Based Chemotherapy

The preferential platin, cisplatin or carboplatin, still remains a matter of debate. While some trials suggested or even proved the superiority of cisplatin-based protocols over their carboplatin counterparts, none of the trials could demonstrate a superiority of carboplatin-based protocols over their cisplatin counterparts. A recent meta-analysis which included 2,968 patients from 9 randomized trials confirmed the advantages of cisplatin-based protocols [4]. Cisplatin-based chemotherapy compared to carboplatin-based chemotherapy resulted in a higher response rate (30 vs. 24%). Carboplatin-based protocols were associated with an increase in mortality in patients treated with third-generation anticancer drugs (HR = 1.11; 95% CI 1.01–1.21) and also in patients with nonsquamous NSCLC (HR = 1.12; 95% CI 1.01–1.23).

The two platins have different toxicity profiles. Cisplatin-based chemotherapy primarily leads to nausea/emesis and potential nephrotoxicity and, therefore, requires efficient antiemetic therapy and adequate hydration. Carboplatin-based protocols primarily lead to hematotoxicity, particularly thrombocytopenia.

In daily practice, cisplatin-based chemotherapy should be preferred in patients with good performance status and adequate organ functions (kidney, heart), whereas carboplatin-based protocols might be an option in patients with reduced organ functions (kidney, heart) or when ease of administration is of major importance.

Elderly Patients and Patients with Reduced Performance Status

Elderly patients and patients with reduced performance status benefit from palliative chemotherapy but they require well-tolerated protocols and enhanced supportive care [5]. The magnitude of the benefit in patients with reduced performance status is often less compared to the benefit in patients with good performance status. In both patient populations, cisplatin-based protocols are often too toxic and should only be used with caution.

Thus, these patients are often treated with a third-generation cytotoxic drug as a single agent. Other options might be carboplatin-based protocols or protocols containing only low doses of cisplatin. However, there is general agreement that more trials involving these special patients are required in order to determine the best treatment options for these patients.

Customized Chemotherapy

An important step forward in the systemic treatment of advanced NSCLC is anticipated through the development of individualized chemotherapy. In this case, chemotherapy is tailored according to patient characteristics and/or tumor features. Chemotherapy based on biomarkers of tumor cells has already been and will further be evaluated within clinical trials. These trials focus on enzymes involved in either the mode of action or metabolism of anticancer drugs. Of particular interest is ERCC1, an enzyme involved in DNA repair. Patients with low ERCC1 levels in their tumors did benefit from adjuvant cisplatin-based chemotherapy, while patients with high levels did not [6]. In a prospective trial in patients with advanced NSCLC, customized chemotherapy based on ERCC1 levels of tumors resulted in a higher response rate but did not increase survival as compared to the control arm [7]. In the customized arm, patients received cisplatin/docetaxel in case of low ERCC1 levels and gemcitabine/docetaxel in case of high ERCC1 levels. In the control arm, all patients received cisplatin/docetaxel. Thus, customized chemotherapy remains experimental and should not be recommended outside a clinical trial.

The customized chemotherapy trials performed so far also highlighted the challenges associated with this approach. Availability of sufficient tumor tissue, particularly when required immediately prior to chemotherapy, remains a major challenge in patients with advanced NSCLC. Other challenges associated with biomarkers include storage of tumor specimens, fixation procedures, and standardization and validation of appropriate laboratory tests [8]. These problems will have to be solved before wide-spread application of customized chemotherapy will become a clinical reality.

Targeted Therapies

Integration of targeted therapies is expected to improve the outcome of chemotherapy in patients with advanced NSCLC but the optimal combination of both treatments remains a greater challenge than anticipated [9]. While administration concurrent with chemotherapy might work for one particular targeted therapy, a sequential approach might be more advantageous in case of another targeted therapy.

Targeted therapies focus on the blockade of the epidermal growth factor receptor (EGFR) function and on the inhibition of angiogenesis. Cetuximab added to cisplatin/vinorelbine increased survival in patients with advanced EGFR-positive NSCLC [10]. Bevacizumab added to chemotherapy improved outcome in selected patients with advanced nonsquamous cell NSCLC [11, 12], although a survival benefit was observed in only one of these trials [11].

Many other trials failed to demonstrate a survival benefit for a targeted agent when combined with palliative chemotherapy in patients with advanced NSCLC [9].

Whether targeted therapies might eventually replace chemotherapy in the first-line setting has also been investigated in selected patients with advanced NSCLC. Gefitinib was compared to carboplatin/paclitaxel in chemo-naive Asian never-smokers (or only light smokers) with adenocarcinomas [13]. With regard to progression-free survival, gefitinib led to a benefit in patients with mutations in the EGFR gene but to inferior outcome in those without mutations. Data on overall survival are pending. Based on these findings, gefitinib as first-line therapy should only be given to patients with proven EGFR mutations in their tumors.

Maintenance Therapy

Patients with advanced NSCLC should initially be treated with up to 6 cycles of platinum-based doublets but patients with stable disease under chemotherapy should not receive more than 4 cycles [1]. Maintenance therapy after initial chemotherapy is a potential strategy to improve outcome. Maintenance therapy often prolongs progression-free survival, but its improvement of overall survival remains to be demonstrated.

Pemetrexed was recently compared to placebo in patients who had at least stable disease after 4 cycles of platinum-based first-line chemotherapy [14]. Patients receiving pemetrexed had longer progression-free survival and overall survival compared to those receiving placebo. This benefit was seen only in patients with nonsquamous NSCLC. Although the trial was planned to study the impact of maintenance therapy, it actually evaluated more the role of early versus delayed second-line chemotherapy than the role of maintenance therapy. Consistent with the findings of the pemetrexed study, early second-line docetaxel chemotherapy compared to docetaxel initiated at the time of progression was recently shown to improve survival [15].

Taken together, maintenance therapy and early second-line chemotherapy are not yet accepted as standards but second-line chemotherapy probably should be initiated earlier than according to current practice.

Systemic Chemotherapy in Patients Progressing after First-Line Chemotherapy

Patients progressing after first-line chemotherapy are treated with docetaxel, pemetrexed or erlotinib. Pemetrexed was shown to have similar efficacy but better tolerability compared to docetaxel [2]. Moreover, a subgroup analysis indicated superior efficacy of pemetrexed in patients with nonsquamous NSCLC. Thus, pemetrexed is currently preferred in patients with nonsquamous NSCLC, whereas docetaxel is preferred in patients with squamous cell NSCLC.

Erlotinib is preferentially given to patients who are likely to respond to these agents, such as never-smokers, females, patients with adenocarcinomas and patients with activating mutations in the epidermal growth factor receptor gene. Such mutations occur in approximately 10–15% of Caucasian patients but are more common in patients of Asian ethnicity with frequencies of up to 60%.

Gefitinib did not increase survival in a large trial compared to placebo [16]. However, gefitinib was recently shown to be noninferior to docetaxel in patients previously treated with chemotherapy [17] and, therefore, will also increasingly be accepted as a treatment option for patients progressing after first-line chemotherapy.

Assessment of Efficacy

There is controversy on the optimal assessment of the outcome of palliative chemotherapy or targeted therapies within clinical trials. Overall survival remains the most relevant endpoint. However, its reliability with regard to the assessment of the efficacy of first-line chemotherapy has been questioned based on the argument that the observed associations between first-line chemotherapy and survival might have been affected by subsequent therapies. Thus, progression-free survival is preferred as the primary endpoint by some investigators. However, progression-free survival is difficult to be assessed in patients with advanced NSCLC where the expected differences in outcome are small. Moreover, the association between progression-free survival and overall survival appears to be rather weak. Response rates are well established but are not the most relevant clinical endpoints in patients with advanced NSCLC and their associations with survival are weak.

In order to obtain clinically useful information, clinical trials should always attempt to assess several efficacy parameters and, whenever possible, should be powered to allow the detection of small but clinically still relevant differences in survival. In those instances in which progression-free survival is chosen as the primary endpoint, its assessment should be within a placebo-controlled trial and accompanied by measures on tumor-related symptoms and quality of life. Efficacy data based on progression-free survival will be more easily accepted when the prolongation of progression-free survival is accompanied by improvements in cancer-related symptoms or quality of life.

In daily practice, doctors should always be aware of the goal of their treatment. In most instances, treatment will aim at improving cancer-related symptoms, increasing survival or improving both symptoms and survival. Doctors should be aware that improvements in survival by chemotherapy have only been proven for first-line and second-lines therapies and that, therefore, the goal of any subsequent treatments can only be relief of cancer-related symptoms.

References

1 Pfister DG, Johnson DH, Azzoli CG, Sause W, Smith TJ, Baker S Jr, Olak J, Stover D, Strawn JR, Turrisi AT, Somerfield MR, American Society of Clinical Oncology: American Society of Clinical Oncology treatment of unresectable non-small-cell lung cancer guideline: update 2003. J Clin Oncol 2004;22:330–353.

2 Hanna N, Shepherd FA, Fossella FV, Pereira JR, De Marinis F, von Pawel J, Gatzemeier U, Tsao TC, Pless M, Muller T, Lim HL, Desch C, Szondy K, Gervais R, Shaharyar, Manegold C, Paul S, Paoletti P, Einhorn L, Bunn PA Jr: Randomized phase III trial of pemetrexed versus docetaxel in patients with non-small-cell lung cancer previously treated with chemotherapy. J Clin Oncol 2004;22:1589–97.

3 Scagliotti GV, Parikh P, von Pawel J, Biesma B, Vansteenkiste J, Manegold C, Serwatowski P, Gatzemeier U, Digumarti R, Zukin M, Lee JS, Mellemgaard A, Park K, Patil S, Rolski J, Goksel T, de Marinis F, Simms L, Sugarman KP, Gandara D: Phase III study comparing cisplatin plus gemcitabine with cisplatin plus pemetrexed in chemotherapy-naive patients with advanced-stage non-small-cell lung cancer. J Clin Oncol 2008;26: 3543–51.

4 Ardizzoni A, Boni L, Tiseo M, Fossella FV, Schiller JH, Paesmans M, Radosavljevic D, Paccagnella A, Zatloukal P, Mazzanti P, Bisset D, Rosell R, CISCA (CISplatin versus CArboplatin) Meta-analysis Group: Cisplatin- versus carboplatin-based chemotherapy in first-line treatment of advanced non-small-cell lung cancer: an individual patient data meta-analysis. J Natl Cancer Inst 2007;99:847–57.

5 Gridelli C, Maione P, Rossi A, Guerriero C, Ferrara C, Del Gaizo F, Colantuoni G, Nicolella D, Napolitano L: Chemotherapy of advanced NSCLC in special patient population. Ann Oncol 2006; 17(suppl 5):v72–78.

6 Olaussen KA, Dunant A, Fouret P, Brambilla E, André F, Haddad V, Taranchon E, Filipits M, Pirker R, Popper HH, Stahel R, Sabatier L, Pignon JP, Tursz T, Le Chevalier T, Soria JC, IALT Bio Investigators: DNA repair by ERCC1 in non-small-cell lung cancer and cisplatin-based adjuvant chemotherapy. N Engl J Med 2006;355: 983–991.

7 Cobo M, Isla D, Massuti B, Montes A, Sanchez JM, Provencio M, Viñolas N, Paz-Ares L, Lopez-Vivanco G, Muñoz MA, Felip E, Alberola V, Camps C, Domine M, Sanchez JJ, Sanchez-Ronco M, Danenberg K, Taron M, Gandara D, Rosell R: Customizing cisplatin based on quantitative excision repair cross-complementing 1 mRNA expression: a phase III trial in non-small-cell lung cancer. J Clin Oncol 2007;25:2747–2754.

8 Eberhard DA, Giaccone G, Johnson BE, Non-Small-Cell Lung Cancer Working Group: Biomarkers of response to epidermal growth factor receptor inhibitors in Non-Small-Cell Lung Cancer Working Group: standardization for use in the clinical trial setting. J Clin Oncol 2008;26: 983—994.

9 Pirker R, Filipits M: Targeted therapies in lung cancer. Curr Pharmac Design 2009;15:188–206.

10 Pirker R, Pereira JR, Szczesna A, von Pawel J, Krzakowski M, Ramlau R, Vynnychenko I, Park K, Yu CT, Ganul V, Roh JK, Bajetta E, O'Byrne K, de Marinis F, Eberhardt W, Goddemeier T, Emig M, Gatzemeier U, FLEX Study Team: Cetuximab plus chemotherapy in patients with advanced non-small-cell lung cancer (FLEX): an open-label randomised phase III trial. Lancet 2009;373:1525–1531.

11 Sandler A, Gray R, Perry MC, Brahmer J, Schiller JH, Dowlati A, Lilenbaum R, Johnson DH: Paclitaxel-carboplatin alone or with bevacizumab for non-small-cell lung cancer. N Engl J Med 2006; 355:2542–2550.

12 Manegold C, von Pawel J, Zatloukal P, Ramlau R, Gorbounova V, Hirsh V, Leighl N, Mezger J, Archer V, Reck M, on behalf of the AVAiL Study Group: A phase III randomised study of first-line bevacizumab combined with cisplatin/gemcitabine (CG) in patients with advanced or recurrent non-squamous, non-small cell lung cancer (NSCLC). Ann Oncol 2008;19(suppl 8):viii1–viii4.

13 Mok TS, Wu YL, Thongprasert S, Yang CH, Chu DT, Saijo N, Sunpaweravong P, Han B, Margono B, Ichinose Y, Nishiwaki Y, Ohe Y, Yang JJ, Chewaskulyong B, Jiang H, Duffield EL, Watkins CL, Armour AA, Fukuoka M: Gefitinib or carboplatin-paclitaxel in pulmomary adenocarcinoma. N Engl J Med 2009;361:947–957.

14 Ciuleanu T, Brodowicz T, Zielinski C, Kim JH, Krzakowski M, Laack E, Wu YL, Bover I, Begbie S, Tzekova V, Cucevic B, Pereira JR, Yang SH, Madhavan J, Sugarman KP, Peterson P, John WJ, Krejcy K, Belani CP: Maintenance pemetrexed plus best supportive care versus placebo plus best supportive care for non-small-cell lung cancer: a randomised, double-blind, phase 3 study. Lancet 2009; Epub ahead of print.

15 Fidias PM, Dakhil SR, Lyss AP, Loesch DM, Waterhouse DM, Bromund JL, Chen R, Hristova-Kazmierski M, Treat J, Obasaju CK, Marciniak M, Gill J, Schiller JH: Phase III study of immediate compared with delayed docetaxel after front-line therapy with gemcitabine plus carboplatin in advanced non-small-cell lung cancer. J Clin Oncol 2009;27:591–598.

16 Thatcher N, Chang A, Parikh P, Rodrigues Pereira J, Ciuleanu T, von Pawel J, Thongprasert S, Tan EH, Pemberton K, Archer V, Carroll K: Gefitinib plus best supportive care in previously treated patients with refractory advanced non-small-cell lung cancer: results from a randomised, placebo-controlled, multicentre study (Iressa Survival Evaluation in Lung Cancer). Lancet 2005;366: 1527–1537.

17 Kim ES, Hirsh V, Mok T, Socinski MA, Gervais R, Wu YL, Li LY, Watkins CL, Sellers MV, Lowe ES, Sun Y, Liao ML, Osterlind K, Reck M, Armour AA, Shepherd FA, Lippman SM, Douillard JY: Gefitinib versus docetaxel in previously treated non-small-cell lung cancer (INTEREST): a randomised phase III trial. Lancet 2008;372:1809–1818.

Robert Pirker, MD
Department of Medicine I, Medical University of Vienna
Währinger Gürtel 18–20
AT–1090 Vienna (Austria)
Tel. +43 1 40400 4422, Fax +1 43 1 40400 4461, E-Mail robert.pirker@meduniwien.ac.at

Heide J, Schmittel A, Kaiser D, Hinkelbein W (eds): Controversies in the Treatment of Lung Cancer.
Front Radiat Ther Oncol. Basel, Karger, 2010, vol 42, pp 164–172

Radiotherapy

Irenäus A. Adamietz

Klinik für Strahlentherapie und Radio-Onkologie der Ruhr-Universität Bochum, Herne, Germany

Abstract

The intrathoracic growth of the tumor causes several severe symptoms as cough, dyspnea, chest pain, hemoptysis, hoarseness, anorexia/nausea, and dysphagia. In patients with manifest or threatening symptoms radiotherapy (RT) as an effective measure should be implemented into the management concept. Palliative RT radiotherapy prefers short hypofractionated schemas (e.g. 10 × 3 Gy, 4 × 5 Gy, 2 × 8 Gy, 1 × 10 Gy). Careful radiation planning supports the precision of palliative RT and reduces significantly the complication rate. A good response and prolonged palliation effects (6–12 months) can be achieved in many cases. However, the minimum biologically equivalent dose should not be less than 35 Gy. RT produces a good outcome in all types of metastases of lung carcinoma. In emergencies like VCSS or spinal cord compression RT should be initiated immediately. The selection of the optimal therapy for locally advanced lung carcinoma with malignant airway obstruction is difficult. Both brachytherapy and percutaneous irradiation are effective, however published results including local a sum of response, functionality and life quality demonstrates more benefit by percutaneous RT. Due to different physical properties of these two methods the combination of brachytherapy and external beam irradiation may be advantageous.

Clinical Manifestations of Advanced Lung Carcinoma

The carcinoma of the lung demonstrates different patterns of growth depending on histological type of disease. Among the various histologic types of the non-small cell lung carcinoma (NSCLC), adenocarcinoma has the slowest doubling time and small cell carcinoma has the fastest [1]. On the other hand, adenocarcinoma has shown higher potential for distant metastasis.

Signs and symptoms referable to the advanced lung tumor vary depending on the location and size of the tumor. Centrally located tumors produce cough, a localized wheeze, hemoptysis, and symptoms and signs of airway obstruction and postobstructive pneumonitis such as dyspnea, fever, and productive cough. Peripheral tumors are more likely to be asymptomatic when they are small and confined within the lung. Occasionally, cough and pleuritic chest pain may be evident. One of the most common neurologic disorders arising from mediastinal involvement is hoarseness owing to entrapment of the recurrent laryngeal nerve [2].

The principal vascular syndrome associated with the extension of lung cancer into the mediastinum is superior vena cava (SVC) syndrome, most commonly caused by invasion of the vein and extrinsic compression by the tumor but also by intraluminal thrombosis. Lung cancer accounts for 65–90% of all cases of SVC syndrome [3].

With apical tumors, the classic Pancoast's syndrome (lower brachial plexopathy, Horner's syndrome, and shoulder pain) may become manifest owing to local invasion of the lower brachial plexus (C8 and T1 nerve roots), satellite ganglion, and chest wall. The tumor may cause symptoms through involvement of the first or second rib or vertebrae and other nerve roots [2].

Approximately 50% of patients with disseminated lung cancer develop pleural effusion during the course of their illness. A pleural effusion may be asymptomatic when small, but it is usually associated with dyspnea, cough, or chest pain. Pericardial involvement arises from direct extension of the tumor or as a result of retrograde spread through mediastinal and epicardial lymphatics. Lung cancer is the single most frequent source of pericardial metastases, accounting for 37% of reported cases [3].

Stage IV metastatic disease will be found in approximately 30–40% of patients with NSCLC [2]. Although lung cancer can metastasize to virtually any organ site, the most common sites of hematogeneous spread that are clinically apparent are the central nervous system (CNS), bones, liver, and adrenal glands. Many of these patients do not have symptoms that can be attributed to a specific distant site. Bone pain seems to be common. Symptoms related to liver involvement (right upper quadrant pain) are less common or nonspecific (nausea, weight loss, anemia). Involvement of the adrenal glands is often asymptomatic, and most adrenal metastases are discovered incidentally during staging evaluation or at autopsy. If symptomatic, it presents with unilateral pain in the ankle, abdomen, or costovertebral angle. Much less commonly, signs or symptoms point to brain and CNS involvement. These can range from nonspecific headache or mental status change to focal or generalized seizures and localized weakness. Epidural and intramedullary spinal cord metastases may be the sole neurologic manifestations of lung cancer.

Palliative Potential of Radiotherapy

The majority of patients who present with locally advanced or metastatic lung cancer are treated with palliative intent, with the goals of relief of pain and other

Table 1. Palliation of special symptoms of advanced NSCLC by radiation treatment (external beam radiation; data from Fairchild et al. [9])

Symptom	CR	PR
Hemoptysis	71.3% (350/491)	80.6% (639/792)
Cough	29.1% (274/941)	50.9% (822/1614)
Chest pain	54.7% (295/539)	64.3% (616/958)

symptoms, and preservation of quality of life (QoL) [4]. Palliative-intent radiotherapy (RT) is effective for improvement of symptoms resulting from intrathoracic disease, such as hemoptysis, cough, chest pain, dyspnea, and airway obstruction, and in approximately one third of patients, improves global QoL (table 1) [4, 5].

Radiation dose can be delivered by percutaneous irradiation or by brachytherapy. The latter one is very effective due to high radiation dose that can be delivered proximally to the radiation source. A disadvantage of brachytherapy is the dose inhomogeneity. The steep decrease of dose rate distally to the radiation source produces inefficient doses in the deeper layers of tumor resulting in the lack of response. External beam radiation provides a good dose homogeneity that enables a sufficient dose application across the entire tumor volume.

The maximal dose that can be delivered to the lung tumor, including the involved lymph nodes, is restricted by the tolerance of normal tissues within the high-dose volume. Within the thorax, the tissues of concern include especially the spinal cord, lung, and esophagus. 3D-CRT enables the spatial dose distribution to be more conformal to the target volume while reducing the dose to normal tissues. This approach, therefore, has the potential to decrease the probability of normal tissue toxicity. Graham et al. [6] have reported increasing rates of radiation pneumonitis with an increasing radiation dose to normal lung tissue.

It is well documented that local control rates have improved with an increasing radiation dose. However, because of the proximity of critical normal structures to the primary tumor, the prescription dose had traditionally been limited to between 60 and 70 Gy. A report by Arriagada et al. [7] revealed a 17% pathologic local control rate after a radiation dose of 65 Gy. From the basic principles advocated by Fletcher [8], it is thought that doses of ≤100 Gy may be required to sterilize the size of tumors frequently treated in bronchogenic carcinoma. Radiation doses required to slow down the growth of the advanced tumor lesion are significantly lower (approximately 25–45 Gy).

However, the optimal dose of percutaneous RT needed to palliate symptoms of advanced lung cancer has not been well defined. Randomized controlled trials comparing different regimens for the amelioration of thoracic symptoms have reported contradictory results for symptom palliation. Even more controversial is what impact, if any, palliative RT has on survival [9].

The meta-analysis by Fairchild et al. [9] confirmed the equivalence of palliation of specific symptoms for a broad range of radiation doses, but report that patients have a statistically lower total symptom score after higher doses of palliative thoracic RT (tables 2, 3). This systematic review provides further evidence of equivalency of specific symptom palliation outcomes (hemoptysis, cough, chest pain), but describes statistically significantly improved total symptom score and overall survival with higher doses of palliative thoracic RT compared with lower doses. They reported a 4.8% absolute increase in overall survival at 1 year, favoring dose schedules of 35 Gy_{10} BED, at the expense of significantly increased esophagitis. Although the authors observed a greater incidence of chest reirradiation after RT with lower doses, the results were not statistically significant.

The value of endobronchial brachytherapy as a palliative treatment for bronchial obstruction is now widely accepted. Initially performed with low-dose-rate sources, endobronchial brachytherapy (EBBT) is now usually delivered with miniaturized high-dose-rate (HDR) iridium sources. This method is recognized as an effective palliative treatment of tumorous endobronchial obstruction. Symptomatic regression has been observed in 60–80% of patients, with shrinkage of the endobronchial tumor in 80%. Toxicity was mild, despite rare late toxicities such as radiation bronchitis and massive hemoptysis [10, 11].

Radiation treatment of preirradiated tumor may also be effective. Reirradiation achieves responses offering the patient another period without or with reduced symptoms. The published response rates in NSCLC are very promising and range between 50 and 90% depending on observed symptom [12, 13].

Treatment Strategies

The treatment strategy in patients with advanced NSCLC should refer to patient needs and his condition. If there are pressing symptomatic needs for palliation, such as significant obstruction of a major airway, severe hemoptysis, superior vena cava obstruction, painful bony metastases in the weight-bearing areas, or symptomatic brain metastases, the initial treatment is radiotherapy with or without chemotherapy. If a patient has evidence of disseminated disease and there is no pressing need for radiotherapy, the approach includes consideration of systemic chemotherapy, or supportive therapy alone if the patient's general condition is not suitable for systemic chemotherapy.

Consideration of RT schedules of at least 35 Gy_{10} BED may therefore be warranted in certain clinical scenarios, provided that patients are informed of the trade-off

Table 2. Selection of randomized clinical trials on palliative radiotherapy in NSCLC demonstrating the applied doses and fractionation schemas (data from Fairchild et al. [9])

Trial	Year	Number of patients	Group A (lower BED)				Group B (higher BED)			
			Gy	number of fractions	duration	BED (Gy_{10})	Gy	number of fractions	duration	BED (Gy_{10})
Simpson et al. [23]*	1985	409	30	10	2 weeks	35.0	40	8	4 weeks	45.0
Teo et al. [24]	1988	291	31.2	4	4 weeks	43.7	45	18	4.5 weeks	42.8
MRC 1991 [25]	1991	374	17	2	8 days	30.7	30	10	2 weeks†	35.0
MRC 1992 [26]	1992	235	10	1	1 day	24.8	17	2	8 days	30.7
Abratt et al. [27]‡	1995	84	35	10	2.5 weeks	40.1	45	15	4 weeks	45.0
MRC 1996 [28]	1996	509	17	2	8 days	30.7	39	13	2.5 weeks§	42.8
Rees et al. [29]	1997	216	17	2	8 days	30.7	22,5	5	1 week	34.2
Nestle et al. [30]//	2000	152	32	16 b.i.d.	10 days	36.0	60	30	6 weeks	45.9
Bezjak et al. [31]	2002	230	10	1	1 day	24.8	20	5	1 week	29.6
Sundstrøm et al. [32]*	2004	421	17	2	8 days	30.7	50	25	5 weeks	39.4
Erridge et al. [33]	2005	149	10	1	1 day	24.8	30	10	2 weeks	35.0
Kramer et al. [34]	2005	303	16	2	8 days¶	28.0	30	10	2 weeks¶	35.0
Senkus-Konefka et al. [35]	2005	100	16	2	8 days	28.0	20	5	1 week	29.6

Within the study, group A was treated with lower equivalent total dose (LD) and group B received higher total dose (HD).
BED = Biologically equivalent dose.
* Intermediate dose arm omitted; higher dose arm was split course delivered 4 days/week with 2-week break.
† Alternate schedule of 27 Gy in 6 fractions.
‡ Delivered 4 days/week.
§ Alternate schedule of 36 Gy in 12 fractions.
// Interfraction interval ≥6 h.
¶ Delivered 4 or 5 days/week.

between the potential advantages (survival benefit, decreased likelihood of reirradiation to the thorax) and disadvantages (higher incidence of esophagitis, greater time investment) of each schedule. Alternatively, patients with intrathoracic symptoms and a short expected survival may achieve a high rate of symptom relief with minimal toxicity and inconvenience with a short course of palliative thoracic radiotherapy [9, 14].

Table 3. Results of clinical trials on palliative radiotherapy in NSCLC demonstrating the difference between efficacy of lower (LD) and higher (HD) radiation doses (compare also table 2; data from Fairchild et al. [9]): percent values

Trial	Year	Number of Patients	Complete remission		Partial remission		1-Year survival		2-Year survival	
			LD	HD	LD	HD	LD	HD	LD	HD
Simpson et al. [23]	1985	409	25.3	27.2	72.6	75.7	22.1	30.1	7.4	8.1%
Teo et al. [24]	1988	291	0.0	0.9	53.9	70.6	16.3	21.7	5.2	5.1
MRC 1991 [25]	1991	374	–	–	–	–	19.8	23.0	4.8	4.8
MRC 1992 [26]	1992	235	–	–	–	–	9.3	13.7	3.4	1.7
Abratt et al. [27]	1995	84	14.0	19.5	67.4	75.6	39.5	36.6	–	–
MRC 1996 [28]	1996	509	–	–	–	–	31.0	35.8	9.0	11.8
Rees et al. [29]	1997	216	–	–	–	–	18.0	21.9	5.4	12.4
Nestle et al. [30]	2000	152	–	–	–	–	35.6	38.0	9.6	8.9
Bezjak et al. [31]	2002	230	–	–	–	–	17.2	27.2	–	–
Sundstrøm et al. [32]	2004	421	–	–	–	–	28.8	32.3	10.3	10.0
Erridge et al. [33]	2005	149	4.7	22.6	76.6	91.9	18.9	28.4	4.1	8.1
Kramer et al. [34]	2005	303	–	–	–	–	10.9	19.9	5.8	9.0
Senkus-Konefka et al. [35]	2005	100	–	–	–	–	26.7	10.9	–	–

Short fractionation has been recommended by many guidelines [15] although a number have cautioned against the use of single fractions for various reasons [16]. Other position papers have not recommended a specific dose fractionation schedule. Although the use of palliative chemotherapy for NSCLC is increasing, RT alone can provide more timely palliation of thoracic symptoms without the morbidity of chemotherapy, and may be the primary or only treatment option for poor-PS patients, or patients who have declined or progressed despite systemic therapy.

According to our experience severity of symptoms, general condition of the patient and the prognosis of disease are the factors with impact on treatment concept. In case of acute bronchial obstruction EBBT should always be considered. In palliative situation a sole irradiation of critical tumor mass is usually sufficient. After successful brachytherapy percutaneous irradiation of the treated tumor lesion prolongs the response to radiation treatment. The reduction of acute side effects can be supported by use of small treatment volumes and 3D treatment planning. Split-course radiotherapy may help to adapt treatment schema to the general condition of the patient.

Bone metastases occur frequently in advanced lung carcinoma. Radiation therapy has been reported to be effective in palliating painful bone metastases, with partial pain relief seen in 80–90% of patients, and complete pain relief in 50% of patients. For patients with a longer life span, there is a greater opportunity for regrowth of the tumor. For patients with a poor performance status, difficulty making multiple trips for treatment, extensive nonosseous metastases, and/or a short life expectancy, the most appropriate treatment is a single fraction of 8 Gy. For patients with a longer life expectancy, bone-only metastases, and good performance status, a longer course of treatment (30 Gy in 10 fractions) may be more appropriate to minimize the risk of retreatment. The use of bisphosphonates with external-beam radiotherapy may further improve the outcome in terms of both pain and bone healing [17].

In brain metastasis the most common primary site is the lung. The initial therapy should promptly start with corticosteroids followed by whole-brain radiotherapy (WBRT), which is the standard of care in patients with brain metastasis [18]. There is still no agreement on the dose and fractionation schedule for WBRT despite numerous studies designed to determine the optimum delivery. Typically, the radiographic and clinical response rates range from 50 to 75%. A total of 30 Gy in 10 fractions continues to be the standard for most patients. Radiosurgery provides a substitute or alternative to conventional surgery. Although no randomized trials have been performed comparing surgery with SRS, the latter appears to provide similar local control rates (in the order of 80–90% only when combined with WBRT) [19].

Palliative radiotherapy has been the standard of care in the treatment of patients with metastatic spinal cord compression (MSCC). Although a total of 30 Gy in 10 fractions is most frequently employed fractionation schedule, multiple fractionation schemes have been reported, which undoubtedly reflects the heterogeneity in the patient population and tumor histology. Rades et al. [20, 21] reported a retrospective series of 1,304 patients with MSCC. All of the groups had similar posttreatment ambulatory rates (63–74%) and motor function improvements (26–31%). However, in-field recurrence rates were much lower for the protracted schedules. They recommend that a single fraction of 8 Gy should be used in MSCC patients with limited survival expectations, and that 30 Gy in 10 fractions should be used for all other patients. For patients receiving radiotherapy for MSCC from NSCLC, 30 Gy in 10 fractions is considered the standard of care. Shorter fractionation schedules, such as 8 Gy × 1 or 4 Gy × 5, should only be reserved for those with clear evidence of progressive disease, refractory to systemic therapy.

The superior vena cava syndrome is produced by extrinsic compression of the SVC or intracaval thrombosis, which is seen in approximately 40–50% of patients with this syndrome. Although it generally is believed that these patients have an extremely poor prognosis, approximately 10–20% survive longer than 2 years. Therefore, in the absence of distant metastasis, aggressive management and support are indicated. RT should be initiated as soon as possible. Patients initially should be given high-dose fractions (3- to 4-Gy tumor dose) for 2 or 3 days, followed by additional daily doses of 1.8–2 Gy to complete the definitive course of RT. The recommended total tumor dose for patients with localized bronchogenic carcinoma is 60–70 Gy in 6–7 weeks. Excellent symptomatic relief (disappearance of dyspnea, edema of the face, and distention of the neck and thoracic veins) has been observed in approximately 20% of patients. Good symptomatic improvement also has been noted in an additional 50% of patients. Only 15% of patients with bronchogenic carcinoma had minimal improvement, and 15% showed no significant response [22].

References

1 Chahinian A, Israel L: Rates and patterns of growth of lung cancer; in Israel L, Chahinian AP (eds): Lung Cancer: Natural History, Prognosis and Therapy. New York, Academic Press, 1976, pp 63–79.

2 Chang JY, Bradley JD, Govindan R, Komaki R: Lung; in Halperin EC, Perez CA, Brady LW (eds): Perez and Brady's Principles and Practice of Radiation Oncology, ed 5. Philadelphia, Wolters Kluwer/Lippincott Wiliams & Wilkins, 2008, pp 1076–1080.

3 Martins SJ, Pereira JR: Clinical factors and prognosis in non-small cell lung cancer. Am J Clin Oncol 1999;22:453–457.

4 Sirzen F, Kjellen E, Sorenson S, Cavallin-Stahl E: A systematic overview of radiation therapy effects in non-small cell lung cancer. Acta Oncol 2003; 42:493–515.

5 Hoegler D: Radiotherapy for palliation of symptoms in incurable cancer. Curr Probl Cancer 1997; 21:129–183.

6 Graham PH, Gebski VJ, Langlands AO: Radical radiotherapy for early nonsmall cell lung cancer. Int J Radiat Oncol Biol Phys 1995;31:261–266.

7 Arriagada R, Bergman B, Dunant A, Le Chevalier T, Pignon JP, Vansteenkiste J: Cisplatin-based adjuvant chemotherapy in patients with completely resected non-small-cell lung cancer. N Engl J Med 2004;350:351–360.

8 Fletcher GH: Clinical dose response curves of human malignant epithelial tumours. Br J Radiol 1973;46:151.

9 Fairchild A, Harris K, Barnes E, et al: Palliative thoracic radiotherapy for lung cancer: a systematic review. J Clin Oncol 2008;26:4001–411.

10 Hennequin C, Bleichner O, Tredaniel J, et al: Long-term results of endobronchial brachytherapy: a curative treatment? Int J Radiat Oncol Biol Phys 2007;67:425–430.

11 Zorlu AF, Selek U, Emri S, Gurkaynak M, Akyol FH: Second line palliative endobronchial radiotherapy with HDR Ir 192 in recurrent lung carcinoma. Yonsei Med J 2008;49:620–624.

12 Gressen EL, Werner-Wasik M, Cohn J, Topham A, Curran WJ Jr: Thoracic reirradiation for symptomatic relief after prior radiotherapeutic management for lung cancer. Am J Clin Oncol 2000;23: 160–163.

13 Kramer GW, Gans S, Ullmann E, van Meerbeeck JP, Legrand CC, Leer JW: Hypofractionated external beam radiotherapy as retreatment for symptomatic non-small-cell lung carcinoma: an effective treatment? Int J Radiat Oncol Biol Phys 2004;58: 1388–1393.

14 Cross CK, Berman S, Buswell L, Johnson B, Baldini EH: Prospective study of palliative hypofractionated radiotherapy (8.5 Gy × 2) for patients with symptomatic non-small-cell lung cancer. Int J Radiat Oncol Biol Phys 2004;58:1098–1105.

15 Timothy AR, Girling DJ, Saunders MI, Macbeth F, Hoskin PJ: Radiotherapy for inoperable lung cancer. Clin Oncol (R Coll Radiol) 2001;13:86–87.

16 Okawara G, Mackay JA, Evans WK, Ung YC: Management of unresected stage III non-small cell lung cancer: a systematic review. J Thorac Oncol 2006;1: 377–393.

17 Adamietz IA: Palliative Radiotherapie; in Bamberg M, Molls M, Sack H (eds): Radioonkologie. München, Zuckschwerdt, 2004, pp 1117–1155.

18 Rades D, Bohlen G, Dunst J, et al: Comparison of short-course versus long-course whole-brain radiotherapy in the treatment of brain metastases. Strahlenther Onkol 2008;184:30–35.

19 Rades D, Kueter JD, Hornung D, et al: Comparison of stereotactic radiosurgery (SRS) alone and whole brain radiotherapy (WBRT) plus a stereotactic boost (WBRT + SRS) for one to three brain metastases. Strahlenther Onkol 2008;184:655–662.

20 Rades D, Rudat V, Veninga T, et al: A score predicting posttreatment ambulatory status in patients irradiated for metastatic spinal cord compression. Int J Radiat Oncol Biol Phys 2008;72:905–908.

21 Rades D, Veninga T, Stalpers LJ, et al: Outcome after radiotherapy alone for metastatic spinal cord compression in patients with oligometastases. J Clin Oncol 2007;25:50–56.

22 Wudel LJ Jr, Nesbitt JC: Superior vena cava syndrome. Curr Treat Options Oncol 2001;2:77–91.

23 Simpson JR, Francis ME, Perez-Tamayo R, et al: Palliative radiotherapy for inoperable carcinoma of the lung: Final report of a RTOG multi-institutional trial. Int J Radiat Oncol Biol Phys 1985;11: 751–758.

24 Teo P, Tai TH, Choy D, et al: Randomized study on palliative radiation therapy for inoperable non small cell carcinoma of the lung. Int J Radiat Oncol Biol Phys 1988;14:867–871.

25 Medical Research Council Lung Cancer Working Party: Inoperable non-small-cell lung cancer: A Medical Research Council randomized trial of palliative radiotherapy with two fractions or ten fractions. Br J Cancer 1991;63:265–270.

26 Medical Research Council Lung Cancer Working Party: A Medical Research Council randomized trial of palliative radiotherapy with two fractions of a single fraction in patients with inoperable non-small-cell lung cancer and poor performance status. Br J Cancer 1992;65:934–941.

27 Abratt RP, Shepherd LJ, Mameena Salton DG: Palliative radiation for stage 3 non-small-cell lung cancer: A prospective study of two moderately high dose regimens. Lung Cancer 1995;13:137–143.

28 Medical Research Council Lung Cancer Working Party: Randomized trial of palliative two-fraction versus more intensive 13-fraction radiotherapy for patients with inoperable non-small-cell lung cancer and good performance status. Clin Oncol (R Coll Radiol) 1996;8:167–175.

29 Rees GJ, Devrell CE, Barley VL, et al: Palliative radiotherapy for lung cancer: Two versus five fractions. Clin Oncol (R Coll Radiol) 1997;9:90–95.

30 Nestle U, Nieder C, Walter K, et al: A palliative accelerated irradiation regimen for advanced non-small-cell lung cancer vs conventionally fractionated 60Gy: Results of a randomized equivalence study. Int J Radiat Oncol Biol Phys 2000;48:95–103.

31 Bezjak A, Dixon P, Brundage M, et al: Randomized phase III trial of single versus fractionated thoracic radiation in the palliation of patients with lung cancer (NCIC CTG SC. 15). Int J Radiat Oncol Biol Phys 2002;54:719–728.

32 Sundstrøm S, Bremnes R, Aasebo U, et al: Hypofractionated palliative radiotherapy (17Gy per two fractions) in advanced non-small-cell lung carcinoma is comparable to standard fractionation for symptom control and survival: A national phase III trial. J Clin Oncol 2004;22:801–810.

33 Erridge SC, Gaze MN, Price A, et al: Symptom control and quality of life in people with lung cancer: A randomized trial of two palliative radiotherapy fractionation schedules. Clin Oncol (R Coll Radiol) 2005;17:61–67.

34 Kramer GW, Wanders SL, Noordijk EM, et al: Results of the Dutch national study of the palliative effect of irradiation using two different treatment schemes for non-small-cell lung cancer. J Clin Oncol 2005;23:2962–2970.

35 Senkus-Konefka E, Dziadziuszko, Bednaruk-Mlynski E, et al: A prospective, randomized study to compare two palliative radiotherapy schedules for non-small-cell lung cancer. Br J Cancer 2005;92: 1038–1045.

Prof. Dr. Irenäus A. Adamietz
Klinik für Strahlentherapie und Radio-Onkologie der Ruhr-Universität Bochum
Hölkeskampring 40
DE–44625 Herne (Germany)
Tel. +49 2323 499 1531, Fax +49 2323 499 306, E-Mail irenaeus.adamietz@rub.de

Heide J, Schmittel A, Kaiser D, Hinkelbein W (eds): Controversies in the Treatment of Lung Cancer.
Front Radiat Ther Oncol. Basel, Karger, 2010, vol 42, pp 173–179

Treatment of Limited Disease Small Cell Lung Cancer

Dirk De Ruysscher

Department of Radiation Oncology (Maastro Clinic), GROW Research Institute, University Medical Center Maastricht, Maastricht, The Netherlands

Abstract

Limited disease small cell lung cancer (LD-SCLC) is a heterogeneous disease, not only for its clinical behavior, but also for is anatomical extension. In very rare, early cases, LD-SCLC might be treated with surgery and chemotherapy, but as the overwhelming majority of patients present with locally advanced disease, the standard of care is concurrent chest radiotherapy with cisplatin and etoposide chemotherapy followed by prophylactic cranial irradiation (PCI). Newer chemotherapeutic drugs as well as targeted agents have not improved the outcome thus far. Given concurrently with chest irradiation, cisplatin combined with etoposide, administered every 21 days for 4–5 cycles have frequently been used. Thoracic radiotherapy should begin as early as possible during the first chemotherapy cycle. A total radiation dose of 45 Gy is recommended, delivered in a short overall treatment time (less than 4 weeks). Accelerated therapy increased absolute 5-year survival rates by 10% compared to longer treatment times, at the expense of an incidence of severe esophagitis of approximately 30%, which is reversible within a few weeks. Hematological complications and late pulmonary damage may occur, but is not more frequent than with less intensive schedules that impair long-term survival. Obviously, patient selection is crucial. Because after combined chemotherapy and thoracic radiotherapy, the remission status of the tumor is difficult to assess because of radiation-induced radiographic changes, patients that show no tumor progression are suitable for PCI. With this treatment, 5-year survival rates of 25% can be achieved in patients with LD-SCLC.

Small cell lung cancer (SCLC) accounts for 10–15% of all lung cancers [1]. Approximately 20% of these patients present with so-called limited disease (LD) and are potentially amendable for treatment with curative intent. SCLC is characterized by rapid growth, with volume doubling times of approximately 30 days and early development of distant metastases [2].

It should be stressed that the definition of LD-SCLC varies across studies and time eras. The first staging system for SCLC was introduced in the 1950s by the

Veterans' Administration Lung Study Group (VALSG) [3]. This still widely used system divided SCLC into two disease subgroups: limited and extensive disease. Limited disease (LD) was characterized by tumors confined to one hemithorax, although local extension and ipsilateral, supraclavicular nodes could also be present if they could be encompassed in the same radiation portal as the primary tumor. No extrathoracic metastases could be present. All other disease was classified as extensive disease (ED). At present, using the tumor, node, metastasis (TNM) staging system, also for SCLC, is advocated [4]. As in clinical trials, the definition of LD-SCLC has been used differently, and inclusion criteria such as the size of the mediastinal lymph nodes along with patient characteristics also vary, outcome comparisons between studies are fraught with error and should therefore only be done with great scrutiny.

Because LD-SCLC is a systemic disease from the onset in the overwhelming majority of the patients, chemotherapy has become an essential part of the treatment.

A logical question is whether the addition of a local treatment affects survival or not. Surgery is in most cases not possible because of the local extend of the tumor or lymph nodes, but might be considered in rare, early stages [5]. For the majority of patients, chest radiotherapy is the most important local therapy.

Two meta-analyses [6, 7] have shown an improvement of 5.4% in absolute survival at two years and three years in patients who received chest irradiation in addition to chemotherapy versus those receiving chemotherapy alone, but the 5-year survival rate remained disappointingly low at 10–15%.

The two meta-analyses provided evidence that chemotherapy should be supplemented with chest irradiation.

At present, the combination of cisplatin and etoposide is standard for SCLC [8]. Therefore, most trials combining chest radiotherapy with chemotherapy have used this doublet.

Thoracic Radiotherapy

Historically, SCLC was considered as being a very radiosensitive tumor, as rapid shrinkage of the tumor is achieved in the majority of patients. However, local tumor failures still occur in over 30% of the patients, even with the best available concurrent chemo-radiation regimen [9]. The view that this tumor is extremely sensitive for radiation should thus be reconsidered.

Important questions to be addressed are: (1) What is the optimal radiation dose and fractionation? (2) What are the target volumes? (3) What is the best timing, sequencing and overall treatment time? These items have been reviewed in De Ruysscher and Vansteenkiste [10].

(1) What is the Optimal Radiation Dose and Fractionation?

The effect of the radiation dose on local tumor control was studied in only one phase III trial, randomizing between 25 Gy in 10 fractions in 2 weeks or 37.5 Gy in 15 fractions in 3 weeks. The local recurrence rate after 2 years was 80% for the low-dose group and 63% for the higher dose ($p < 0.05$). However, these doses are still low and not representative of current clinical practice.

We therefore have to rely on nonrandomized, retrospective and prospective data to evaluate the effect of higher doses on local control. It seems that in sequential schedules, i.e. chemotherapy followed by chest irradiation, it seems that the major improvement in local control is achieved when the dose is increased from 35 to 40 Gy, with possibly a modest gain of 10% with a further escalation to 50 Gy. However, because the data come from non-randomized studies employing a wide variety of other treatment parameters such as the irradiated volume, the overall treatment time and the type and sequence of chemotherapy, these findings are very difficult to interpret.

In RTOG 97–12, a phase I study, it was established that the maximal tolerated dose of accelerated radiation, delivered with concurrent cisplatin and etoposide, was 61.2 Gy in 5 weeks [11].

Phase III trials are underway to determine the optimal dose and fractionation. In all of them, chest irradiation is delivered concurrently with the first or the second chemotherapy cycle.

(2) What Are the Target Volumes?

The volume to be treated was investigated in only one randomized trial. In this Southwest Oncology Group (SWOG) study, 466 patients with LD-SCLC after induction chemotherapy were randomized according to their response. In a rather complex design, using sequential chemo-radiation, postchemotherapy margins appeared safe. This has been confirmed in several pro-and retrospective series.

In NSCLC, elective irradiation of mediastinal lymph nodes has gradually been replaced by the treatment of pathological nodes on CT or PET only [12]. By doing so, radiation volumes could be reduced and hence toxicity diminished. In LD-SCLC, only one prospective study has been carried out in which only CT-positive mediastinal lymph nodes were included in the gross tumor volume (GTV) [13]. Twenty-seven patients were treated with concurrent carboplatin, etoposide and chest irradiation (45 Gy delivered in 30 BID fractions). Three patients (crude rate 11%, 95% CI 2.4–29%), developed an isolated nodal failure, all of them in the ipsilateral supraclavicular fossa. Because of the higher than expected isolated recurrence rates, the study was terminated early. Because

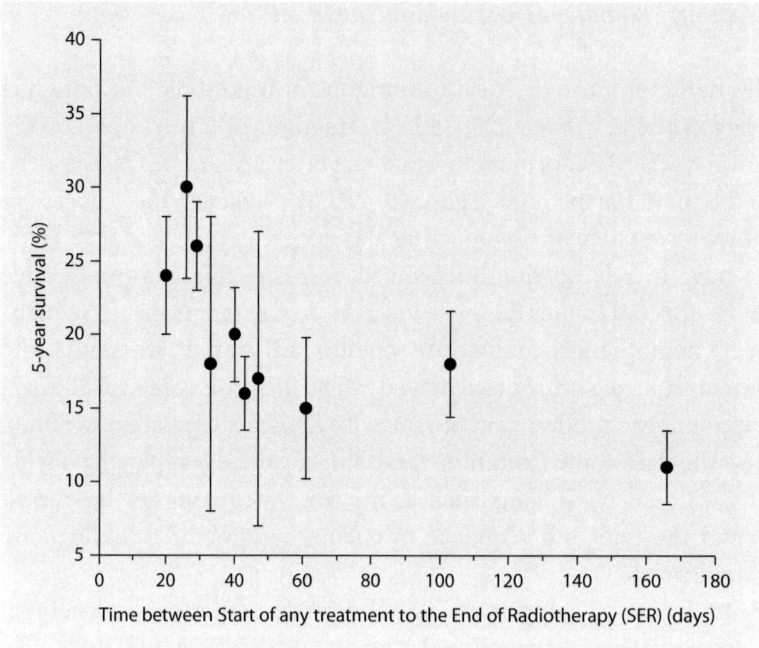

Fig. 1. Survival at 5 years as a function of the SER (Start of *any* treatment to the End of Radiotherapy) [17]. Each dot represents a single trial ± SE.

^{18}F-deoxyglucose PET scans have also in SCLC a higher accuracy than CT scans, irradiation of only PET positive nodes would be a possibility to omit elective nodal irradiation in the future [14].

At present, the safety of selective nodal irradiation in NSCLC should not be extrapolated to patients with LD-SCLC until more data are available. In the mean time, elective nodal irradiation should only be omitted in clinical trials.

(3) What Is the Best Timing, Sequencing and Overall Treatment Time?

Many phase III studies have investigated the timing of chest radiation in LD-SCLC [reviewed in 9, 15]. When all studies were considered, the delivery of early versus late thoracic irradiation did not influence the survival. However, when the most active chemotherapy regimen (platinum-based) were administered concomitantly with chest radiotherapy, long-term survival was increased at the expense of a higher incidence of severe, though transient esophagitis. At 5 years, the survival was significantly higher when chest radiotherapy was given early, i.e. within 30 days after the initiation of chemotherapy, representing a 5-year survival rate of 20.2% for early versus 13.8% for late thoracic radiotherapy. In a pivotal phase III study [16], decreasing the overall treatment time of chest radiotherapy from 5 weeks (2 Gy QD) to 3 weeks (1.5 Gy BID), whilst keeping the total radiation dose to 45 Gy, increased the 5-year survival from 16 to 26%.

Early, concurrent chemotherapy with accelerated radiation may result in approximately 30% grade 3 acute esophagitis, which contrasts with about 15% in early, concurrent, nonaccelerated radiotherapy and approximately 5% in sequential schedules. Interestingly, lung toxicity was not different according to the timing of radiotherapy.

Because a time-interaction between chest radiation and chemotherapy was suspected, an integrated approach was proposed [17]. It was hypothesized that accelerated repopulation was triggered by the first dose of any effective cytotoxic agent and that in order to obtain local tumor control, the last tumor clonogen should be killed by the end of radiotherapy. It follows from these two assumptions that the long-term survival should decrease with increasing time between the Start of *any* treatment to the End of Radiotherapy (SER). A meta-analysis of published data showed superior long-term survival if the SER was kept below 30 days in LD-SCLC (fig. 1).

These results are consistent with accelerated proliferation of tumor clonogens triggered by radiotherapy and/or chemotherapy. As expected, accelerated treatments also cause more toxicity in rapidly proliferating tissues such as the esophageal mucosa.

In conclusion, for limited-stage small cell lung cancer, current evidence supports the early administration of thoracic radiotherapy with concurrent cisplatin and etoposide chemotherapy.

Patient Selection

Because accelerated, concurrent chemotherapy and radiotherapy leads to more acute toxicity, at a time patients are susceptible for infections and organ dysfunction, patient selection is crucial. This is reflected in the inclusion and exclusion criteria in clinical trials and several guidelines. In general, concurrent chemo-radiation is restricted to younger (maximum 75 years) patients, in a good general condition (e.g. WHO performance status 0–1), without significant co-morbidities and with adequate organ function. However, in a prospective population-based study including 711 patients, only about 40% of patients were eligible for concurrent chemo-radiation [18]. Already about one fourth of patients with locally advanced lung cancer were 75 years or older, and comorbidity was very frequent. Even in patients less than 75 years, the comorbidity incidence was 278 (52.9%) 0, 188 (35.7%) 1, and 56 (11.4%) 2 or more. Less toxic alternatives are needed for these patients. At present, sequential chemotherapy and chest radiation is a realistic option.

Future Perspectives

Small cell lung cancer remains a challenging disease with most patients dying from distant metastases, and still a significant proportion with persistent local tumor. A better integration of systemic treatment with thoracic irradiation is still needed, as well as innovative drugs and sophisticated thoracic and cranial irradiation techniques. At present, targeted drugs failed to improve the prognosis of patients with SCLC, but as times goes by, there is a very high probability that this situation will change. Possibilities include anti-angiogenesis drugs and hypoxic cell sensitizers. Moreover, although at the time of writing, small-cell lung cancer stem cells have not been identified, selectively targeting these cells has a high therapeutic potential. The same applies for the integration of molecular imaging data into radiotherapy treatment planning. Lastly, identification of predictive and/ or prognostic factors on an individual patient basis may allow selecting the right patient for the best fitted treatment.

References

1 Jemal A, Siegel R, Ward E, Hao Y, Xu J, Murray T, Thun MJ: Cancer statistics, 2008. CA Cancer J Clin 2008;58:71–96.

2 Brigham BA, Bunn PA Jr, Minna JD, Cohen MH, Ihde DC, Shackney SE: Growth rates of small cell bronchogenic carcinomas. Cancer 1978;42:2880–2886.

3 Zelen M: Keynote address on biostatistics and data retrieval. Cancer Chemother Rep 1973;4:31–42.

4 Shepherd FA, Crowley J, Van Houtte P, Postmus PE, Carney D, Chansky K, Shaikh Z, Goldstraw P: International Association for the Study of Lung Cancer International Staging Committee and Participating Institutions. The International Association for the Study of Lung Cancer lung cancer staging project: proposals regarding the clinical staging of small cell lung cancer in the forthcoming (seventh) edition of the tumor, node, metastasis classification for lung cancer. J Thorac Oncol 2007;2:1067–1077.

5 Eberhardt W, Korfee S: New approaches for small-cell lung cancer: local treatments. Cancer Control 2003;10:289–296.

6 Pignon JP, Arriagada R, Ihde DC, Johnson DH, Perry MC, Souhami RL, Brodin O, Joss RA, Kies MS, Lebeau B, et al: A meta-analysis of thoracic radiotherapy for small-cell lung cancer. N Engl J Med 1992;327:1618–1624.

7 Warde P, Payne D: Does thoracic irradiation improve survival and local control in limited-stage small-cell carcinoma of the lung? A meta-analysis. J Clin Oncol 1992;10:890–895.

8 Sundstrøm S, Bremnes RM, Kaasa S, Aasebø U, Hatlevoll R, Dahle R, Boye N, Wang M, Vigander T, Vilsvik J, Skovlund E, Hannisdal E, Aamdal S; Norwegian Lung Cancer Study Group: Cisplatin and etoposide regimen is superior to cyclophosphamide, epirubicin, and vincristine regimen in small-cell lung cancer: results from a randomized phase III trial with 5 years' follow-up. J Clin Oncol 2002;20:4665–4672.

9 Pijls-Johannesma M, De Ruysscher D, Vansteenkiste J, Kester A, Rutten I, Lambin P: Timing of chest radiotherapy in patients with limited stage small cell lung cancer: a systematic review and meta-analysis of randomised controlled trials. Cancer Treat Rev 2007;33:461–473.

10 De Ruysscher D, Vansteenkiste J: Chest radiotherapy in limited-stage small cell lung cancer: facts, questions, prospects. Radiother Oncol 2000; 55:1–9.
11 Komaki R, Swann RS, Ettinger DS, Glisson BS, Sandler AB, Movsas B, Suh J, Byhardt RW: Phase I study of thoracic radiation dose escalation with concurrent chemotherapy for patients with limited small-cell lung cancer: Report of Radiation Therapy Oncology Group (RTOG) protocol 97–12. Int J Radiat Oncol Biol Phys 2005;62:342–350.
12 Belderbos JS, Kepka L, Spring Kong FM, Martel MK, Videtic GM, Jeremic B: Report from the International Atomic Energy Agency (IAEA) consultants' meeting on elective nodal irradiation in lung cancer: non-small-Cell lung cancer (NSCLC). Int J Radiat Oncol Biol Phys 2008;72:335–342.
13 De Ruysscher D, Bremer RH, Koppe F, Wanders S, van Haren E, Hochstenbag M, Geeraedts W, Pitz C, Simons J, ten Velde G, Dohmen J, Snoep G, Boersma L, Verschueren T, van Baardwijk A, Dehing C, Pijls M, Minken A, Lambin P: Omission of elective node irradiation on basis of CT-scans in patients with limited disease small cell lung cancer: a phase II trial. Radiother Oncol 2006;80: 307–312.
14 van Loon J, Offermann C, Bosmans G, Wanders R, Dekker A, Borger J, Oellers M, Dingemans AM, van Baardwijk A, Teule J, Snoep G, Hochstenbag M, Houben R, Lambin P, De Ruysscher D: 18FDG-PET based radiation planning of mediastinal lymph nodes in limited disease small cell lung cancer changes radiotherapy fields: a planning study. Radiother Oncol 2008;87:49–54.
15 Fried DB, Morris E, Poole C, et al: Systematic review evaluating the timing of thoracic radiation therapy in combined modality therapy for limited-stage small-cell lung cancer. J Clin Oncol 2004;22:4837–4845.
16 Turrisi AT 3rd, Kim K, Blum R, Sause WT, Livingston RB, Komaki R, Wagner H, Aisner S, Johnson DH: Twice-daily compared with once-daily thoracic radiotherapy in limited small-cell lung cancer treated concurrently with cisplatin and etoposide. N Engl J Med 1999;340:265–371.
17 De Ruysscher D, Pijls-Johannesma M, Bentzen SM, Minken A, Wanders R, Lutgens L, Hochstenbag M, Boersma L, Wouters B, Lammering G, Vansteenkiste J, Lambin P: Time between the first day of chemotherapy and the last day of chest radiation is the most important predictor of survival in limited-disease small-cell lung cancer. J Clin Oncol 2006;24:1057–1063.
18 De Ruysscher D, Botterweck A, Dirx M, Pijls-Johannesma M, Wanders R, Hochstenbag M,. Dingemans AC, Bootsma G, Geraedts W, Simons J, Pitz C, Lambin P: Eligibility for concurrent chemotherapy and radiotherapy of locally advanced lung cancer patients: a prospective, population-based study. Ann Oncol 2009;20:98–102.

Dirk De Ruysscher, MD, PhD
Department of Radiation Oncology (Maastro Clinic), GROW Research Institute, University Medical Center Maastricht
Dr. Tanslaan 12
NL–6229 ET Maastricht (The Netherlands)
Tel. +31 88 445 57 00, Fax +31 88 445 57 73, E-Mail dirk.deruysscher@maastro.nl

Heide J, Schmittel A, Kaiser D, Hinkelbein W (eds): Controversies in the Treatment of Lung Cancer.
Front Radiat Ther Oncol. Basel, Karger, 2010, vol 42, pp 180–186

Radiochemotherapy in Extensive Disease Small Cell Lung Cancer ED-SCLC

Branislav Jeremic[a] · Francesc Casas[b] · Luhua Wang[c] · Branislav Perin[d]

[a]Division of Human Health (NAHU), Applied Radiobiology and Radiotherapy (ARBR) Section, International Atomic Energy Agency (IAEA), Vienna, Austria; [b]Department of Radiation Oncology, University Clinic, Barcelona, Spain; [c]Chinese Medical Academy of Sciences, Beijing, China; [d]Institute of Lung Disease, Sremska Kamenica, Serbia

Abstract

Patients with extensive disease small cell lung cancer (ED-SCLC) represent approximately one-third of all SCLC patients. For these patients, chemotherapy (CHT) is the standard treatment of choice. With CHT given alone, however, there is not a high risk of distant progression, but also progression within the thorax and brain frequently occurs, even in patients achieving a response to CHT. To improve poor figures obtained with CHT alone and address important issue of intrathoracic tumor control and it relationship to overall survival, thoracic radiation therapy (TRT) was introduced with a curative intent in a prospective randomized trial by Jeremic et al (1988–1993). In that trial CHT alone was compared with CHT followed by TRT, and in both groups by a prophylactic cranial irradiation. This trial showed that TRT can offer an improvement on local control that leads to an improvement in overall survival. Toxicity was acceptable, while multivariate analysis identified number of metastasis as an independent prognosticator of outcome. Based on the data of this trial, researchers in the USA and Europe will undergo two prospective trials addressing the issue of TRT in ED-SCLC.

Chemotherapy (CHT) is the standard treatment option for patients with extensive disease small cell lung cancer (ED-SCLC). With this approach median survival time is 9–12 months and 5-year survivals are 1–3% [1–3]. In spite of the fact that up to 90% of patients experience objective response following initial CHT, the prognosis for patients with ED-SCLC remains poor. Most of them eventually relapse, leading to one of the most frustrating challenges in thoracic oncology.

This is especially so since approaches such as maintenance CHT after 4–6 cycles of induction CHT [4–6] and higher doses of CHT [7, 8] did not prove to be beneficial in this setting.

In addition, patterns of failure in patients with ED-SCLC treated with CHT alone show that besides distant progression, local progression remains very frequent event. It is therefore, that thoracic radiation therapy (TRT) and/or prophylactic cranial irradiation (PCI) could be of a benefit in suitable patients. Those would likely be the ones who experience some form of response to CHT, having reasonable chances to have prolonged periods of survival.

While RT is well established in limited disease (LD) SCLC [9–11], the usefulness of RT in ED-SCLC is much more open to debate. More than 20 years ago, a large retrospective review of literature showed that RT reduced the frequency of initial chest failure, but complete response (CR) rates, overall response rates (ORR), MST, and 2-year disease-free survival (DFS) were identical for patients treated with CHT alone and those treated with CHT and TRT [12]. However, the majority of studies from that report originated in 1960s and 1970s. Therefore, they cannot be considered as the optimal RT today, regarding total tumor dose (TD), dose per fraction, and timing as well as rather primitive treatment planning. In addition, when one explores the effectiveness of TRT in ED-SCLC, the systemic character of ED-SCLC that may obscure possible effects of RT on survival (established on a local level), especially in adequately chosen subgroup of patients suitable for 'curative' role of RT should not be forgotten. Other issues concerning RT, like irradiation to sites of systemic tumor or the role of prophylactic cranial irradiation (PCI), were also controversial.

Trying to focus on the issues of possible improvement in local (intrathoracic) tumor control and its subsequent impact, if any, on overall survival in favourable patient population, we tested the role of TRT in a prospective randomized trial designed late 1987 which run from 1988 to 1993 [3].

RT in ED-SCLC Trial

Eligibility criteria included naïve patients with ED-SCLC defined as the tumor beyond the confines of the hemithorax, mediastinum, and ipsilateral or contralateral supraclavicular nodes. Patients with tumors that could not be encompassed within a tolerable RT field were also considered as having ED-SCLC, as well as those having an 'isolated' pleural effusion with positive cytology, while those with negative cytology in an 'isolated' pleural effusion were found ineligible for this study. Patients had to have a Karnofsky performance status (KPS) score of ≥70, age 18–70 years, and adequate hematological, renal, and hepatic function (unless due to liver metastases). No recent or concurrent severe, uncontrolled cardiovascular or pulmonary disease was allowed nor were central nervous system metastases or other abnormality when substantially impairing mental status allowed.

Staging procedures included chest X-rays and tomography, bronchoscopy, bone marrow biopsy, brain, bone and liver radionuclide scans, and abdominal ultrasonography. CT scans of the thorax, brain, and abdomen were highly recommended as well as pulmonary function tests and were actually performed in all patients treated from 1989.

Eligible patients were treated with 3 cycles of standard-dose cisplatin/etoposide (PE) regimen given at 3-week intervals: P, 80 mg/m^2, day 1, and E, 80 mg/m^2, days 1–3. After 3 cycles of PE, complete patient reevaluation and restaging was performed, using the procedures outlined above. Patients achieving complete response at local and distant levels (CR/CR) and those achieving partial response (PR) within the thorax accompanied with the CR elsewhere (PR/CR) were randomized to receive either accelerated hyperfractionated radiation therapy (ACC HFX RT) and concurrent low-dose daily chemotherapy (CHT) consisting of carboplatin and etoposide (CE), 50 mg each, given on each RT day, followed by prophylactic cranial irradiation (PCI) and then by additional 2 cycles of PE (group I) or 4 additional cycles of PE and PCI (group II). Patients achieving worse response, i.e. those achieving CR or PR within thorax, but only a PR elsewhere (CR/PR – group III; PR/PR – group IV), were treated with 2 additional PE cycles followed by the same ACC HFX RT/CE and in case of CR at distant level, also PCI. Those with SD or PD (group V) were either observed until death (treated with supportive care only) or treated with orally administered etoposide, 50 mg/m^2, days 1 – 21, every 28 days to a total of 6 cycles or until further progression (on oral etoposide).

RT was administered with 6–10 MV photons from linear accelerators in groups I–IV. Target volume included all gross disease and ipsilateral hilum with a 2 cm margin, and the entire mediastinum with a 1-cm margin. Both supraclavicular fossae were routinely irradiated, AP–PA fields were used to deliver 36 Gy in 24 fractions in 12 treatment days over 2.5 weeks, after which combination of an anterior, lateral, and/or posterior oblique fields were used to give additional 18 Gy in 12 fractions in 6 treatment days. Total tumor dose (TD) was 54 Gy in 36 fractions in 18 treatment days in 3.5 weeks. Doses were specified at mid-depth at the central axis for parallel – opposed fields, and at the intersection of the central axes for oblique techniques. The maximum dose was 36 Gy to the spinal cord and the entire heart, 54 Gy for the esophagus, and 18 Gy for the contralateral lung. Two daily fractions of 1.5 Gy were used.

During ACC HFX RT, 50 mg of CBDCA and 50 mg of VP 16 were both given on each RT day between the two daily fractions (3–4 h after the first one, i.e. 1–2 h before the second one).

PCI was administered to the whole brain with TD 25 Gy in 10 daily fractions in 2 weeks via two parallel – opposed lateral fields in groups I and II. Patients in groups III and IV also received PCI, but only in cases achieving CR at distant level. Palliative RT with 30 Gy in 10 daily fractions was offered to patients with metastatic tumors when appropriate.

Patients were fully examined at the end of their treatment (groups I–IV), every month for 6 months after the end of the treatment, every 2 months for 2 years thereafter, and every 4–6 months thereafter. Restaging at time of progression was made by using the diagnostic tools outlined above.

Patients were evaluated for response after 3 cycles of PE (week 9), then after either ACC HFX RT or 2 additional PE cycles (week 15), and at the end of treatment (week 21).

CHT-induced toxicity was evaluated using the criteria of the Eastern Cooperative Oncology Group (ECOG) and that attributable to ACC HFX RT by the Radiation Therapy Oncology Group/European Organization for the Research and Treatment of Cancer (RTOG/EORTC).

Of a total of 210 patients entered this four patients were excluded from analysis due to occurrence of second (bladder) cancer, voluntary discontinuation of their treatment within the first cycle of CHT, stroke, and myocardial infarction, the former two occurring during the first week of treatment and the latter two occurring before the onset of treatment. A total of 206 patients were fully evaluable for toxicity and survival. There was no difference in the distribution of various variables between the five treatment groups. For all 206 patients, the median survival time (MST) was 9 months, and the yearly survival rates at 1, 2, 3, 4, and 5 years were 38, 19, 9.7, 4.9 and 3.4%, respectively. Since the only randomized part of the whole study included patients in groups 1 and 2, further data and the discussion are limited to these patients.

Patients in group I achieved best results that were significantly better than those in group 2: better outcome was observed in patients treated with combined CHT and ACC HFX RT when compared to those treated with CHT only ($p = 0.041$), with 5-year survival rates of 9.1 and 3.7% for groups I and II, respectively. Local recurrence-free survival (LRFS) was also better in group I than in group II, with median time to local recurrence (MTLR) of 30 and 22 months, respectively, and 5-year local recurrence-free survival of 20% and 8.1%, respectively ($p = 0.062$). Distant metastasis-free survival was similar between the two groups. Although group II patients treated with CHT only achieved longer median time to distant metastasis than group I patients treated with combined CHT/RT (16 vs. 14 months, respectively), they had poorer 5-year distant metastasis-free survival (DMFS: 14 vs. 27%), and the difference was not significant ($p = 0.35$). Because LRFS was only marginally insignificant and DMFS was not significantly different between groups I and II, we then performed first relapse-free survival (FRFS) analysis which showed that patients in group I achieved better results than those in group II regarding both median time to first relapse (MTFR) (13 vs. 9 months, respectively) and 1–5 year FRFS ($p = 0.045$).

Interestingly, analysis of response rates shows the local CR rate in groups I and II at weeks 9, 15, and 21. At week 9 after 3 cycles of induction PE, there was unexpectedly high CR rate at distant sites (52%). At that time there was no difference between the two groups in the local CR rate between the two groups, but at week 15 when either ACC HFX RT/CE (group I) or 2 additional cycles of PE (group II) were administered, the CR rate was significantly higher in group I than in group II ($p = 0.000007$), and it persisted until week 21 ($p = 0.00005$). Actual CR rates for the groups I and II were 96% and 66%, respectively. Interestingly, the 4th and 5th cycles of CHT add nothing to response achieved after ACC HFX RT was added to 3 cycles of PE. Furthermore, the 6th and 7th cycles of PE in the CHT-alone group brought only a few percent increase in RR, altogether questioning the duration (number of cycles) of CHT.

Of acute high-grade (≥3) treatment-related toxicity, hematological toxicity was more frequent in group II than in group I, but the difference was not significant and that was the case for all groups regarding leukopenia, trombocytopenia, and anemia. There was no difference between groups I and II regarding incidence of high-grade infection ($p = 0.64$). Due to more cycles of CHT administered to patients in group II, nausea and vomiting were significantly more frequent in that group than in group I ($p = 0.0038$), as was the case with alopecia ($p = 0.000003$). High-grade kidney toxicity was observed only in group II. Acute high-grade (≥3) RT-induced esophageal toxicity was observed only in patients that received RT. On the other hand, RT-induced high-grade bronchopulmonary toxicity was infrequent and, therefore, the difference between these groups was not significant ($p = 0.082$).

This was the very first prospective randomized study that evaluated curative TRT in ED-SCLC. It showed that TRT may play an important role in ED-SCLC. In an effort to learn more about the study results and gather some basic information for future studies, we also performed a multivariate analysis of the most common pretreatment prognostic factors in these patients. This analysis showed that besides KPS and weight loss, number of metastases significantly and independently predicted improved overall survival. Patients with only one metastasis had better outcome than those with ≥2 metastases, showing that metastatic tumor burden should be taken into account in future studies. Finally, overall good results should be attributed, at least in a part, to the fact that approximately 90% of all patients in that study had 1–2 metastases.

Future Approaches

After a gap of almost 10 years following the publication of this landmark study (i.e. 20 years since its start!), investigators over the world finally started with preparations for additional studies of TRT in ED-SCLC. The Radiation Therapy Oncology Group (RTOG) in the US plans a study (RTOG 0835) in which patients with ED-SCLC and no brain metastasis, having ECOG PS0–2 will be enrolled. Patients would have to achieve either CR or PR, with brain restaging done and with 0–1 residual sites of extrathoracic disease present at the time of restaging. Radiotherapy part of the study would include TRT of 45 Gy in 15 fractions, PCI of 25 Gy in 10 fractions, while 45 Gy in 15 fractions will be given to metastatic lesions. Major objectives of the trial would include (1) overall median and 1-year survival, (2) recurrence patterns and time to failure, as well as (3) acute and late toxicity of radiation therapy. Similarly, the Dutch Lung Cancer Study Group plans a Chest Radiotherapy in ED-SCLC Trial (CREST) with the primary endpoint being overall survival. Secondary endpoints would include pattern of relapse and toxicity. In CREST trial, patients with ED-SCLC without brain metastasis or pleural metastasis will undergo CHT. Those achieving any response to 4–6 cycles of chemotherapy will be randomized to PCI and no TRT versus those to be treated with PCI and TRT (30 Gy in 10 fractions) given only if the toxicity of the required fields will not be prohibitive. It is expected that these two studies provide data that will be supplementary to the data obtained during the study of Jeremic et al. [3] and help optimize both treatment approach with RT and identification of suitable patients for TRT.

Conclusions

After many years of silence for radiation oncologists, the field of ED-SCLC seems again to be an interesting and exciting field for clinical research. Recent data on the effectiveness of PCI in ED-SCLC [13] and renewed interest in TRT in ED-SCLC bring the focus of radiation oncologists worldwide to the issue of place and role of TRT in ED-SCLC. Every effort should be undertaken to help promote these studies, support them by enrolling patients in order to have them finished as soon as possible as to bring important answers in this disease.

References

1 Bunn PA Jr, Cohen MH, Ihde DC, Fossieck BE Jr, Matthews MJ, Minna JD: Advances in small cell bronchogenic carcinoma: a commentary. Cancer Treat Rep 1977;61:333–342.

2 Beck LK, Kane MA, Bunn PA Jr: Innovative and future approaches to small cell lung cancer treatment. Semin Oncol 1988;15:300–314.

3 Jeremic B, Shibamoto Y, Nikolic N, Milicic B, Milisavljevic S, Dagovic, A, Aleksandrovic J, Radosavljevic-Asic G: The role of radiation therapy in the combined modality treatment of patients with extensive disease small-cell lung cancer (ED SCLC): a randomized study. J Clin Oncol 1999;17:2092–2099.

4 Bunn PA Jr.: Clinical experience with carbolatin (paraplatin) in lung cancer. Semin Oncol 1992; 19(suppl 2): 1–11.

5 Splinter TAW: Chemotherapy of small cell lung cancer (SCLC): duration of treatment. Lung Cancer 1989;5:186–196.

6 Schiller JH, Adak S, Cella D, DeVore RF 3rd, Johnson DH: Topotecan versus observation after cisplatin plus etoposide in extensive-stage small-cell lung cancer: E7593 – a phase III trial of the Eastern Cooperative Oncology Group. J Clin Oncol. 2001, 19:2114–22.

7 Ihde DC, Mulshine JL, Kramer BS, Steinberg SM, Linnoila RI, Gazdar AF, Edison M, Phelps RM, Lesar M, Phares JC: Prospective randomized comparison of high-dose and standard-dose etoposide and cisplatin chemotherapy in patients with extensive-stage small cell lung cancer. J Clin Oncol 1994;12:2022–2034.

8 Leyvraz S, Pampallona S, Martinelli G, Ploner F, Perey L, Aversa S, Peters S, Brunsvig P, Montes A, Lange A, Yilmaz U, Rosti G, Solid Tumors Working Party of the European Group for Blood and Marrow Transplantation: A threefold dose intensity treatment with ifosfamide, carboplatin, and etoposide for patients with small cell lung cancer: a randomized trial. J Natl Cancer Inst 2008, 100: 533–41.

9 Murray N, Coy, Pater J, Hodson I, Arnold A, Zee BC, Payne D, Kostashuk EC, Evans WK, Dixon P.: Importance of timing for thoracic irradiation in the combined modality treatment of limited stage small cell lung cancer. J Clin Oncol 1993;11:336–344.

10 Jeremic B, Shibamoto Y, Acimovic L, Milisavljevic S: Initial versus delayed accelerated hyperfractionated radiation therapy and concurrent chemotherapy in limited small cell lung cancer. J Clin Oncol 1997;15:893–900.

11 Takada M, Fukuoka M, Kawahara M, Sugiura T, Yokoyama A, Yokota S, Nishiwaki Y, Watanabe K, Noda K, Tamura T, Fukuda H, Saijo N: Phase III study of concurrent versus sequential thoracic radiotherapy in combination with cisplatin and etoposide for limited-stage small-cell lung cancer: results of the Japan Clinical Oncology Group study 9104. J Clin Oncol 2002;20:3054–3060.

12 Bunn PA, Ihde DC: Small cell bronchogenic carcinoma: a review of therapeutic results; in Livingston RB (ed): Lung Cancer. Boston, Martin Nijhoff, 1981, pp 169–208.

13 Slotman B, Faivre-Finn C, Kramer G, Rankin E, Snee M, Hatton M, Postmus P, Collette L, Musat E, Senan S, EORTC Radiation Oncology Group and Lung Cancer Group: Prophylactic cranial irradiation in extensive small-cell lung cancer. N Engl J Med 2007 357:664–672.

Branislav Jeremic, MD, PhD
Institute of Lung Disease
Institutski put 4
RS–21204 Sremska Kamenica (Serbia)
Tel. +381 65 4146663, E-Mail nebareje@gmail.com

Heide J, Schmittel A, Kaiser D, Hinkelbein W (eds): Controversies in the Treatment of Lung Cancer.
Front Radiat Ther Oncol. Basel, Karger, 2010, vol 42, pp 187–192

Radiotherapy for Extensive Stage Small Cell Lung Cancer

B.J. Slotman

Department of Radiation Oncology, VU University Medical Center, Amsterdam, The Netherlands

Abstract

Small cell lung cancer is an aggressive form of lung cancer with a poor prognosis. Most patients present with extensive stage of the disease. To reduce the high risk of brain metastases, prophylactic cranial irradiation has been shown to be very effective. Prophylactic cranial irradiation should now routinely be used for all patients who have responded to chemotherapy. Thoracic radiotherapy is often reserved for palliation. However, the high incidence of residual disease after chemotherapy and the reported beneficial effect of radiotherapy in a single study has led to two clinical trials which will soon open and address the question whether thoracic radiotherapy also has a role in responding patients with extensive stage small cell lung cancer.

Introduction

Small cell lung cancer (SCLC) accounts for 10–15% of all newly diagnosed lung cancers [1]. Most patients have extensive stage (ES-SCLC) at presentation. The progression of the disease is generally rapid, and without treatment, median survival is only a few months. Although the prognosis has been improved by the use of chemotherapy, long-term survival remains disappointing. The 2-year survival of patients with ES-SCLC has increased from 1.5% in 1973 to 4.6% by 2000 [1]. In this article, the role of prophylactic cranial radiotherapy and thoracic irradiation in patients with ES-SCLC is discussed. The use of palliative radiotherapy for local or distant progression (e.g. bone metastases) is not part of this paper.

Brain Metastases

Brain metastases are very common in SCLC. They are detected in about 20% of the patients at diagnosis [2]. During the course of the disease, the incidence of brain metastases increases considerably, and at autopsy they are found in 80% of cases [3]. The risk of brain metastases is higher in patients with extensive stage than in those with limited stage SCLC [4, 5]. Maintenance chemotherapy fails to reduce the incidence of brain metastases [6]. Results of treatment for brain metastases are poor. The response rate after whole brain irradiation without chemotherapy in patients with brain-only relapse of SCLC is only 50% [7]. Various studies have shown that response to systemic is also very poor [8, 9]. The combination of chemotherapy and radiotherapy improves the response rate, but has no effect on survival [10]. Despite local and/or systemic treatment, many patients still suffer from the serious effects of brain metastases [11] and the majority of patients with symptomatic brain metastases die with, or due to, active brain disease [12].

Prophylactic Cranial Irradiation

Prophylactic cranial irradiation (PCI) has been used to reduce the risk of symptomatic metastases. Initial studies focused on patients with a complete response after chemotherapy, since these patients had the best prognosis and the possible largest benefit from PCI. In a number of randomized trials, it was shown that PCI is able to significantly reduce the risk of brain metastases [13–15]. Two meta-analyses confirmed this and additionally showed that PCI resulted in improved survival [16, 17]. In their meta-analysis, Auperin et al. [16] showed a reduction from 59% to 33% in the risk of brain metastases and an improvement of 3-year survival from 15 to 21%. Although PCI has the potential of inducing neurotoxicity, the avoidance of concomitant chemotherapy and use of low fraction dose schedules have reduced this considerably. No increase in late neuropsychological side effects was observed in randomized trials [13–15]. Another study revealed that even with moderate neurotoxicity, PCI was still considered beneficial for long-term survivors [18].

Some studies which evaluated the role of PCI also included some patients with ES-SCLC with a complete response. However, only one study specifically addressed this topic [19]. In this study performed within the European organization for Research and Treatment of Cancer (EORTC), patients with ES-SCLC who had responded to chemotherapy were randomized between PCI or no further therapy. Contrast-enhanced CT and/or MRI scan of the brain was not required at baseline, but was only performed when signs and/or symptoms suggestive for brain metastases were present. The use of PCI resulted in a reduction

Table 1. Effect of prophylactic cranial irradiation on brain metastases-free survival, progression-free survival and overall survival (adapted from Slotman et al. [19])

	PCI arm %	Control arm %	HR (95% CI)	Significance
1 year brain metastases-free survival	85.4	59.6	0.27 (0.16–0.44)	p<0.001
6 months progression-free survival	23.4	15.5	0.76 (0.59–0.96)	P=0.02
1 year overall survival	27.1	13.3	0.68 (0.52–0.88)	P=0.003

of the risk of symptomatic brain metastases at 1 year of 40.4% in the control arm to 14.6% in the patients which received PCI, corresponding to a hazard ratio of 0.27 [19]. In addition, the study showed a significant benefit of PCI for failure-free and overall survival. Survival at 1 year from randomization, i.e. about 4 months after diagnosis, was 27.1% for the PCI group, compared to 13.3% for patients in the controls arm (table 1) [19]. In this study, most patients received a PCI scheme of 20 Gy in 5 fractions (66%), others received 25–30 Gy in 8–12 fractions. Treatment was well tolerated, with very few patients experiencing grade 3 acute and/or or late toxicity. Although acute side effects resulted in negative influences on some quality of life scales shortly after PCI [20], there was no overall effect in the analysis of global quality of life up to 9 months [19]. A nationwide study in the United Kingdom recently showed that after the publication of the these study results, PCI is now routinely used in patients with ES-SCLC who responded to chemotherapy in about 90% of the centers [21]. The question of the optimal dose for PCI is unresolved. In LS-SCLC, a dose-response relationship was reported up to (radiobiologically equivalent) doses of 30–35 Gy (in 2-Gy fractions), but not for higher doses, provided that radiotherapy was started early after chemotherapy [22]. However, the results of a recent multigroup study failed to show a significant benefit of PCI doses of 36 Gy, either delivered in 18 daily fractions or in 24 twice daily fractions, over 25 Gy in 10 daily fractions [23]. The risk of brain metastases was 29% for the standard dose and 23% for the higher dose group. Interestingly, the study showed an unexplained statistically significant higher rate of chest relapse (40% for the standard dose and 48% for the high-dose arms) and poorer survival (42% for the standard dose and 37% for the high-dose group).

In view of the short survival of patients with ES-SCLC, PCI schemes for this group of patients should preferably be short. As the rate of extracranial progression is around 90% in these patients [19], in future studies, emphasis should preferably be put on this rather than on the dose-response relationship for PCI in ES-SCLC.

Table 2. Summary of the results of the study by Jeremic et al. [24]

Distant response	Thoracic response	Thoracic radiotherapy	Overall survival			Local relapse-free survival	
			median	3 years %	5 years %	median	3 years %
CR	CR or PR	yes	17 months	22	9	30 months	43
CR	CR or PR	no	11 months	13	4	22 months	30
PR	CR	yes	8 months	3	0	12 months	13
PR	PR	yes	6 months	0	0	12 months	0

Thoracic Radiotherapy

Although thoracic radiotherapy has a definite role in the treatment of patients with limited stage SCLC, in ES-SCLC it is has traditionally been reserved for patients who need local palliation. The lack of interest in thoracic radiotherapy in ES-SCLC can be attributed to the systemic nature of this disease and the rapid progression rate in many patients. There is only one study in which the role of thoracic radiotherapy in patients with ES-SCLC has been addressed systematically.

Jeremic et al. [24] treated 206 patients with 3 cycles of chemotherapy, consisting of cisplatin and etoposide. Patients (n = 109) with a complete response at distant sites and a complete or partial response in the thorax were randomized to either chemotherapy alone or accelerated hyperfractionated radiotherapy. The radiotherapy of 54 Gy in 36 fractions over 18 days was given concurrently with carboplatin and etoposide [24]. Thoracic radiotherapy was also given to all patients who has a partial response at distant sites, without randomization. The use of thoracic radiotherapy in patients with a complete response at distant sites resulted in a significant improvement of survival. Median survival was 17 months for patients who received thoracic radiotherapy, compared to only 11 months for those who only received chemotherapy [24]. Survival at 3 and 5 years was 22% and 9% for the thoracic radiotherapy group and 13% and 4% for the chemotherapy-only group, respectively (table 2) [24]. However, this single-center study alone has not resulted in the routine use of thoracic radiotherapy in ES-SCLC.

The Dutch Lung Cancer Study Group has initiated a randomized controlled trial of thoracic radiotherapy versus observation for patients with ED-SCLC who have responded to chemotherapy. In this trial, patients (18–75 years age) with ES-SCLC who have responded to chemotherapy and have a WHO score of 0–2 will be randomized to receive thoracic radiotherapy plus PCI or PCI only. No strict response

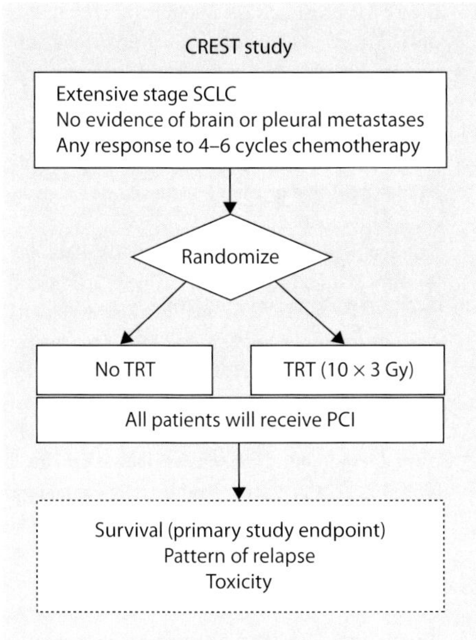

Fig. 1. Design of the CREST trial.

criteria are given, but the radiotherapy volume should be encompass able by acceptable radiation fields to prevent excessive toxicity. The radiation scheme for thoracic radiotherapy will be 30 Gy in 10 fractions. For PCI, radiation schemes of 20 Gy in 5 fractions and 30 Gy in 10 fractions can be used. The primary endpoints of this study is overall survival. Secondary endpoints include pattern of relapse and toxicity (fig. 1). In addition, the RTOG is planning a phase II trial to determine the role of consolidation extracranial radiotherapy (thoracic and other extracranial metastatic sites) alongside PCI after a response to systemic chemotherapy [pers. commun.].

References

1 Govindan R, Page N, Morgensztern D, et al: Changing epidemiology of small-cell lung cancer in the United States Over the Last 30 Years: analysis of the surveillance, epidemiologic, and end results database. J Clin Oncol 2006;24:4539–4544.
2 Seute T, Leffers P, Ten Velde GPM, Twijnstra A: Neurologic disorders in 432 consecutieve patients with small cell lung carcinoma. Cancer 2004;100: 801–806.
3 Nugent JL, Bunn PA Jr, Matthews MJ, et al: CNS metastases in small cell bronchogenic carcinoma: increasing frequency and changing pattern with lengthening survival. Cancer 1979;44:1885–1893.
4 Glantz MJ, Choy H, Yee L: Prophylactic cranial irradiation in small cell lung cancer: rationale, results and recommendations. Semin Oncol 1997; 24:477–483.
5 Van Oosterhout AG, Van de Pol M, Ten Velde G, Twijnstra A: Neurologic disorders in 203 consecutive patients with small cell lung cancer: results of a longitudinal study. Cancer 1996;77:1434–1441.
6 Schiller JH, Adak S, Cella D, DeVore RF III, Johnson DH: Topotecan versus observation after cisplatin plus etoposide in extensive-stage small-cell lung cancer: E7593 – a phase III trial of the Eastern Cooperative Oncology Group. J Clin Oncol 2001;19:2114–2122.

7 Postmus PE, Haaxma-Reiche H, Gregor A, et al: Brain-only metastases of small cell lung cancer; efficacy of whole brain radiotherapy: an EORTC phase II study. Radiother Oncol 1998;46:29–32.

8 Postmus PE, Haaxma-Reiche H, Sleijfer DTh, et al: High dose etoposide for brain metastases of small cell lung cancer: a phase II study. Br J Cancer 1989;5:254–256.

9 Postmus PE, Smit EF, Haaxma-Reiche H, et al: Teniposide for brain metastases of small cell lung cancer: a phase II study. J Clin Oncol 1995;13:660–665.

10 Postmus PE, Haaxma-Reiche H, Smit EF, et al: Treatment of brain metastases of small-cell lung cancer: comparing teniposide and teniposide with whole brain radiotherapy: a phase III study of the EORTC Lung Cancer Cooperative Group. J Clin Oncol 2000;18:3400–3408.

11 Felletti R, Souhami RL, Spiro SG, et al: Social consequences of brain or liver relapse in small cell carcinoma of the bronchus. Radiother Oncol 1985; 4:335–339.

12 Hardy J, Smith I, Cherryman G, et al: The value of computed tomography (CT) scan surveillance in the detection and management of brain metastases in patients with small cell lung cancer. Br J Cancer 1990;62:684–686.

13 Arriagada R, Monnet I, Riviere A, et al: Prophylactic cranial irradiation for patients with small cell lung cancer in complete remission. Eur J Cancer 1995;31A(suppl 5):83.

14 Arriagada R, LeChevalier T, Borie F, et al: Prophylactic cranial irradiation for patients with small-cell lung cancer in complete remission. J Natl Cancer Inst 1995;87:183–190.

15 Gregor A, Cull A, Stephens RJ, et al: Prophylactic cranial irradiation is indicated following complete response to induction therapy in small cell lung cancer: results of a multicentre randomized trial (UKCCCR and EORTC). Eur J Cancer 1997;33: 1752–1758.

16 Auperin A, Arriagada R, Pignon JP, et al: Prophylactic cranial irradiation for patients with small-cell lung cancer in complete remission. N Engl J Med 1999;341:476–484.

17 Meert AP, Paesmans M, Berghmans T, et al: Prophylactic cranial irradiation in small cell lung cancer: a systematic review of the literature with meta-analysis. BMC Cancer 2001;1:5.

18 Lee JJ, Bekele BN, Zhou X, Cantor SB, Komaki R, Lee JS: Decision analysis for prophylactic cranial irradiation for patients with small-cell lung cancer. J Clin Oncol 2006;24:3597–603.

19 Slotman BJ, Faivre-Finn C, Kramer GW, Rankin E, Snee M, Hatton M, Postmus P, Colette L, Musat E, Senan S: Prophylactic cranial irradiation in small cell lung cancer. N Engl J Med 2007;357:664–672.

20 Slotman BJ, Mauer ME, Bottomley A, Faivre-Finn C, Kramer GW, Rankin EM, Snee M, Hatton M, Postmus PE, Collette L, Senan S: Prophylactic cranial irradiation in extensive disease small-cell lung cancer: short-term health-related quality of life and patient reported symptoms: results of an international phase III randomised controlled trial. J Clin Oncol 2009;27:78–84.

21 Bayman N, Lorigan P, Blackhall F, Thatcher N, Faivre-Finn C: Current trends in prophylactic cranial irradiation (PCI) for extensive-disease small cell lung cancer (EDSCLC): results of a UK survey. J Clin Oncol 2008;26(suppl):abstr 19040.

22 Suwinski R, Lee SP, Withers HR: Dose-response relationship for prophylactic cranial irradiation in small cell lung cancer. Int J Radiat Oncol Biol Phys 1998;40:797–806.

23 Le Péchoux C, Dunant A, Senan S, Wolfson A, Quoix E, Faivre-Finn C, Ciuleanu T, Arriagada R, Jones R, Wanders R, Lerouge D, Laplanche A, Prophylactic Cranial Irradiation (PCI) Collaborative Group: Standard-dose versus higher-dose prophylactic cranial irradiation (PCI) in patients with limited-stage small-cell lung cancer in complete remission after chemotherapy and thoracic radiotherapy (PCI 99-01, EORTC 22003-08004, RTOG 0212, and IFCT 99-01): a randomised clinical trial. Lancet Oncol 2009;10:467–474.

24 Jeremic B, Shibamoto Y, Nikolic N, et al: Role of radiation therapy in the combined-modality treatment of patients with extensive disease small-cell lung cancer: a randomized study. J Clin Oncol 1999;17:2092–2099.

B.J. Slotman, MD, PhD
Department of Radiation Oncology, VU University Medical Center
De Boelelaan 1117
NL–1081 HV Amsterdam (The Netherlands)
Tel. +31 20 4440414, Fax +31 20 4440410, E-Mail bj.slotman@vumc.nl

Heide J, Schmittel A, Kaiser D, Hinkelbein W (eds): Controversies in the Treatment of Lung Cancer.
Front Radiat Ther Oncol. Basel, Karger, 2010, vol 42, pp 193–197

Controversies in the Treatment of Advanced Stages of Small Cell Lung Cancer

Alexander Schmittel

Department of Haematology and Oncology, Charité, Campus Benjamin Franklin, Berlin, Germany

Abstract

Small cell lung cancer is a highly proliferative tumor with the potential of early hematogeneous spread. At the time of first diagnosis more than 80% of patients present with distant metastases. Although response rate to chemotherapy is high with >50% confirmed objective responses, the majority of patients relapse within several months after first-line chemotherapy. The combination of cisplatin plus etoposide has become standard chemotherapy. In contrast to early stages, equal efficacy of cisplatin and carboplatin in combination with etoposide has been suggested in advanced disease in two randomized trials in the 1990s. Newer agents like the topoisomerase I inhibitors topotecan and irinotecan have been investigated for first line treatment. Two phase III studies demonstrated similar efficacy of topotecan when compared to etoposide. Results of first line therapy with irinotecan are more contradictory. A first trial demonstrated superiority of irinotecan/cisplatin over etoposide/cisplatin in a Japanese population. However, two subsequent North American phase III trials showed equivalent efficacy. Recently a Scandinavian phase III trial found superiority of irinotecan/carboplatin over etoposide/carboplatin. Prophylactic cranial irradiation (PCI) after first line chemotherapy has become standard of care in advanced stages, because a randomized phase III trial of the EORTC demonstrated a survival benefit. Second-line therapy in relapsed disease improves survival. A randomized trial showed similar efficacy of topotecan when compared to anthracyline containing chemotherapy, with an improvement of cancer related symptoms in the topotecan arm.

First-Line Chemotherapy

Chemotherapy is the treatment of choice in extensive disease small cell lung cancer (SCLC). Response rates are high with 50–90% of patients showing confirmed partial or complete responses. Given the high probability of response chemotherapy also is the first choice in individuals with superior vena cava syndrome.

In a meta-analysis containing 19 randomized trials with a total of 4054 patients superiority of cisplatin over non-cisplatin-based chemotherapy had clearly been shown [1]. Similar efficacy of carboplatin and cisplatin had been demonstrated in two smaller randomized trials, which included unselected patients with SCLC [2, 3]. Therefore, cisplatin or carboplatin plus etoposide have become standard therapy and most groups administer 4–6 cycles of chemotherapy.

One of the most controversial questions in treatment of extensive disease SCLC is whether or not modern topoisomerase-I inhibitors like topotecan or irinotecan are superior to etoposide:

Two prospectively randomized phase III trials compared topotecan + ciplatin versus etoposide + cisplatin. The North American trial randomized 784 patients to oral topotecan + cisplatin versus intravenous etoposide + cisplatin. This trial showed noninferiority of topotecan/cisplatin combination and a slightly but statistically longer PFS with etoposide/cisplatin [4]. The second study demonstrated a significant improvement of response rate and progression-free survival in favor of intravenous topotecan/cisplatin; however, overall survival analysis showed no difference between the arms. Hematologic toxicity was higher in the topotecan arm [5]. Since no overall survival benefit could be demonstrated topotecan has not become standard therapy in the first line.

The role of irinotecan in the treatment of SCLC is even more controversial at the moment:

Initial evidence for superiority of irinotecan over etoposide came from a Japanese randomized phase III trial, which was terminated early after an interim analysis showed a benefit for combined irinotecan-cisplatin over etoposide-cisplatin [6]. Response rate, progression-free and overall survival favored irinotecan therapy; however, because this trial included only 154 patients and all patients were Asians, confirmatory studies were initiated in the US and Europe. Both US studies compared various schedules and doses of cisplatin-etoposide with cisplatin-irinotecan [7, 8]. Median survival, progression-free survival and response rates did not differ between the two arms in both trials. One possible reason for contradictory results observed between the Japanese and US trials, and the higher toxicity of irinotecan observed in the Japanese study might be due to racial variations in the UDP-glucuronosyltransferase 1 leading to increased concentrations of irinotecan and its metabolites in Japanese patients [9].

Two European trials have compared etoposide with irinotecan in combination with carboplatin. Preliminary results of a phase II European trial showed improved progression-free survival in favor of irinotecan-carboplatin [10]. The final results of the phase III trial will be available in 2009.

The binational, multicenter, randomized phase III trial performed in Scandinavia compared intravenous irinotecan with oral etoposide both in combination with carboplatin (area under the curve, 4) [11]. The primary end point of the study was overall survival, and favored the irinotecan arm. Quality of life analysis revealed a trend towards prolonged palliation in the irinotecan arm [11].

A fundamental difference of the European phase III study compared with the Japanese and US trials is that 47% of patients had a performance status >3 and 35% were >70 years old. Conversely, in the Japanese trial and the US trial published by Hanna et al. only included a highly selected patient population with a performance status of 0–2 and the SWOG study included patients with a performance status of 0 or 1 [6–8]. The use of oral etoposide and the dose reductions in selected patients represent limitations of the study. Well-known interpatient variations in bio-availability, pharmacodynamics as well as compliance for oral etoposide might lead to underdosing or significant toxicity in certain patients. Therefore, oral etoposide cannot be recommended for first-line therapy and neither as an ideal control arm for a randomized trial [12]. In addition, 33% dose reduction was performed in all patients with a performance status >3 or age >70 years, which might represent underdosing in the control arm; however, it has been established that elderly patients tolerate chemotherapy similar to younger patients, and generally accepted reasons for dose reductions are comorbidity and poor performance status only.

Taking into account the weaknesses of this trial and the results of the US trials – neither of which could confirm the Japanese data – substitution of etoposide by irinotecan can not be recommended at this time. The final results of the second European trial are awaited.

For years the question of dose escalation had been a matter of debate in SCLC. Finally a randomized trial comparing conventional chemotherapy to high-dose chemotherapy supported by autologous stem cell transplantation could not show a benefit from dose escalation [13].

Prophylactic Cranial Irradiation after First-Line Chemotherapy

The randomized phase III trial performed by the EORTC (08993–22993) compared prophylactic cranial irradiation (PCI) to observation in patients with stable disease or response to first line chemotherapy. PCI was associated with a significantly reduced risk to develop symptomatic brain metastases and with an improved survival for the PCI group. One-year survival after randomization was 27.1 versus 13.3% ($p = 0.003$) [14]. Therefore PCI has become standard therapy for patients with disease stabilization or remission after first line chemotherapy.

Second-Line Chemotherapy

Most patients with SCLC extensive disease will progress shortly after the end of chemotherapy. In case of disease progression within 3 months after the end of first-line therapy efficacy of second-line therapy is rather low and the disease is usually termed 'refractory'. If progression occurred 3 or more months after chemotherapy the disease is usually called 'sensitive'. Sensitive disease is associated with a higher response rate to subsequent therapy.

Various studies investigated topotecan for second-line therapy. Topotecan showed similar activity when compared to an anthracycline-based therapy in patients with sensitive disease. Response rates and survival analysis were similar in both arms, however, symptom control assessment favored topotecan [15].

Another phase III trial compared second line therapy with oral topotecan to best supportive care. This study showed a survival benefit in favor of oral topotecan although the response rate was 7% only [16].

Therefore topotecan or anthracycline-based combination chemotherapy has become the standard of care for patients with acceptable performance status in the second-line setting.

Re-treatment with first-line regimen is recommended in the rare situation of patients with progression more than 6–12 months after first-line chemotherapy.

References

1 Pujol JL, Carestia L, Laures JP: Is there a case for cisplatin in the treatment of small-cell lung cancer? A meta-analysis of randomized trials of a cisplatin-containing regimen versus a regimen without this alkylating agent. Br J Cancer 2000; 83:8–15.

2 Skarlos DV, Samantas E, Kosmidis P, et al: Randomized comparison of etoposide-cisplatin vs. etoposide-carboplatin and irradiation in small-cell lung cancer. Ann Oncol 1994;5:601–607.

3 Lassen U, Kristjansen PE, Osterlind K, Bergman B, Sigsgaard TC, Hirsch FR, Hansen M, Dombernowsky P, Hansen HH: Superiority of cisplatin or carboplatin in combination with teniposide and vincristine in the induction chemotherapy of small-cell lung cancer: a randomized trial with 5 years follow up. Ann Oncol 1996;7:365–371.

4 Eckhardt JR, von Pawel J, Papai Z, Tomova A, Tzekova V, Crofts TE, Brannon S, Wissel P, Ross G: Open-label, multicenter, randomized, phase III study comparing oral topotecan/cisplatin versus etoposide/cisplatin as treatment for chemotherapy-naive patients with extensive-disease small cell lung cancer. J Clin Oncol 2006;24:2044–2051.

5 Heigener DF, Freitag L, Eschbach C, Huber RM, Fink T, Hummler S, Banik N, Wolf W: Topotecan/cisplatin (TP) compared to cisplatin/etoposide (PE) for patients with extensive disease-small cell lung cancer (ED- SCLC): final results of a randomised phase III trial. J Clin Oncol 2008;26 (suppl):abstr 7513.

6 Noda K, Nishiwaki Y, Kawahara M, et al: Irinotecan plus Cisplatin compared with etoposide plus cisplatin for extensive small lung cancer. N Engl J Med 2002;346:85–91.

7 Hanna N, Bunn PA Jr, Langer C, Einhorn L, Guthrie T Jr, Beck T, Ansari R, Ellis P, Byrne M, Morrison M, Hariharan S, Wang B, Sandler A: Randomized phase III trial comparing irinotecan/cisplatin with etoposide/cisplatin in patients with previously untreated extensive-stage disease small-cell lung cancer. J Clin Oncol 2006;24:2038–2043.

8 Natale RB, Lara PN, Chansky K, Crowley JJ, Jett JR, Carleton JE, Kuebler JP, Lenz HJ, Mack PC, Gandara DG: A randomized phase III trial of cisplatin + irinotecan (IP) with etoposide/cisplatin (EP) in patients (pts) with previously untreated extensive stage small cell lung cancer (E-SCLC). J Clin Oncol 2008;26(suppl):abstr 7512.

9 Beutler E, Gelbart T, Demina A: Racial variability in the UDP-glucuronosyltransferase 1 (UGT1A1) promoter: a balanced polymorphism for regulation of bilirubin metabolism? Proc Natl Acad Sci USA 1998;95:8170–8174.
10 Schmittel A, Fischer von Weikersthal L, Sebastian M, Martus P, Schulze K, Hortig P, Reeb M, Thiel E, Keilholz U: A randomized phase II trial of irinotecan plus carboplatin versus etoposide plus carboplatin treatment in patients with extended disease small-cell lung cancer. Ann Oncol 2006; 17:663–667.
11 Hermes A, Bergman B, Bremnes R, Ek L, Fluge S, Sederholm C, Sundstrøm S, Thaning L, Vilsvik J, Aasebø U, Sörenson S: Irinotecan plus carboplatin versus oral etoposide plus carboplatin in extensive small-cell lung cancer: a randomized phase III trial. J Clin Oncol 2008;26:4261–4267.
12 Souhami RL, Spiro SG, Rudd RM, Ruiz de Elvira MC, James LE, Gower NH, Lamont A, Harper PG: Five-day oral etoposide treatment for advanced small-cell lung cancer: randomized comparison with intravenous chemotherapy. J Natl Cancer Inst 1997;89:577–580.
13 Leyvraz S, Pampallona S, Martinelli G, Ploner F, Perey L, Aversa S, Peters S, Brunsvig P, Montes A, Lange A, Yilmaz U, Rosti G: A threefold dose intensity treatment with ifosfamide, carboplatin, and etoposide for patients with small cell lung cancer: a randomized trial. . J Natl Cancer Inst. 2008;100:533–541.
14 Slotman B, Faivre-Finn C, Kramer G, Rankin E, Snee M, Hatton M, Postmus P, Collette L, Musat E, Senan S: Prophylactic cranial irradiation in extensive small-cell lung cancer. N Engl J Med 2007;357:664–672.
15 von Pawel J, Schiller JH, Shepherd FA, Fields SZ, Kleisbauer JP, Chrysson NG, Stewart DJ, Clark PI, Palmer MC, Depierre A, Carmichael J, Krebs JB, Ross G, Lane SR, Gralla R: Topotecan versus cyclophosphamide, doxorubicin, and vincristine for the treatment of recurrent small-cell lung cancer. J Clin Oncol 1999;17:658–67.
16 O'Brien MER, Ciuleanu T, Tsekov H, Shparyk Y, Čučević B, Juhasz G, Ross GA, Dane G, Crofts T: Survival benefit of oral topotecan plus supportive care versus supportive care alone in relapsed, resistant SCLC. Lung Cancer 2005;49(suppl 2):157.

Alexander Schmittel, MD
Department of Haematology and Oncology, Charité, Campus Benjamin Franklin
Hindenburgdamm 30
DE–12203 Berlin (Germany)
Tel. +49 30 8445 3090, Fax +49 30 8445 4468, E-Mail Alexander.schmittel@charite.de

Heide J, Schmittel A, Kaiser D, Hinkelbein W (eds): Controversies in the Treatment of Lung Cancer.
Front Radiat Ther Oncol. Basel, Karger, 2010, vol 42, pp 198–205

Complementary and Alternative Medicine in Lung Cancer Patients: A Neglected Phenomenon?

O. Micke[a,b,g] · J. Büntzel[c,g] · K. Kisters[d,g] · U. Schäfer[e,g] · P. Micke[f] · R. Mücke[e,g]

[a]Department of Radiotherapy and Radiation Oncology, Franziskus Hospital, Bielefeld, [b]Department of Radiotherapy, Radiation Oncology, Münster University Hospital, Münster, [c]Department of Otolaryngology, Südharz Hospital, Nordhausen, [d]Department of Internal Medicine I, St Anna Hospital, Herne, and [e]Department of Radiotherapy, Lippe Hospital, Lemgo, Germany; [f]Department of Genetics and Pathology, Uppsala University, Uppsala, Sweden; [g]German Working Group Trace Elements and Electrolytes in Radiation Oncology – AKTE, Bielefeld, Germany

Abstract

Study on the use of complementary and alternative medicine (CAM) in lung cancer patients has been widely neglected. Therefore, we initiated a study on the use of CAM in lung cancer patients in addition to radiation treatment. Overall, 120 patients from 3 institutions were interviewed by a standardized questionnaire. Besides the tumor parameters and the use of CAM, the reason for the use, patient information of the medication, the information sources and the subjective condition of the patient. Altogether, 54% of the patients reported using CAM (66% of female patients, 52% of male patients). The most frequently used CAM measures were vitamin combinations (17%), mistletoe (15%), and selenium (12%). A total of 52% reported the wish to support the tumor treatment as a reason for using CAM and 27% had a 'better feeling' using CAM. 50% of CAM was bought by the patients themselves and 50% were prescribed by their family physicians. The use of CAM is frequent in lung cancer patients. Our results suggest that it is very important to obtain information on the CAM use of patients and, particularly in controlled clinical trials, to prospectively document it.

Lung cancer ranks 3rd of the most frequent tumor diseases in men and women in Germany. In death statistics, it ranks place 1 in men and place 3 in women, reflecting the overall persistently devastating prognosis of the patients. About 45,000 new patients per year are diagnosed with lung cancer in Germany [1].

In recent years, complementary and alternative medicine (CAM) has experienced an increasing popularity in particular among patients with life-threatening diseases such as cancer [2–6]. Therefore, as Burstein [7] already stated in 2000 in the *Journal of Clinical Oncology*, the use of CAM has become the norm in most tumor patients. Patients with lung and other poor-outlook cancers are particularly vulnerable to heavily promoted claims for unproved or disproved alternatives or complements to conventional tumor treatment [8].

The difference between 'complementary' and 'alternative' therapies is important and essential to recognize [8], because it can have far-reaching consequences for the patient.

Complementary and alternative medicine was defined by the US National Center for Complementary and Alternative Medicine (NCCAM) as diverse medical and health care systems, practices, and products that are not presently considered to be part of conventional medicine [9].

To define CAM more specifically, *complementary medicine* is used *together with* conventional medicine (also termed mainstream, orthodox, or regular medicine).

In contrast, *alternative medicine* is considered to *replace* conventional medicine. Other terms for CAM used in the medical literature include unconventional, nonconventional, unproven, or irregular medicine [9, 10]. Alternative therapies are typically promoted as literal, viable options for cancer treatment. Unfortunately, these are unproven products and regimens, often completely ineffective against cancer, that draw patients with unsubstantiated, often fanciful, claims of easy cure [8]. This is especially problematic in oncology, when delayed treatment can diminish the chances of remission and cure [11].

Over time, some complementary therapies are proven safe and effective. These become integrated into mainstream care, producing integrative oncology, a synthesis of the best of mainstream cancer treatments and rational, data-based, adjunctive complementary therapies [8]. Such an integration is currently evolving more and more [4, 13–15].

Most complementary therapies are not specific to a particular cancer diagnosis. Instead, they are used typically to treat symptoms shared by patients across most cancer diagnoses [8]. Most CAM practices can be loosely grouped into five categories according to the National Institutes of Health (NIH) National Center for Complementary and Alternative Medicine (table 1). The therapies in these categories are quite mixed; some are helpful, others are humbug. There is also considerable overlap among the categories. For example, traditional Chinese medicine uses biologically active botanicals and acupuncture. Yoga has mind-body and manipulative components and Ayurvedic principles in theory. Some interventions, such as music therapy, do not fit easily into a category [9, 16].

Wherever CAM is provided and used, it is essential to know which interventions work, which do not work, and which are likely to be harmful [16].

Table 1. Categories and examples of complementary and alternative therapies according to the National Center for Complementary and Alternative Medicine (NCCAM) [9]

Category	Examples
Biologically based practices	herbal remedies, vitamins, other dietary supplements
Mind-body techniques	meditation, guided imagery
Manipulative and body-based practices	massage, reflexology
Energy therapies	magnetic field therapy
Ancient medical systems	traditional Chinese medicine, Ayurvedic medicine, acupuncture

In oncology centers worldwide (including developing countries), the frequencies of CAM use vary between 32 and 83% [2, 3, 6, 18–21]. Breast cancer patients are most likely to use CAM compared to other tumor diagnoses [2, 3, 6, 10, 12, 18, 21, 22].

However, the CAM use in lung cancer patients has been widely neglected up to now. We could identify in Medline (Pubmed) just a single study focusing complementary and alternative medicine in Lung cancer patients [23]. The relation between radiotherapy and complementary and alternative therapies has been not examined until now.

Therefore, the German Working Group Trace Elements and Electrolytes in Radiation Oncology – AKTE initiated an explorative study on the use of CAM in lung cancer patients in addition to radiation treatment.

Methods

The study population consisted of 120 patients with histologically confirmed lung cancer (non-small cell lung cancer) from three different institutions in Germany (one university hospital and three community hospitals) referred for curative (n = 42) or palliative radiotherapy (n = 78). There were 38 female and 72 male patients. The median age was 57 years (range: 32–81 years).

Patients with a Karnofsky performance status (KPS) of less than 70% were excluded from the study, since they were not considered to be fully independent in their medical decisions.

The study was conducted as a semistructured face-to-face interview based on a standardized questionnaire checklist, which was based on the experiences of other studies [10, 21].

Patients were interviewed before the beginning of radiation treatment by an experienced staff member. Study participants were classified as either CAM users or CAM nonusers according to whether or not they had used at least one CAM therapy during the past 4 weeks.

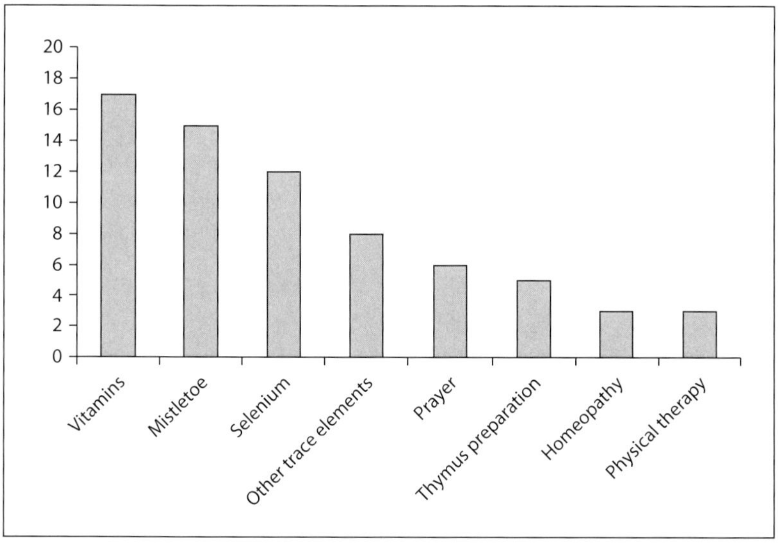

Fig. 1. Percentage of the most frequently used CAM therapies (percentage of all therapies reported).

Demographic variables included age, gender, highest educational degree, smoking, and alcohol drinking habits. The histology of disease, stage, and specific characteristics of the primary tumors and metastases, as well as current and previous treatments, were also recorded.

Besides the reason for the use, information on the receipt of the medication, the information sources and the subjective condition under CMA treatment were interrogated.

Results

All study patients suffered from a non-small cell lung cancer with the following tumor stages: stage II, 18; stage III, 60; stage IV, 42.

Altogether, 54% of the patients reported using CAM (66% of female patients, 52% of male patients). The most frequent used CAM measures were vitamin combinations (17%), mistletoe (15%), selenium (12%), other trace element combinations (8%), prayer (6%), thymus preparations (5%), homeopathy (3%) and other physical treatment (3%) (fig. 1).

The multivariate analysis (logistic regression) revealed a statistical significant correlation of CAM use to more advanced tumor stage, treatment intention (curative/palliative) female gender, higher education, smoking and drinking behavior.

Simplified it can stated that the typical CAM use is a young female nonsmoking patient, with a more advanced disease, and higher educational level without alcohol consumption.

A total of 52% reported the wish to support the tumor treatment as a reason for using CAM and 27% had a 'better feeling' using CAM.

Half of CAM was bought by patients themselves and 50% were prescribed by their family physicians. Sources of CAM supply predominantly were pharmacies and drugstores. Information sources were mostly the family physician (46% of the cases) and other patients or local cancer support groups (24% of cases).

Overall, 55% of patients described an improvement of their subjective condition after using CAM.

Discussion

In general, the use of CAM in lung cancer patients has been widely neglected up to now. We could identify just one study in literature which had concentrated on this topic [23]. They studied the use of CAM to control symptoms in 189 women living with non-small cell lung cancer. Forty-four percent of patients (84 women) used CAM therapies. Women who were younger, experienced more symptoms, and lived on the West Coast or South (versus Northeast) were more likely to use CAM. The CAM therapies used were predominantly prayer (34.9%) and meditation (11.6%), which is very different to our results in German patients. This marked difference once again clearly manifested the different spiritual and socioreligious background of patients in Europe, in particular Central Europe, and the United States. This distinct sociocultural imprint makes it very difficult and sometimes impossible to compare results on CAM use, notably spiritual ones between the different continents [24–26].

The use of CAM therapies in Lung cancer patients is generally disregarded and often estimated to be very low [4]. The frequency is often compared to head and neck cancer patients concluding from the similar risk factors and the similar gender distribution to be 10–30%. Our study exhibited a CAM use of more than 50% of patients, which is far higher than expected and must not be ignored.

On the other hand, expectations towards CAM are quite high. Patients hope to improve their quality of life, alleviate symptoms, prolong life, cure their disease and boost their immune system [7]. But the promised positive effects are mostly not proven and the proposed underlying molecular mechanisms are commonly mere speculation, making CAM therapies unattractive for academic clinical research. Additionally, self-treatment is most often not reported by the patients or verbalized by the treating oncologist, although it is very common among cancer patients. Consequently, there is only limited information about the type of CAM, the frequency of use, the source and the expenses as well as the patients' attitudes and beliefs about such therapies [10]. Multivariate analysis revealed age, gender, stage, disease extent as well as educational level, smoking and drinking behavior to be relevant predictors for CAM use. These findings also reflect clinical experience that younger patients with progressive disease and poor prognosis apply 'every method available' [19]. Several studies support these findings [2, 3, 10, 12, 16–21].

Using a semiquantative, nonvalidated subjective score, an improvement in quality of life was claimed by 55% of all patients, most frequently by supplementation with vitamins, selenium and mistletoe preparations. Comparable beneficial effects were also reported in other studies [19, 27, 28]. However, it is important to mention that there are also studies demonstrating the negative effects of CAM use, including depression, anxiety and lower quality of life [2, 29].

Although side effects were seldom reported and most CAM therapies can be regarded as harmless, potentially perilous CAM-drug interactions can occur [17, 30–33]. The concurrent use of antioxidants can diminish or enhance the effects of chemotherapy [33–35]. Excessive consumption of vitamins A, D and B_6, zinc and selenium can lead to increased toxicity, e.g. skin sensitization during radiotherapy or blood pressure swings [36, 37]. With regard to herbal remedies patients are often not aware that due to the lack of quality control these natural drugs contain different, not documented chemicals, in varying amounts [38].

Therefore, the responsible physician must be aware of these possible interactions and, in case of doubt, replace or stop the CAM treatment as necessary.

Remarkably, the growing role of the internet as an information source on CAM is under-represented with only 8% internet use. However, in light of the growing interest of laypersons concerning the use of the World Wide Web as an information source on CAM, it is imperative to ameliorate the quality of health information for consumers on the World Wide Web, because it seems to become the major information source of the 21st century [39, 40].

Conclusions

Complementary therapies have an increasingly important role in the control of symptoms associated with cancer and cancer treatment [2].

The use of CAM is more frequent in lung cancer patients than expected [21]. Therefore, it important to take the possibility of a covert CAM use into account when treating lung cancer patients.

Nota bene, it is fundamental to identify these patients in order to avoid interactions with conventional treatment schedules, wasting time and money, and getting a bias in clinical trials, in addition to giving the support that patients request. Only with detailed knowledge about the effects, side effects, safety, indications, efficacy, needs, and cost-effectiveness balance of CAM can oncologists give their patients the information they expect, and prevent patients having to depend upon unqualified sources. To evaluate the value or potential hazards of such treatment, further studies are clearly warranted.

References

1 Robert Koch-Institut und die Gesellschaft der epidemiologischen Krebsregister in Deutschland e. V. (eds): Krebs in Deutschland 2003–2004. Häufigkeiten und Trends, ed 6, revised. Berlin, 2008.

2 Burstein HJ, Gelber S, Guadagnoli E, Weeks JC: Use of alternative medicine by women with early-stage breast cancer. N Engl J Med 1999;340:1733–1739.

3 Ernst E, Cassileth BR: The prevalence of complementary/alternative medicine in cancer: a systematic review. Cancer 1998;83:777–782.

4 Micke O, Büntzel J: Complementary and alternative medicine in tumor patients. A dilemma in modern oncology. Onkologe 2008;14:73–80.

5 Risberg T, Kolstad A, Bremnes Y, Holte H, Wist EA, Mella O, Klepp O, Wilsgaard T, Cassileth BR: Knowledge of and attitudes toward complementary and alternative therapies; a national multicentre study of oncology professionals in Norway. Eur J Cancer 2004;40:529–535.

6 Risberg T, Lund E, Wist E: Use of non-proven therapies: differences in attitudes between Norwegian patients with non-malignant disease and patients suffering from cancer. Acta Oncol 1995; 34:893–898.

7 Burstein HJ: Discussing complementary therapies with cancer patients: what should we be talking about? J Clin Oncol. 2000;18:2501—2504.

8 Cassileth BR, Deng GE, Gomez JE, Johnstone PA, Kumar N, Vickers AJ: Complementary therapies and integrative oncology in lung cancer: ACCP evidence-based clinical practice guidelines, ed 2. Chest. 2007;132(3 suppl):340S–354S.

9 NCCAM: What is complementary and alternative medicine (CAM)? National Center for Complementary and Alternative Medicine (NCCAM), National Institutes of Health, 2009. http://nccam.nih.gov/health/whatiscam/overview.htm.

10 Schönekaes K, Micke O, Mücke R, Büntzel J, Glatzel M, Bruns F, Kisters K: Use of complementary/alternative therapy methods by patients with breast cancer. Forsch Komplementarmed Klass Naturheilkd 2003;10:304–308.

11 Cassileth BR, Deng G: Complementary and alternative therapies for cancer. Oncologist 2004;9:80–89.

12 Büntzel J, Glatzel M, Bruns F, KistersK, Micke O, Mücke R: Selenium supplementation in head and neck surgery. Trace Elem Electrolytes 2008;25:221.

13 Ernst E, Cassileth BR: How useful are unconventional cancer treatments? Eur J Cancer 1999;35: 1608–1613.

14 Micke O, Büntzel J, Bruns F, Glatzel M, Hunger R, Kisters K, Mücke R: Clinical elementology in oncology: experiences and proposals from Germany. Trace Elem Electrolytes 2008;25:221.

15 Barnes PM, Bloom B, Nahin RL: Complementary and Alternative Medicine Use Among Adults and Children: United States, 2007. National Health Statistics Reports; No 12. Hyattsville, National Center for Health Statistics, 2008.

16 Micke O, Mücke R, Schönekaes K, Büntzel J: Complementary and alternative medicine in radiotherapy patients – more harm than expected? In regard to D'Amico et al: Self-administration of untested medical therapy for treatment of prostate cancer can lead to clinically significant adverse events. Int J Radiat Oncol Biol Phys 2002; 54:1311–1313.

17 Richardson MA, Sanders T, Palmer JL, Greisinger A, Singletary S: Complementary/alternative medicine use in a comprehensive cancer center and the implications for oncology. J Clin Oncol 2000; 8:2505–2514.

18 Söllner W, Maislinger S, DeVries A, Steixner E, Rumpold G, Lukas P: Use of complementary and alternative medicine by cancer patients is not associated with perceived distress or poor compliance with standard treatment but with active coping behavior: a survey. Cancer 2000;89:873–880.

19 Vapiwala N, Mick R, Hampshire MK, Metz JM, DeNittis AS: Patient initiation of complementary and alternative medical therapies (CAM) following cancer diagnosis. Cancer J 2006;12:467–474.

20 Micke O, Bruns F, Glatzel M, Schönekaes K, Micke P, Mücke R, Büntzel J: Predictive factors for the use of complementary and alternative medicine (CAM) in radiation oncology. Eur J Integ Med 2009;1:22–30.

21 Boon H, Stewart M, Kennard MA, Gray R, Sawka C, Brown JB, McWilliam C, Gavin A, Baron RA, Aaron D, Haines-Kamka T: Use of complementary/alternative medicine by breast cancer survivors in Ontario: prevalence and perceptions. J Clin Oncol 2000;18:2515–2521.
22 Wells M, Sarna L, Cooley ME, Brown JK, Chernecky C, Williams RD, Padilla G, Danao LL: Use of complementary and alternative medicine therapies to control symptoms in women living with lung cancer. Cancer Nurs 2007;30:45–55.
23 Bass DB, Stewart-Sicking J: Christian Spirituality in Europe and North America since 1700- SO. Blackwell Companion to Christian Spirituality 2007;139–155.
24 Sloan RP: Religion, medical science, and the rise of subjectivity. Eur J Integ Med 2009;1:1–7.
25 Micke O, Büntzel J, Mücke R, Glatzel M: Spirituality in radiation oncology – from belief to bedside: a new focus for research? Eur J Integ Med 2008;1(suppl):11.
26 Boon H, Brown J, Gavin A: What are the experiences of women with breast cancer as they decide whether to use complementary/alternative medicine? West J Med 2000;173:39.
27 Astin JA: Why patients use alternative medicine: results of a national study. JAMA 1998;279:1548–1553.
28 Verhoef MJ, Hagen N, Pelletier G, Forsyth P: Alternative therapy use in neurologic diseases: use in brain tumor patients. Neurology 1999;52: 617–622.
29 Ernst E: Intangible risks of complementary and alternative medicine. J Clin Oncol 2001;19:2365–2366.
30 Jungi WF: Risks of alternative cancer treatment. Onkologie 1986;9:231–234.
31 Markman M: Safety issues in using complementary and alternative medicine. J Clin Oncol 2002; 20:39S–41S.
32 Lamson DW, Brignall MS: Antioxidants in cancer therapy; their actions and interactions with oncologic therapies. Altern Med Rev 1999;4:304–329.
33 Lamson DW, Brignall MS: Antioxidants in cancer therapy; their actions and interactions with oncologic therapies. Altern Med Rev 1999;4:304–329.
34 Labriola D, Livingston R: Possible interactions between dietary antioxidants and chemotherapy. Oncology (Huntingt) 1999;13:1003–1008;
35 Lagman R, Walsh D: Dangerous nutrition? Calcium, vitamin D, and shark cartilage nutritional supplements and cancer-related hypercalcemia. Support Care Cancer 2003;11:232–235.
36 Snodgrass SR: Vitamin neurotoxicity. Mol Neurobiol 1992;6:41–73.
37 Ernst E: Harmless herbs? A review of the recent literature. Am J Med 1998;104:170–178.
38 Schmidt K, Ernst E: Assessing websites on complementary and alternative medicine for cancer. Ann Oncol 2004;15:733–742.
39 Bruns F, Mücke R, Büntzel J, Kisters K, Micke O: Trace elements supplementation in radiation oncology: an empirical study assessing the quality of health information for consumers on the World Wide Web in Germany. Trace Elem Electrolytes 2005;22:311–315.

Priv.-Doz. Dr. med. Oliver Micke
Department of Radiotherapy and Radiation Oncology, Franziskus Hospital
Kiskerstrasse 26
DE–33615 Bielefeld (Germany)
Tel. +49 521 5891801, Fax +49 521 5891804, E-Mail strahlenklinik@web.de

Author Index

Subject Index